Community-Acquired Respiratory Infections

INFECTIOUS DISEASE AND THERAPY

Series Editor

Burke A. Cunha

Winthrop-University Hospital
Mineola, and
State University of New York School of Medicine
Stony Brook, New York

1. Parasitic Infections in the Compromised Host, *edited by Peter D. Walzer and Robert M. Genta*
2. Nucleic Acid and Monoclonal Antibody Probes: Applications in Diagnostic Methodology, *edited by Bala Swaminathan and Gyan Prakash*
3. Opportunistic Infections in Patients with the Acquired Immunodeficiency Syndrome, *edited by Gifford Leoung and John Mills*
4. Acyclovir Therapy for Herpesvirus Infections, *edited by David A. Baker*
5. The New Generation of Quinolones, *edited by Clifford Siporin, Carl L. Heifetz, and John M. Domagala*
6. Methicillin-Resistant *Staphylococcus aureus*: Clinical Management and Laboratory Aspects, *edited by Mary T. Cafferkey*
7. Hepatitis B Vaccines in Clinical Practice, *edited by Ronald W. Ellis*
8. The New Macrolides, Azalides, and Streptogramins: Pharmacology and Clinical Applications, *edited by Harold C. Neu, Lowell S. Young, and Stephen H. Zinner*
9. Antimicrobial Therapy in the Elderly Patient, *edited by Thomas T. Yoshikawa and Dean C. Norman*
10. Viral Infections of the Gastrointestinal Tract: Second Edition, Revised and Expanded, *edited by Albert Z. Kapikian*
11. Development and Clinical Uses of Haemophilus b Conjugate Vaccines, *edited by Ronald W. Ellis and Dan M. Granoff*
12. *Pseudomonas aeruginosa* Infections and Treatment, *edited by Aldona L. Baltch and Raymond P. Smith*
13. Herpesvirus Infections, *edited by Ronald Glaser and James F. Jones*
14. Chronic Fatigue Syndrome, *edited by Stephen E. Straus*
15. Immunotherapy of Infections, *edited by K. Noel Masihi*
16. Diagnosis and Management of Bone Infections, *edited by Luis E. Jauregui*
17. Drug Transport in Antimicrobial and Anticancer Chemotherapy, *edited by Nafsika H. Georgopapadakou*

18. New Macrolides, Azalides, and Streptogramins in Clinical Practice, *edited by Harold C. Neu, Lowell S. Young, Stephen H. Zinner, and Jacques F. Acar*
19. Novel Therapeutic Strategies in the Treatment of Sepsis, *edited by David C. Morrison and John L. Ryan*
20. Catheter-Related Infections, *edited by Harald Seifert, Bernd Jansen, and Barry M. Farr*
21. Expanding Indications for the New Macrolides, Azalides, and Streptogramins, *edited by Stephen H. Zinner, Lowell S. Young, Jacques F. Acar, and Harold C. Neu*
22. Infectious Diseases in Critical Care Medicine, *edited by Burke A. Cunha*
23. New Considerations for Macrolides, Azalides, Streptogramins, and Ketolides, *edited by Stephen H. Zinner, Lowell S. Young, Jacques F. Acar, and Carmen Ortiz-Neu*
24. Tickborne Infectious Diseases: Diagnosis and Management, *edited by Burke A. Cunha*
25. Protease Inhibitors in AIDS Therapy, *edited by Richard C. Ogden and Charles W. Flexner*
26. Laboratory Diagnosis of Bacterial Infections, *edited by Nevio Cimolai*
27. Chemokine Receptors and AIDS, *edited by Thomas R. O'Brien*
28. Antimicrobial Pharmacodynamics in Theory and Clinical Practice, *edited by Charles H. Nightingale, Takeo Murakawa, and Paul G. Ambrose*
29. Pediatric Anaerobic Infections: Diagnosis and Management, Third Edition, Revised and Expanded, *Itzhak Brook*
30. Viral Infections and Treatment, *edited by Helga Rübsamen-Waigmann, Karl Deres, Guy Hewlett, and Reinhold Welker*
31. Community-Acquired Respiratory Infections: Antimicrobial Management, *edited by Charles H. Nightingale, Paul G. Ambrose, and Thomas M. File, Jr.*

Additional Volumes in Production

Community-Acquired Respiratory Infections

Antimicrobial Management

edited by

Charles H. Nightingale

Hartford Hospital
Hartford
and University of Connecticut School of Pharmacy
Storrs, Connecticut, U.S.A.

Paul G. Ambrose

Cognigen Corporation
Buffalo, New York, U.S.A.

Thomas M. File, Jr.

Northeastern Ohio Universities College of Medicine
Rootstown
and Summa Health System
Akron, Ohio, U.S.A.

MARCEL DEKKER, INC. NEW YORK • BASEL

Library of Congress Cataloging-in-Publication Data
A catalog record for this book is available from the Library of Congress.

ISBN: 0-8247-4698-8

This book is printed on acid-free paper.

Headquarters
Marcel Dekker, Inc., 270 Madison Avenue, New York, NY 10016, U.S.A.
tel: 212-696-9000; fax: 212-685-4540

Distribution and Customer Service
Marcel Dekker, Inc., Cimarron Road, Monticello, New York 12701, U.S.A.
tel: 800-228-1160; fax: 845-796-1772

Eastern Hemisphere Distribution
Marcel Dekker AG, Hutgasse 4, Postfach 812, CH-4001 Basel, Switzerland
tel: 41-61-260-6300; fax: 41-61-260-6333

World Wide Web
http://www.dekker.com

The publisher offers discounts on this book when ordered in bulk quantities. For more information, write to Special Sales/Professional Marketing at the headquarters address above.

Current printing (last digit):

10 9 8 7 6 5 4 3 2 1

PRINTED IN THE UNITED STATES OF AMERICA

Preface

Even in this age of modern medicine, community-acquired respiratory tract infections continue to plague mankind. Most recently, with the outbreak of the severe acute respiratory syndrome (SARS) virus, we have seen the potential danger these infections pose in our increasingly global world.

In this publication our objective is to address the current and emerging issues and problems facing the clinician in the treatment of community-acquired respiratory tract infections. One of these problems is the lack of rapid diagnostic tools, which may result in treatments that focus around empirical therapy. An issue of concern is the increased reporting of antibiotic-resistant organisms, indicating that some antimicrobial agents have limited utility. This in turn increases the pressure on the clinician to prescribe newer and newer medications.

The question becomes how much of this is a real issue and how much involves the marketing strategies of drug manufacturers. Out of necessity, issues related to drug choice and doses and dosing regimens become important considerations. Concurrently, most modern approaches to dosage and dosage issues involve incorporating the pharmacodynamic properties of antibiotics into the decision-making process. In addition, the pressures of managed care to see as many patients as possible in the shortest period of time present real challenges for the practitioner.

The book reviews each important community-acquired disease state and focuses on the objectives described above. The discussion of antibiotics is from two perspectives: clinical use and pharmacodynamics, for use in prescribing doses and dosing regimens based on the most recent information.

Recognized experts in the pharmacology and pharmacodynamics of antibiotics have contributed chapters on specific classes of antibiotics. Specialists in infectious disease and experts in the treatment of community-acquired respiratory infections have written the clinical chapters. These chapters focus on clinical presentation, diagnostic modalities, and treatment.

This book is a practical guide for the treatment of the most common community-associated respiratory infections. In addition to the medical aspects of the treatment of patients, the book provides the pharmacodynamic basis for some of the treatment drug choices, especially for the dose and dosing regimen. It incorporates the most recent data and combines it with proven clinical approaches. Antimicrobial recommendations from practice management guidelines have been included whenever appropriate. This material will be useful and practical for clinicians in the management of patients with community-acquired respiratory infections.

This book is a collaborative effort of pharmacologists, clinical pharmacists, and physicians that will be invaluable to all. In particular, it should be of interest and service to family practitioners, general internists, infectious disease specialists, pulmonologists, and pharmacists.

Charles H. Nightingale
Paul G. Ambrose
Thomas M. File, Jr.

Contents

Contributors

Sandra G. Adams, M.D. The University of Texas Health Science Center at San Antonio and The South Texas Veterans Health Care System, San Antonio, Texas, U.S.A.

Paul G. Ambrose, Pharm.D. Cognigen Corporation, Buffalo, New York, U.S.A.

David R. Andes, M.D. University of Wisconsin, Madison, Wisconsin, U.S.A.

Vincent T. Andriole, M.D. Yale University School of Medicine, New Haven, Connecticut, U.S.A.

Antonio Anzueto, M.D. The University of Texas Health Science Center at San Antonio and The South Texas Veterans Health Care System, San Antonio, Texas, U.S.A.

William R. Bishai, M.D., Ph.D. John Hopkins School of Medicine, Baltimore, Maryland, U.S.A.

Ann L. N. Chapman, M.D., Ph.D. Royal Hallamshire Hospital, Sheffield, England

Blaise L. Congeni, M.D. Northeastern Ohio Universities College of Medicine, Rootstown, and Children's Hospital Medical Center of Akron, Akron, Ohio, U.S.A.

William A. Craig, M.D. University of Wisconsin, Madison, Wisconsin, U.S.A.

Scott F. Dowell, M.D. U.S. Centers for Disease Control and Prevention and Thai Ministry of Public Health, Nonthaburi, Thailand

George L. Drusano, M.D. Albany Medical College, Albany, New York, U.S.A.

Thomas M. File Jr., M.D. Northeastern Ohio Universities College of Medicine, Rootstown, and Summa Health System, Akron, Ohio, U.S.A.

Naomi R. Florea, Pharm.D. Hartford Hospital, Hartford, Connecticut, U.S.A.

James A. Hadley, M.D. University of Rochester Medical Center, Rochester, New York, U.S.A.

Paul B. Iannini, M.D. Danbury Hospital, Danbury, and Yale University School of Medicine, New Haven, Connecticut, U.S.A.

Joseph L. Kuti, Pharm. D. Hartford Hospital, Hartford, Connecticut, U.S.A.

Matthew E. Levison, M.D. Drexel University College of Medicine, Medical College of Pennsylvania Hospital, Philadelphia, Pennsylvania, U.S.A.

Robert C. Owens, Jr., Pharm.D. Maine Medical Center, Portland, Maine, U.S.A.

Michael S. Niederman, M.D. Winthrop University Hospital, Mineola, and State University of New York at Stony Brook, Stony Brook, New York, U.S.A.

Charles H. Nightingale, Ph.D. Hartford Hospital, Hartford, and University of Connecticut School of Pharmacy, Storrs, Connecticut, U.S.A.

Sandra L. Preston, Pharm.D. Albany Medical College, Albany, New York, U.S.A.

Richard Quintiliani, M.D. Hartford Hospital, Hartford, and University of Connecticut School of Medicine, Farmington, Connecticut, U.S.A.

Harley A. Rotbart, M.D. University of Colorado Health Science Center, Denver, Colorado, U.S.A.

James S. Tan, M.D. Northeastern Ohio Universities College of Medicine, Rootstown, and Summa Health System, Akron, Ohio, U.S.A.

Martin J. Wood, M.D.† Heartlands Hospital, Birmingham, England

† Deceased.

Community-Acquired Respiratory Infections

1

Overview of Community-Acquired Respiratory Tract Infections

Thomas M. File, Jr.
Northeastern Ohio Universities College of Medicine, Rootstown
and Summa Health System
Akron, Ohio, U.S.A.

INTRODUCTION

Community-acquired respiratory tract infections (CRTIs) are a leading cause of morbidity and mortality in the United States and worldwide, and they are associated with substantial health care costs. In addition, CRTIs are the most common reason for the use of antimicrobial agents, much of which use is inappropriate. In recent years, the management of these infections has been challenged by the escalation of antimicrobial resistance among predominant pathogens.

Optimal treatment outcomes for CRTIs depend on appropriate and prompt initiation of antibiotic therapy when indicated. Appropriate therapy for these infections presents a significant challenge to practicing clinicians in the light of rising time constraints and the increasing pressure for treatment to be cost-effective. Ultimately, the best outcomes for patients depend on several factors, which include the establishment of an accurate diagnosis, the consideration of likely pathogens and their patterns of resistance, and the selection of an appropriate antibiotic based on efficacy, pharmacology, and tolerability. Promoting the appropriate use of antibiotics through the development and application of treatment guidelines and educational efforts aimed at clinicians as well as patients should help curb unnecessary prescribing and misuse of antibiotics, decrease treatment costs, and increase patient satisfaction. This chapter is designed to provide an overview of the overall impact of CRTIs and to identify important difficulties in the diagnosis and treatment of patients suffering from such diseases.

IMPACT OF CRTIs

Morbidity and Mortality

Community respiratory tract infections are the most common type of infection managed by health care providers and they are of great consequence [1,2]. Although many of these infections are of relatively mild severity, some may be associated with significant morbidity or mortality. The widespread morbidity and mortality caused by CRTIs are serious problems for society. Acute respiratory tract infections are the greatest single cause of death in children worldwide (4.3 million deaths in 1992) [2]. Lower respiratory tract infections and influenza are responsible for most deaths caused by infectious disease in the United States.

According to the National Center for Health Statistics (NCHS) of the Centers for Disease Control and Prevention, there were more than 200 million episodes of respiratory disorders (including infections and other conditions such as asthma) reported in the United States in 1996 [3]. During the years 1980 through 1996, respiratory tract infections (including upper respiratory tract infections, otitis, and lower respiratory tract infections) accounted for 16% of all outpatient visits to physicians [4]. The rate of visits for outpatient care ranged from 74/1000 population per year for lower respiratory tract infections and influenza to 200/1000 population per year for upper respiratory tract infection. The NCHS reported morbidity due to respiratory infections in 1996 led to 152 days lost from school per 100 youths, and 99 days lost from work per 100 employed persons [3]. In addition, recent indicators of overall burden of respiratory infections suggest that the morbidity and mortality rates attributed to some of these infections is increasing as well, in part because of the proportion of attributed hospitalizations [5]. Many factors, such as the emergence of acquired immune deficiency syndrome [AIDS] and increased antibiotic resistance, probably contribute to this increase.

Upper CRTIs

The most frequent CRTIs are acute upper respiratory tract viral respiratory infections (VRIs) which encompass a range of illnesses with the common cold being most widespread. Children have an average of three to eight colds annually; incidence decreases with age to an average of about two to four colds a year by adulthood [6]. In 1996, data from a survey by the NCHS reported 62 million cases of colds required some form of treatment [7]. Gonzales et al. reported there were 25 million office visits to primary care providers in 1998 for upper respiratory tract infections, most of which were viral in etiology [8].

For otitis media and otitis externa, an average of 19,000 outpatient visits per year occurred from 1980 to 1996 [4]. For children younger than 15 years, acute otitis media was the most frequent diagnosis in physician's office practice. This disease is less common in older children and adults; however, it can still be a significant cause of illness in older patients as well.

Sinusitis is one of the most common health care complaints among adults in the United States, with a minimum of 35 million cases diagnosed by physicians annually [9]. However, because many episodes are unreported, many patients suffer without seeking care from a physician.

Lower RTIs

The prevalence of chronic bronchitis and chronic obstructive pulmonary disease (COPD) is increasing worldwide. An estimated 20–30 million persons in the United States suffer from these conditions [10–13]. While for the past few years all the other leading causes of death in the United States, such as heart disease, stroke, and cancer, have been declining, the number of deaths due to COPD has actually increased over the same time period by 22% [14]. Much of the morbidity, mortality, and cost expended for COPD is associated with patients who present with difficult-to-treat cases and/or multiple recurrences of infectious exacerbation.

In the United States, approximately 4–5 million cases of community-acquired pneumonias (CAP) occur each year, accounting for 10 million physician visits, approximately 500,000 hospitalizations, and approximately 45,000 deaths [15]. Mortality has ranged from 2% to 30% among hospitalized patients; mortality is less than 1% for patients who are not hospitalized. CAP occurs more commonly in children under the age of 5 years and in adults over the age of 65 years. The incidence of CAP for persons between the ages of 5 and 60 years has been reported to be between 100 and 500 per 100,000 population [16]. In a series of studies, Foy and coworkers examined the incidence of pneumonia by age in a prepaid medical care group that had a population of 180,000 when the study ended in February 1975 [16]. The overall annual rate of pneumonia was 12 per 1,000 population per year. Rates were highest in the 0–4 years age group at 12 to 18 per 1,000 population. Between the ages of 5 and 60 years, the rate ranged from 1 to 5 per

TABLE 1 Employer Payments in 1997 per Beneficiary, by Type of Respiratory Infection, and Employer Overall Costs

	Costs per beneficiary, $								Aggregate Employer Costs, $[b]
	Health care costs								
Respiratory Infections	Inpatient	Outpatient	Prescription drug	Office	Other[a]	Disability costs	Absenteeism costs	Total costs	Overall costs
Symptoms of the respiratory system (n = 24,851)	3,098	1,822	883	602	157	776	507	7,845	194,956,095
Acute upper respiratory infections of multiple or unspecified sites (n = 13,874)	613	688	455	356	81	297	301	2,791	38,722,334
Acute tonsillitis and acute pharyngitis (n = 13,706)	448	628	350	315	72	156	211	2,180	29,879,080
Acute bronchitis (n = 10,852)	1,114	951	682	441	114	474	443	4,219	45,784,588
Acute sinusitis (n = 9,856)	700	889	674	449	88	335	429	3,564	35,126,784

Chronic sinusitis (n = 7,368)	990	1,200	787	516	102	404	456	4,455	32,824,440
Chronic bronchitis (n = 5,296)	2,054	1,168	820	518	168	668	478	5,874	31,108,704
Strep throat and scarlet fever, chronic pharyngitis and nasopharyngitis, chronic diseases of the tonsils and adenoids (n = 4,464)	498	886	409	371	75	179	224	2,642	11,793,888
Pneumonia (n = 4,036)	6,316	1,902	973	604	242	1,016	491	11,544	46,591,584
Acute nasopharyngitis (acute cold) and acute laryngitis (n = 2,041)	940	787	455	449	95	252	301	3,279	6,692,439
Influenza (n = 1,514)	1,315	1,038	680	437	112	621	525	4,728	7,158,192
Unique individuals in respiratory infections sample (n = 63,890)	1,459	1,047	598	413	97	437	346	4,397	280,924,330

[a] Includes care at patient's home, nursing/extended care facility, psychiatric day-care facility, substance abuse treatment facility, and independent clinical laboratories.
[b] Aggregate employer costs is calculated by multiplying total costs by the number of beneficiaries with a specific condition.
Source: Ref. 21.

1,000 population. In 1987, Houston et al. retrospectively evaluated the incidence of pneumonia (nursing home and community-associated) in elderly patients and residents 65 years of age or older in Homestead County, Minneapolis, Minnesota [17]. The overall incidence rate for an initial episode of pneumonia was 3,032 per 100,000 population; this rate rose to 7,923 per 100,000 population among residents aged 85 or older. In a prospective study of all adult patients (≥18 years of age) hospitalized for CAP in two counties in Ohio during 1991 (Ohio Community Based Pneumonia Incidence Study) Marston et al. reported an incidence of 280 cases per 100,00 population [18]. The rate was 962 cases per 100,000 for persons older than 65 years of age. In this study, the incidence was higher among blacks than whites and higher among males than females. The incidence of CAP (like most CRTIs) is highest in the winter months and during influenza epidemics.

The mortality of CAP has not changed significantly over the past 2 decades in part due to the increased number of patents at risk for CAP (i.e., elderly patients and patients with multiple comorbid conditions). In a prospective study of prognostic factors of CAP due to bacteremic pneumococcal disease in five countries, mortality ranged from 6% in Canada to 20% in the United States and Spain (13% in the United Kingdom and 8% in Sweden) [19]. Independent predictors of death were age greater than 65, nursing home residence, presence of chronic lung disease, high APACHE score, and need for mechanical ventilation. Differences in disease severity and frequency of underlying conditions were factors for different outcomes. In a subsequent study, Mortensen et al. found approximately half of the CAP deaths were due to worsening of preexisting conditions [20].

Cost of RTIs

Patients with respiratory tract infections represent an important financial burden on society. In one study, the estimated cost to employers of patients with respiratory tract infections in the United States in 1997 was $112 billion, including costs of medical treatment and time lost from work [21]. Patients with pneumonia, "symptoms of the respiratory system," and chronic bronchitis averaged the highest costs at $11,544, $7,845, and $5,874 per employee, respectively (Table 1).

Costs associated with the common cold have been estimated to exceed $3.5 billion per year in the US [6]. Sinusitis is also a substantial economic burden, associated with high health care costs and reduced quality of life. In a recent study, 26.7 million patient visits were attributed to sinusitis and related airway disorders, at a cost of $5.78 billion [22]. Cases in adults accounted for most of the overall costs.

The cost of treating CAP and acute exacerbations of chronic bronchitis (AECB) is also high. One study found that the total direct cost, in 1995 dollars, of treating pneumonia patients younger than 65 years of age in the United States was $3.6 billion per year and was $4.8 billion for patients 65 years or older [23]. Another study estimated the annual cost to employers for employees with pneumonia was five times higher than for employees without pneumonia [24]. In a recent estimate, the direct costs of COPD in the United States were $14.5 billion; much of this is due to the management of AECB [25]. The largest proportion of these costs, $7.8 billion, was related to hospitalization, with the second most significant cost factor being drugs at $5.1 billion. Antibiotic costs made up 6.5% of these drug costs (approximately $330 million), and therefore only a small proportion of the total costs.

GENERAL APPROACH TO ANTIMICROBIAL THERAPY OF CRTIs

Respiratory tract infections are the reason for most antibiotic use. Approximately three-quarters of all outpatient antimicrobials used in the United States are for respiratory tract infections [26]. However, a large proportion of these prescriptions are unnecessary because many of the treated conditions (i.e., common cold, acute bronchitis, acute uncomplicated rhinosinusitis) have a predominantly viral etiology, and antibacterial therapy has not been shown to have a beneficial impact. The Centers for Disease Control and Prevention estimates that approximately 59% of the approximately 100 million courses of antibiotics prescribed by office-based physicians are unnecessary [27]. The common colds and related VRI syndromes are among the most frequent reasons for inappropriate antibiotic use; this increases the costs of illness unnecessarily and contributes to the increasing prevalence of antibiotic-resistant pathogens. Thus, the progress previously made in dealing with the most common bacterial cause of respiratory tract infections, *Streptococcus pneumoniae*, is now associated with a global explosion of drug resistance that has made treatment decisions very difficult.

The appropriate management of CRTIs poses multiple challenges for the clinician. Prescribers are faced with an ever-increasing selection of antimicrobial agents from which to choose the most appropriate therapy for their patients (Table 2). The likelihood of achieving a successful outcome is influenced by a number of factors involving the patient, the pathogen, and the drug. A primary consideration is whether antimicrobial agents are warranted in the first place. This involves differentiating viral from bacterial etiology to the best extent possible: such knowledge is critical in order to

TABLE 2 Commonly Used Antimicrobials for Community Respiratory Tract Infections (antibacterials and antivirals for infections associated with immunocompetent hosts)

Antibacterials
β-Lactams
Penicillin VK
Amoxicillin/Ampicillin
Amoxicillin/clavulanate
Ampicillin/sulbactam
Oral cephalosporins (i.e., cefuroxime, loracarbef, ceprozil, cefpodoxime, ceftibutin, cefdinir)
Parenteral cephalosporins (i.e., cefuroxime, cefotaxime, ceftriaxone)
Macrolides
Erythromycin, dirithromycin, clarithromycin, azithromycin
Ketolides
Telithromycin
Clindamycin
Tetracyclines
Tetracycline, doxycycline
Trimethoprim/sulfamethoxazole
Fluoroquinolones
Ofloxacin, ciprofloxacin, levofloxacin, sparfloxacin, gatifloxacin, moxifloxacin, gemifloxacin
Others: Linezolid, vancomycin
Antivirals
Acyclovir, valacyclovir, famciclovir
Amantadine, rimantadine, zanamavir, oseltamavir

determine whether patients require antibiotic therapy. Bacterial infections warrant antimicrobial therapy, whereas viral infections do not require antibiotics. Viral illness generally resolves within a week, whereas bacterial infections typically worsen and can be accompanied by clinical signs of infection.

If antimicrobial agents are warranted, the clinician then must decide which of the many agents available is most appropriate for each individual patient. Many factors need to be considered, which include likely pathogens, severity of illness, patient age, safety profile, concomitant medications, comorbidities, antimicrobial activity, pharmacokinetic/pharmacodynamic parameters, clinical experience, ease of administration, local epidemiological considerations, and concern for development of resistance (Table 3).

Antibiotics, when used appropriately, are effective in eradicating pathogens causing bacterial RTIs, leading to more rapid resolution of infection and improvement of symptoms. For example, in patients with acute com-

Table 3 Factors for Consideration of Antimicrobial Choice for CRTIs

Antimicrobial activity against most likely pathogens
Epidemiological considerations: Age, comorbid conditions, travel, animal-exposure, etc.
Safety profile (adverse effects and drug interactions)
Pharmacokinetic/pharmacodynamic parameters
Potential for resistance
Cost

munity-acquired bacterial sinusitis, Gwaltney and coinvestigators showed that antibiotics improved symptoms and decreased or eradicated bacteria from the maxillary sinus [28]. Recovery also is more rapid in children with acute sinusitis who are treated with antimicrobials compared with those treated with placebo [29]. Antibiotics also can help avoid complications, such as in patients with bacterial acute otitis media (AOM). Treatment of bacterial AOM with an antibiotic that provides coverage for the most common pathogens can help avoid the potential consequences of untreated or incorrectly treated disease, including hearing impairment and delayed speech development [30]. Antibiotics also can help prevent the progression of disease from acute to chronic manifestations.

The Challenge of Identifying the Causative Pathogens

Myriad microorganisms can cause CRTIs, including bacteria and viruses. However, a handful of most likely microorganisms are responsible for the majority of infections (Table 4). Viruses such as rhinoviruses are undoubtedly responsible for the majority of mild CRTIs. The most frequent and clinically significant bacterial pathogen associated with CRTIs is *S. pneumoniae*, which is the most common bacterial pathogen for CAP, otitis, and sinusitis and a common cause of AECB. *Hemophilus influenzae* is also an important cause of CAP, AECB, sinusitis, and otitis. The so-called atypical pathogens such as *Mycoplasma*, *Legionella*, and *Chlamydia* species are emerging as increasingly recognized causes of CAP and occasionally of AECB. *Septococcus pyogenes* and viruses are the most common microorganisms associated with tonsillitis/pharyngitis. Gram-negative bacilli and *Staphylococcus aureus* may be the cause of CRTI in selected patients especially those with multiple comorbid conditions. Mycobacteria, fungi, and so forth may be associated with CRTIs (especially CAP), based on epidemiological considerations.

At the time of patient presentation to the physician, the microbial etiology of the infection is generally unknown. No convincing association

Table 4 Microbial Etiology of Common Community Respiratory Tract Infections (relative percentages)

Pathogen	Common cold	*Pharyngitis*	Otitis media	Sinusitis	AECB	CAP
S. pneumoniae			25–65	35	10–15	20–60
H. influenzae			20–40	20–30	20–35	10
S. pyogenes		15–30	1–6	2–4		
M. pneumoniae		1			<10	1–30
C. pneumoniae					<10	5–20
L. pneumophila						1–5
S. aureus				2–8	<10	3–5
Gram negative				0–10	<10	3–10
Virus	100%	35–40	10–30	4–25	30	10–20

AECB = Acute exacerbations of chronic bronchitis.
CAP = Community-acquired pneumonias.

has been demonstrated between individual symptoms, physical findings or laboratory test results, and specific etiology in most cases of CRTIs. While there may be epidemiological associations with a variety of specific pathogens, physicians cannot reliably predict the etiology based on the initial clinical manifestations. Furthermore, for most CRTIs there is at present no test that offers a simple, rapid, cost-effective, accurate means of identifying the causative pathogen at the initial point of service (i.e., clinicians' office). With the exception of the rapid group A streptococcus test for pharyngitis, techniques to identify the causative pathogen are often insensitive or generally unavailable in most clinical settings. Subsequently, therapy is usually initiated empirically using antimicrobials with activity against the most likely causative pathogens.

Challenge of Differentiating Viral from Bacterial RTI

A significant challenge to clinicians is to distinguish which patients with symptoms of a community respiratory infection warrant antimicrobial therapy. Often clinical findings are not definitive with this process. Establishing the correct diagnosis—whether viral or bacterial infection—is key to limiting the use of unnecessary antibacterial agents. It is estimated that as many as 50 million antibiotic prescriptions a year could be avoided if clinicians differentiated between viral and true bacterial RTIs [30,31]. However, for the clinician faced with a patient exhibiting cough, nasal congestion, postnasal drip, nasal discharge, or pressure or pain over the sinuses, differentiating viral from bacterial illness may present a challenge. Symptoms often overlap, and it is acknowledged that bacterial infections may follow viral disease. Antibiotics do not eradicate viruses and do not shorten the course of viral illness. In fact, when antibiotics are given for viral infections, the result may be subsequent infection with resistant bacteria because previous antibiotic exposure may provide a selective advantage for resistant bacteria [32]. Furthermore, antibiotic use can affect others, fostering the carriage of resistant organisms among children in day-care centers and to other family members [33,34].

As previously indicated, there is a lack of rapidly available, cost-effective diagnostic tests that reliably differentiate self-limiting viral infection from bacterial infection. However, practice guidelines can offer pragmatic criteria for better antimicrobial usage. Thus, although initially suffering from a viral infection, 60% of patients with symptoms of sinusitis persisting for 10 days have a bacterial infection [35]. Restriction of antibiotics to only those patients would significantly reduce unnecessary prescribing. In addition, the restriction of antibiotic therapy in otitis media to those children with acute bacterial disease and avoidance in otitis media with effusion could reduce unnecessary use by two-thirds [36]. Moreover, there is little evidence that antibiotic therapy influences the outcome of acute bronchitis or milder exacerbation of chronic bronchitis, and prescribing could again be dramatically reduced [37]. Thus, more precise discrimination of probable viral versus bacterial CRTIs could improve the quality of therapy.

Although acute pharyngitis is most commonly viral in etiology, an important bacterial pathogens is *S. pyogenes* (group A streptococcus). It is therefore important to differentiate streptococcal from viral etiology in order to direct the most appropriate therapy. The concerns for complications of group A streptococcal infection (i.e., acute rheumatic fever and glomerulonephritis) are other reasons for appropriate diagnosis. The severity of illness due to *S. pyogenes*, as well as the presenting symptoms and signs, varies greatly. In most cases, differentiation of streptococcal etiology from viral etiology is not reliably accurate on clinical grounds alone. The presence of pharyngeal exudate and tender adenopathy may help in the diagnosis, but these findings are not specific or sensitive. The challenge for the clinician is to specify the etiology so that appropriate therapy can be administered. A variety of empirical approaches have been recommended but remain controversial. Guidelines by the Infectious Diseases Society of America and the Pediatric Red Book recommend cultures or antigen testing to allow the best utilization of antimicrobial agents [38,39].

For otitis media (OM), it is also important to differentiate between true acute otitis media (AOM) and otitis media with effusion (OME), because OME does not warrant antibiotic use. AOM is diagnosed when fluid is present in the middle ear and is accompanied by signs or symptoms of acute illness (e.g., ear pain, otorrhea, or fever). In contrast, clinical signs of infection do not accompany OME, which also involves fluid in the middle ear.

Several factors may help clinicians distinguish between viral and bacterial rhinosinusitis. For example, viral illness is usually self-limiting, lasting 2 to 7 days [40]. In contrast, bacterial infections typically worsen after a week or do not resolve after 7 to 10 days. Although a thick, discolored nasal discharge is often seen in patients with CRTIs, this sign is not a definitive indication that a bacterial infection is present. In these patients, it may be prudent to reserve antibiotics unless the condition persists beyond 7 to 10 days. Acute bacterial rhinosinusitis (ABRS) is usually preceded by a viral upper CRTI. Clinical judgment is used to distinguish between viral illness and ABRS. Some of the key clinical symptoms of viral and bacterial disease are listed in Table 5.

AECB due to bacterial infection—which may account for up to 50% of AECB and warrants antibacterial therapy—is very difficult to differentiate from exacerbation due to nonbacterial etiologies (i.e., viruses, pollutants, allergens). However, it is important that the clinician try to distinguish AECB from acute viral bronchitis, which does not require antimicrobial therapy. AECB is defined as an illness in a patient with chronic bronchitis

Table 5 Symptoms Associated with Viral and Bacterial Rhinosinusitis

Viral illness (usually lasting 2–7 days)	ABRS (persisting beyond 5–7 days)
Sneezing	Purulent nasal drainage
Rhinorrhea	Fatigue
Nasal congestion	Nasal congestion
Hyposmia/anosmia	Hyposmia/anosmia
Sore throat	Maxillary facial pain
Postnasal drip	Postnasal drip
Fever	Fever
Cough	Cough
Ear fullness	Ear fullness/pressure
Facial pressure	Facial pain/pressure (especially unilateral and focused)
Myalgia	
	Note: Worsening of symptoms after 7 days may indicate bacterial infection

ABRS = acute bacterial rhinosinusitis.
Source: Ref. 27.

(defined as a productive cough for at least 3 months for 2 consecutive years), which is characterized by an increase in at least one of three cardinal symptoms: dyspnea, sputum volume, or sputum purulence [41,42]. Acute bronchitis is generally used to describe a transient (usually <15 days) respiratory illness that occurs among patients without chronic lung inflammatory conditions and is characterized by cough (with or without sputum, fever, or substernal discomfort) and in the absence of radiographic findings of pneumonia [43]. Timely and accurate diagnosis and treatment of AECB remain challenges to clinicians because of the indefinite beginnings and uncertain treatment modalities of the condition. Because patients with AECB have chronic bronchitis as an underlying disease and because the definition of AECB is subjective, it is sometimes difficult to determine when an exacerbation has begun or ended.

The appropriateness of antimicrobial therapy in AECB is controversial, particularly in the light of current trends in resistance. However, because recurrent episodes of AECB can impair pulmonary function and can severely impact quality of life, many clinicians choose to treat the condition with antibiotics in order to address those cases that are bacterial in origin. To help decide whether antimicrobial therapy is warranted, clinicians are encouraged to stratify patients by the type of exacerbation and by the presence of risk factors associated with poor outcome. Randomized, placebo-controlled trials have shown that antibiotic treatment is beneficial in selected patients with AECB [44]. Specifically, studies show that patients with more severe exacerbation (type I) are more likely to experience benefit than those with less severe disease. Patients with type I exacerbation have all three cardinal symptoms: increased dyspnea, increased sputum volume, and increased sputum purulence; patients with type II exacerbation have two symptoms, and patients with type III have only one. In comparison, patients with moderate exacerbation (type II) experienced less benefit from antibiotics compared with those who received placebo, and patients with mild episodes (type III) did not appear to benefit from antibiotic treatment compared with the placebo group. In one study, patients with AECB who received antibiotic therapy had a more rapid return of peak flow, were more likely to achieve clinical success, and experienced clinical failure less frequently than patients given placebo [44]. Other studies also have shown the benefit of antibiotic therapy in AECB [45]. A clinical practice guideline for management of AECB formulated by the American College of Physicians–American Society of Internal Medicine and the American College of Chest Physicians was recently published; this position paper recommends the use of antibiotics in patients with severe exacerbation (such as type I) of COPD [46]. In addition to stratification by type, high-risk patients for poor outcome of AECB have been identified: these include patients with a history of repeated infections (>4 per year), comorbid illnesses (such as diabetes, asthma, coronary heart disease), or marked airway obstruction (<50% FEV_1) [47].

In patients with AECB of bacterial origin, antibiotics may have a long-term benefit of decreasing the amount of bacteria chronically colonizing the airway once the patient is clinically stable, thus helping to prevent progression to parenchymal lung infection [48]. Antibiotic treatment may also prevent progressive airway injury due to persistent infection and may prolong the duration between exacerbations.

The challenge facing the clinician in establishing a diagnosis of CAP is to distinguish it from less serious respiratory infections such as acute bronchitis. Table 6 lists characteristics associated with both conditions [49–51]. A definitive diagnosis of CAP cannot be based on clinical symptoms alone; a chest x-ray is necessary to determine the presence of pneumonia.

Challenge of Resistance

The discovery of potent antimicrobial agents was one of the greatest contributions to medicine in the 20th century. Unfortunately, the emergence of antimicrobial-resistant pathogens now threatens these advances. Over the past decade, antibiotic resistance has increased markedly among common respiratory pathogens, most notably in *S. pneumoniae* isolates, and, to a lesser extent, *Haemophilus influenzae* and *Moraxella catarrhalis*. Figure 1 illustrates the varying degrees of resistance to penicillin of *S. pneumoniae* over recent years. A parallel and equally troubling development has been the rise of cross-resistance involving other β-lactam and non–β-lactam antibacterial agents as well (e.g., cephalosporins, macrolides, clindamycin, tetracycline, chloramphenicol, trimethoprim/sulfamethoxazole, and, to a lesser extent, fluoroquinolones) [52].

TABLE 6 Characteristics of Acute Bronchitis and CAP

Acute Bronchitis	CAP
Transient duration (<15 days) in patients without chronic lung disease	Cough
Cough ± sputum	Sputum production
Substernal discomfort	Dyspnea
±Fever	Fever
>90% viral	Altered breath sounds
No chest x-ray evidence of pneumonia	Rales
	Chest x-ray evidence of pneumonia

CAP = community-acquired pneumonia.
Source: Ref. 49.

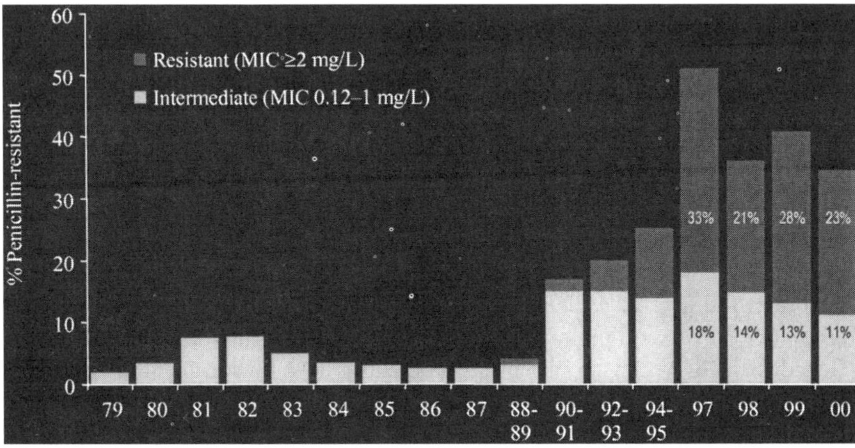

FIGURE 1 Emergence of penicillin-resistant *S. pneumoniae* in respiratory specimens. (From Refs. 52–58.)

Inappropriate use of antibiotics has contributed to the development of drug resistance among the most common bacterial pathogens in RTIs—*S. pneumoniae, H. influenzae,* and *M. catarrhalis*. The increase in resistance is a result of several factors, but a major factor driving resistance is the overall volume of antimicrobial prescribing—particularly for indications that do not warrant such therapy. Thus, it is vitally important that judicious use of antimicrobials be encouraged in order to curb this overuse and, it is hoped, minimize emergence of resistance.

Among respiratory pathogens, drug-resistant *S. pneumoniae* (DRSP) is of the greatest concern because it is the dominant cause of CAP. Surveillance studies indicate that the prevalence of DRSP continues to increase worldwide [53–58]. In two recent multinational studies, the worldwide prevalence of penicillin-resistant and macrolide-resistant *S. pneumoniae* ranged from 17.7% to 22.3% and 26.4% to 31.8%, respectively [57,58]. The dominant factor in the emergence of DRSP in one U.S. study has been human-to-human spread of relatively few clonal groups that harbor resistance determinants to multiple classes of antibiotics (including cephalosporins, macrolides, doxycycline, trimethoprim/sulfamethoxazole) [59].

Despite the rapid increase in DRSP, the clinical relevance for the outcome of some CRTIs remains controversial depending on the class of antimicrobial agent considered. The impact of *S. pneumoniae* drug resistance on morbidity and mortality associated with meningitis is well documented, and mounting evidence suggests that such resistance may also explain the decreased clinical and bacteriological response rates now seen in otitis media as well [60]. The clinical relevance of penicillin-resistant *S. pneumoniae* appears to vary depending on the level of resistance and the site of infection. For CAP, intermediate resistance (MIC 0.1–1.0 μg/mL) has not been shown to be associated with a detrimental outcome; however, this same level of resistance can be significant for otitis [61]. Until recently, however, studies of patients with CAP had failed to establish an independent association between drug-resistant *S. pneumoniae* and clinical outcome. Most studies suggest that current levels of β-lactam resistance do not generally result in treatment failures for patients with CAP [61]. Based on established pharmacokinetic/pharmacodynamic principles, adequate serum and tissue levels should be achieved with parenteral β-lactams or oral amoxicillin to effectively treat the majority of CAP due to DRSP. An analysis of nine controlled trials of a high-dose oral formulation of amoxicillin-clavulanate found a good clinical response for respiratory infections (mostly in outpatients) caused by *S. pneumoniae* with penicillin MICs up to 8 μg/mL [62]. Although most studies have not demonstrated an adverse effect of β-beta lactam resistance on the outcome of pneumococcal pneumonia, most clinicians remain concerned that increased morbidity and mortality will be seen as the proportion of resistant strains and their MICs increase. Moreover, in two controlled studies of pneumococcal bacteremia, one found an increased risk of mortality in patients with high-level resistance (penicillin MIC $\geq$ 4 μg/ml) and another showed an increased risk of suppurative complications for nonsusceptible infections [63,64]. Risk factors for penicillin-resistant *S. pneumoniae* have been identified (i.e., age $<$ than 2 years or $>$ 65 years, β-lactam therapy within 3 months, alcoholism, medical comorbidities, immunosuppressive illness or therapy, and exposure to a child in a day-care center), although it is not clear these are specific enough for individual patients to be clinically reliable [65].

The clinical relevance of macrolide-resistant *S. pneumoniae* (MRSP) may be dependent on the type of resistance expressed by a particular strain. The most common mechanisms of resistance include methylation of a ribosomal target encoded by *erm* gene and efflux of the macrolides by cell membrane protein transporter, encoded by *mef* gene [66]. *S. pneumoniae* strains with mef are resistant at a lower level (with MICs generally 1 to 16 μg/mL) than erm-resistant strains; and it is possible that such strains (particularly with MIC $<$ 8 μg/mL) may be inhibited if sufficiently high levels of macrolide can be obtained within infected tissue (such as may occur with newer macrolides—clarithromycin or azithromycin) [67–71]. However, there is recent evidence that the MICs of these strains are increasing, and this may affect the efficacy of these macrolides [72]. The mef-resistant strains are usually susceptible to clindamycin. Most erm-resistant isolates have an MIC above 32 μg/mL for erythromycin and are considered high-level resistant for all macrolides and clindamycin. Until recently, reports treatment of failure in CAP treated with macrolides have been rare, particularly for patients at low risk for drug-resistant strains. However, since 2000, anecdotal reports and one controlled study have documented failures due to MRSP in patients treated with an oral macrolide who subsequently required admission to the hospital with *S. pneumoniae* bacteremia [73–76]. Currently *mef*-associated resistance predominates in North America. *Erm*-associated resistance predominates in Europe and is common in Japan.

Although the worldwide prevalence of pneumococcal resistance to the newer fluoroquinolones (levofloxacin, gatifloxacin, moxifloxacin) remains low (less than 2%), in some countries resistance has increased markedly [77–79]. The overall prevalence of fluoroquinolone resistance (levofloxacin >4 μg/mL) in Hong Kong in 2000 had increased to 13.3% due to the dissemination of a fluoroquinolone-resistant clone [78]. Treatment failures have already been reported mostly in patients who have previously been treated with fluoroquinolones [80,81]. Risk factors for levofloxacin resistance were identified as prior exposure to a fluoroquinolone, nursing home residence, nosocomial infection, and COPD [82].

In the light of the emerging resistance of the pneumococcus to existing drugs, alternative agents need to be considered. Although glycopeptides (i.e., vancomycin, teicoplanin) are nearly certain to provide antibiotic coverage for DRSP, they are not active against other key respiratory pathogens (i.e., atypicals, *H. influenzae*) and there is a strong reason not to use these drugs until needed because of fear of emergence of other resistant organisms (i.e., VRE, VRSA). Other agents effective against DRSP include quinupristin/dalfopristin, linezolid, and the ketolides. The focus of therapy of quinupristin/dalfopristin and linezolid is more for nosocomial infections (and particularly for VRE or MRSA). The ketolides (telithromycin is the first to be marketed) are a novel addition to the macrolide group of antibacterials and have in vitro efficacy against key respiratory pathogens (including penicillin- and erythromycin-resistant strains) [83].

Principles of Appropriate Antimicrobial Use

Because of the increase in resistance it is increasingly important that recommendations for judicious use of antibiotics for RTI be encouraged. It is hoped that when sound principles are applied to select an appropriate empirical agent, the costs associated with incorrect prescribing and multiple courses of antibiotics can be avoided. Principles of appropriate therapy should be promoted and utilized by prescribing clinicians in order to result in the best outcomes for patients and reduce the emergence of antibiotic resistance. Several core principles of antibiotic therapy that should provide optimal benefit for patients as well as minimize resistance are listed in Table 7 [84].

TABLE 7 Principles of Appropriate Antimicrobial Use

1. Use antibacterial therapy only in those patients with bacterial infection.
2. Utilize diagnostic and other measures to reduce prescribing.
3. Therapy should maximally reduce or eradicate the bacterial load.
4. Use antimicrobial agents with optimal pharmacodynamics to achieve eradication.
5. Use locally relevant resistance data in the decision process.
6. Antimicrobial acquisition cost may be insignificant compared with therapeutic failure.

Source: Ref. 84.

Reduction of Unnecessary Antimicrobials

Because inappropriate prescribing is the major influence on developing resistance, antimicrobial therapy should be limited to infections in which bacteria are the predominant cause. This principle certainly seems self-evident, but it is one to which adherence seems very difficult. The reasons for overprescribing antibiotics are multifactorial. Patients may consult clinicians, expecting an antibiotic to be prescribed for an acute respiratory infection for which the etiology is most likely viral; as a result, clinicians may feel pressured to write antibiotic prescriptions to satisfy patients and to maintain good doctor-patient relationships. Receiving an antibiotic reinforces the patients' perception that antibiotics are warranted in similar situations. Thus, patients may continue to consult clinicians each time similar symptoms occur, expecting that antibiotics are again needed. Clinicians also may prescribe antibiotics as a rapid means of treating patients' symptoms rather than taking the time to educate patients that antibiotics are not always necessary, especially if a viral infection is suspected. However, clinicians should recognize that patient satisfaction is not compromised by the absence of an antibiotic prescription, provided patients understand the reasons. Hamm et al. demonstrated that patient satisfaction was influenced by patient perceptions that the clinician spent enough time discussing the illness and by patient knowledge about the treatment choice [85]. Moreover, clinicians may prescribe antibiotics as part of a defensive approach to avoid the potential sequelae of not prescribing for patients with bacterial infection.

Unfortunately, most patients and many clinicians view "unnecessary" antibiotic prescribing as at worst a neutral intervention (i.e., cannot harm, but may help). It is imperative patients understand this is not the case. In fact, the unnecessary use of antibacterials has several possible harmful effects in addition to selection of resistance, such as increased cost and exposure to unnecessary adverse reactions. Decreasing excess antibiotic use is an important strategy for combating the increase in community-acquired antibiotic-resistant infections. Several studies have documented a benefit of combining physician intervention and patient education that has resulted in decreased use of antimicrobials and reduction of resistance [86–88].

Additional Principles of Appropriate Antimicrobial Usage

Antibiotics that maximize bacterial eradication improve both short and longer term clinical outcomes, reduce overall costs—particularly those relating to treatment failure and consequent hospital admission—and assist in the minimization of resistance emergence and dissemination. There is accumulating evidence to indicate bacterial eradication as the primary goal of antibiotic therapy and the main determinate of therapeutic outcome [89]. However, spontaneous clinical recovery, common in mild to moderate CRTIs, may mask differences in bacterial effectiveness of antibiotics and allow suboptimal agents to continue to be prescribed. Thus, agents with poor bacteriological efficacy can appear clinically almost as good as those with optimal efficacy: the "Pollyanna effect" [90]. These small differences, which may seem insignificant in small series, may translate to significant numbers of failures in larger populations treated with suboptimal therapy. Antibiotic therapy that allows bacterial persistence risks not only poorer clinical outcome but also resistance selection.

Pharmacodynamic (PD) properties can differentiate between antibiotic classes, often between members of the same class, in their ability to eradicate pathogens at drug concentrations attainable during therapy. Integration of minimum inhibitory concentrations (MIC) with pharmacokinetic (PK) parameters provides pharmacodynamic (PD) indices, which are valuable tools with which to predict clinical and bacterial outcomes. Antimicrobial therapy is intended to provide a concentration of the agent that exceeds the concentration needed to inhibit the infecting organism. Traditionally, the MIC, which defines the minimum amount of an antimicrobial necessary to inhibit the growth of a microbe, has been used to describe the in vitro activity of an agent against a specific organism. Microorganisms are identified as susceptible, intermediate, or resistant on the basis of specific MIC levels. These levels, or breakpoints, are generally determined by reference to levels of the drug achieved in human serum, rather than the concentration of the drug attained at the infection site. These breakpoint values may not correlate with recent clinical data. In contrast, pharmacodynamic breakpoints are based on the pharmacokinetic evaluation of antibiotic concentrations (usually using serum concentrations because they are readily measured) as well as the consideration for how different antimicrobials exert their antibacterial action (i.e., time-dependent or concentration dependent killing), and correlated with clinical data on bacteriologic cure. Antibiotics that exhibit time-dependent pharmacodynamic effects are clinically successful when the serum concentration exceeds the MIC for 40% to 50% of the dosing interval [91]. For the β-lactams and the macrolides, clarithromycin and erythromycin, efficacy depends on the amount of time the serum drug concentration exceeds the MIC of the agent. In contrast, the efficacy of the fluoroquinolones is concentration-dependent, with the pharmacodynamic breakpoint dependent on the ratio of the total concentration of the agent to the MIC of the agent against the pathogen. The PK/PD breakpoints primarily rely on the drug concentration achieved in serum that correlates well for infections such as otitis. For pneumonia, the pharmacokinetics of agents in the endothelial lining fluid may be an appropriate marker of clinical effect. However, as of yet clinical trial data have not yet supported or disproved this hypothesis.

Strategies of appropriate empirical therapy should take into account the relative risks for drug-resistant strains. For example, whenever a prescription is written for a CRTI, the prescriber should inquire about factors associated with increased risk of DRSP—recent antimicrobial therapy (within 3 months), recent hospitalization (within 30 days) and whether or not a child who attends a day-care center resides within the household. If there is increased risk for DRSP, it is certainly appropriate to choose empirical therapy with agents likely to be effective against such pathogens (i.e., new fluoroquinolones, ketolides, or high-dose amoxicillin-containing agents).

Acquisition costs of different antimicrobials may be insignificant compared with the cost associated with therapeutic failure or adverse effects. Drug acquisition costs are a primary consideration only if there are no significant differences in treatment outcomes between agents; potential for selection of resistance; and incidence of significant treatment-related adverse events. Thus, a more expensive agent may be much more cost-effective if it is associated with greater efficacy or better tolerance than a less expensive generic comparator. Alternately, a shorter course of equal efficacy may minimize cost. If shorter courses result in similar results, they are clearly preferable. Inappropriate therapy of CRTI is expensive. In a study of LRTI, more effective antimicrobial therapy cost an average of US $8821 per episode compared with US $14754 when treatment was less effective [92]. Treatment failure far exceeds the acquisition costs of any antibiotic; and hospitalization is the key cost-driver. Thus, antibiotics that reduce the risk of hospitalization or reduce the length of stay in the hospital will be more cost-effective; and agents that achieve improved bacterial eradication also have the potential to improve long-term clinical outcomes and reduce overall costs and, perhaps, limit resistance emergence and dissemination.

The Value of Guidelines

The use of clinical practice guidelines can be an effective means of changing behavior, such as promoting the appropriate use of antibiotics [93]. Effective clinical guidelines should improve patient care while enhancing cost savings. However, cost savings should not be the primary motivating factor. For example, a recent report described a government intervention intended to decrease costs by reducing the use of "more-expensive," second-line antimicrobials [94]. As a result, costs increased through the occurrence of adverse outcomes in patients with OM, sinusitis, lower RTI, and AECB.

To maximize effectiveness and applicability, antibiotic use guidelines should be evidence-based. The guidelines should also reflect data on resistance, recognizing that local patterns of resistance often differ across geographic regions. Hence, effective guidelines should be readily adaptable for implementation locally. Primary objectives of guidelines for treating CRTIs should be to discourage antibiotic use to treat viral illness, to outline diagnostic criteria, and to avoid the use of ineffective antimicrobials.

Unfortunately, a meta-analysis of relevant studies has shown that there are numerous barriers to adherence to practice guidelines (Table 8) [95]. For example, clinicians may not be aware of all of the available guidelines or may not be well versed in how to apply specific recommendations appropriately. In addition, clinicians may not agree with some or all of the recommendations made or, as a general principle, may resist the concept of guidelines. If clinicians are doubtful that they can perform the task called for in the guidelines or harbor a belief that the recommendations will be unsuccessful, they probably will not follow the guidelines. Time constraints or health care organization requirements may impose restrictions that hamper the clinician's ability to implement the guidelines. Furthermore, the clinician may not have control over some changes called for in guidelines, such as the acquisition of new resources to perform diagnostic tests. Patient preferences for alternatives not recommended in guidelines also may obstruct adherence to clinical practice guidelines. To be successful, educational efforts and interventions aimed at improving adherence to practice guidelines—such as use of checklists and reminder systems—should address all of the identified barriers.

Educational Strategies to Promote Rational Antibiotic Use

Issuing guidelines on appropriate antibiotic use for treatment of different types of infections is only the first step in ensuring that rational principles are adopted and followed in clinical practice. Educational strategies aimed at enhancing clinician awareness of guidelines and encouraging their implementation is necessary. Educational materials promoting the implementation of

TABLE 8 Barriers to Clinician Adherence to Clinical Practice Guidelines

Barrier	Explanation
Lack of awareness	Clinician unaware that the guidelines exist
Lack of familiarity	Clinician aware of guidelines but unfamiliar with specifics
Lack of agreement	Clinician does not agree with a specific recommendation made in guideline or is averse to the concept of guidelines in general
Lack of self-efficacy	Clinician doubts whether he/she can perform the behavior
Lack of outcome expectancy	Clinician believes the recommendations will be unsuccessful
Lack of motivation	Clinician is unable/unmotivated to change previous practices
Guideline-related barriers	Guidelines are not easy or convenient to use
Patient-related barriers	Clinician may be unable to reconcile guidelines with patient preferences
Environmental-related barriers	Clinician may not have control over some changes (e.g., time, resources, organizational constraints)

Source: Ref. 95.

practice guidelines and emphasizing their benefits could be developed and provided to clinicians. Translation of guidelines into practice also must involve educational efforts geared toward patients. Patients need to understand that antibiotics are not appropriate for the treatment of viral infections. They also must be educated about the need to take antibiotics as directed and for the entire duration prescribed. Public health campaigns can help to spread the word, and traditional print and audiovisual patient education materials also may be useful.

Educational efforts aimed at providers and patients already have proved successful in promoting the rational use of antibiotics in community-acquired upper RTIs. In a study in rural Alaska, the education of health care workers and the community concerning appropriate antimicrobial use in children with community-acquired upper RTIs was associated with a 22% reduction in the number of antibiotic prescriptions in children younger than 5 years and with a 28% decrease in penicillin-resistant pneumococcal nasopharyngeal isolates compared with the two control regions not provided with the educational intervention [96].

In addition to educational campaigns, there is no substitute for the few moments taken by the treating clinician to explain fully why antibiotics are not necessary or why they are being prescribed. This approach helps patients realize that their condition is being taken seriously. The investment in time and personal attention can increase patient satisfaction with the selected treatment and can help ensure that patients comply with therapy.

CRTIs PREVENTION

Measures to reduce the prevalence of bacterial CRTIs by the use of preventive vaccines are very relevant to the appropriate use of antimicrobials. Pneumococcal and influenza vaccines should reduce the incidence of bacterial infections (secondary infections in the case of influenza vaccine) and thereby reduce the use of antibiotics. Preliminary data indicate dramatic reductions in hospitalization and mortality from use of these vaccines, suggesting an associated reduced necessity of antimicrobial prescribing [97]. Despite controversies over efficacy of the polysaccharide pneumococcal vaccine (PPV), both PPV and the influenza vaccines are recommended according to current guidelines by the Centers for Disease Control and Prevention (at ages 65 and 50, respectively, for immunocompetent adults without other risk factors) [98,99]. In a recent meta-analysis of 14 trials totaling more than 48,000 patients, PPV prevented definite pneumonia by 71% and mortality by 32% (but not all-cause death) [100]. However, there was no benefit seen for patients aged 55 years or more. A significant advance has been the development and licensure of the pneumococcal conjugate vaccine in infants. The benefits of this vaccine over the PPV have yet to be demonstrated in adults. In addition to preventive vaccines, smoking cessation should also reduce the burden of CRTIs, and it is worth the effort to provide counseling.

CONCLUSIONS

Community respiratory tract infections are the most common reason for antimicrobial usage. However, much of this use is inappropriate. It is, therefore, a significant challenge for the practicing physician to distinguish which CRTIs warrant antibiotics. The challenge to use antibiotics for CRTIs appropriately is great because of the large number of potential respiratory pathogens, the large number of drugs available, and the increasing resistance of the former to the latter. A working knowledge of the antimicrobial and pharmacologic properties as well as the safety profile of the available agents will provide the clinician a sound basis on which to make decisions regarding the use of antimicrobials for CRTIs. Antibiotic therapy with the appropriate agent shortens the course of the illness, lowers the risk of complications due to untreated disease, helps to prevent disease progression and airway impairment, and avoids the added cost of multiple courses of antibiotics.

REFERENCES

1. File TM Jr. The epidemiology of respiratory tract infections. Seminars in Reps Infections 2000; 15(No.3):184–194.
2. Enarson DA, Chretien J. Epidemiology of respiratory infectious diseases. Curr Opin Pulm Med 1999; 5:128–135.
3. Vital and Health Statistics. Current estimates from the national health interview survey, 1996. Series 10, No. 200. Atlanta, GA: Centers for Disease Control and Prevention, National Center for Health Statistics, October 1999.
4. Armstrong GL, Pinner RW. Outpatient visits for infectious diseases in the United States, 1980 through 1996. Arch Intern Med 1999; 159:2531–2536.
5. Simonsen L, Conn LA, Pinner RW, et al. Trends in infectious disease hospitalizations in the United States, 1980–1994. Arch Intern Med 1998; 158: 1923–1928.
6. Hayden FG. Introduction: emerging importance of the rhinovirus. Am J Med 2002; 112(6A):1S–3S.
7. Adams PF, Hendershot GE, Marano MA. Current estimates from the National Health Interview Survey, 1996. Hyattsville MD: National Center for Health Statistics. Vital Health Stat 10. 1999:No. 200.
8. Gonzales R, Malone D, Maselli J, Sande MA. Excessive antibiotics use for respiratory infections in the United States. Clin Infect Dis 2001; 33:757–762.
9. Gwaltney MJ Jr. Acute community-acquired sinusitis. Clin Infect Dis 1996; 23:1209–1225.
10. Woolcock AJ. Epidemiology of chronic airways disease. Chest 1989; 96(suppl 3):302S–306S.
11. Murphy TF, Sethi S. Bacterial infection in chronic obstructive pulmonary disease. Am Rev Respir Dis 1992; 146:1067–1083.
12. Ball P. Epidemiology and treatment of chronic bronchitis and its exacerbation. Chest 1995; 10:43S–52S.
13. Anzueto A. Acute exacerbation of chronic bronchitis. J Crit Illness 1999; 14 (suppl):S27–S33.
14. Murphy SL. Deaths: final data for 1998. National vital statistics reports from the Centers for Disease Control and Prevention, National Center for Health Statistics, National Vital Statistics System. National Center for Health Statistics, 2000.
15. Bartlett JG, Breiman RF, Mandell LA, et al. Community-acquired pneumonia in adults: guidelines for management. Clin Infect Dis 1998; 26:811–838.
16. Foy HM, Cooney MK, Allan I, et al. Rates of pneumonia during influenza epidemics in Seattle, 1964 to 1975. JAMA 1979; 241:253.
17. Houston MS, Silverstein MD, Suman VJ. Community-acquired lower respiratory tract infection in the elderly: a community-based study of incidence and outcome. J Am Board Fam Pract 1995; 8:347–356.

18. Marston BJ, Plouffe JF, File TM Jr, et al. Incidence of community-acquired pneumonia requiring hospitalization: results of a population-based active surveillance study in Ohio. Arch Intern Med 1997; 157:1709–1718.
19. Kalin M, Ortvist A, Almela M, et al. Prospective study of prognostic factors in community-acquired bacteremic pneumococcal disease in 5 countries. J Inf Dis 2000; 182:840–847.
20. Mortensen EM, Coley CM, Singer DE, et al. Arch Intern Med 2002; 162:1059–1064.
21. Birnbaum HG, Morley M, Greenberg PE, Colice GL. Economic burden of respiratory infections in an employed population. Chest 2002; 122:603–611.
22. Ray NF, Baranjuk JN, Thamer M, et al. Healthcare expenditures for sinusitis in 1996. Contributions of asthma, rhinitis, and other airway disorders. J Allergy Clin Immunol 1999; 103:408–414.
23. Neiderman MS, McCombs JS, Unger AN, et al. The cost of treating community-acquired respiratory infection. Clin Ther 1998; 21:576–591.
24. Birnbaum H, Morley M, Greenberg P, et al. Economic burden of pneumonia in an employed population. Arch Intern Med 2001; 161:2725–2731.
25. Niederman MS, McCombs JS, Unger AN, Kumar A, Popovian R. Treatment costs of acute exacerbation of chronic bronchitis. Clin Ther 1999; 21:576–591.
26. McCaig LF, Hughes JM. Trends in antimicrobial drug prescribing among office-based physicians in the United States. JAMA 1995; 273:214–219.
27. File TM Jr, Hadley JA. Rational use of antibiotics to treat respiratory tract infections. Am J Manag Care 2002; 8:713–727.
28. Gwaltney JM Jr, Scheld WM, Sande MA, Sydnor A. The microbial etiology and antimicrobial therapy of adults with acute community-acquired sinusitis: a fifteen-year experience at the University of Virginia and review of other selected studies. J Allergy Clin Immunol 1992; 90:457–462.
29. Wald ER, Chiponis D, Ledesma-Medina J. Comparative effectiveness of amoxicillin and amoxicillin-clavulanate potassium in acute paranasal sinus infections in children: a double-blind, placebo-controlled trial. Pediatrics 1986; 77:795–800.
30. Bluestone CD, Klein JO. Otitis media in infants and children. 2d ed. Philadelphia, PA: WB Saunders Co, 1995:145–240.
31. Dowell SF, Schwartz B, Phillips WR, and The Pediatric URI Consensus Team. Appropriate use of antibiotics for URIs in children, part II: Cough, pharyngitis and the common cold. Am Fam Physician 1998; 58:1335–1342.
32. Dowell SF, Schwartz B. Resistant pneumococci: protecting patients through judicious use of antibiotics. Am Fam Physician 1997; 55:1647–1654.
33. Mainous AG III, Evans ME, Hueston WJ, Titlow WB, McCown LJ. Patterns of antibiotic-resistant *Streptococcus pneumoniae* in children in a day-care setting. J Fam Pract 1998; 46:142–146.
34. Cherian T, Steinhoff MC, Harrison LH, Rohn D, McDougal LK, Dick J. A cluster of invasive pneumococcal disease in young children in child care. JAMA 1994; 271:695–697.
35. Gwaltney JM Jr, Scheld WM, Sande MA, Sydnor A. The microbial etiology and antimicrobial therapy of adults with acute community-acquired sinusitis: a

fifteen year experience at the University of Virginia and review of selected studies. J of Allergy and Clin Immunology 1992; 90:457–461.
36. Dowell SF, Marcy SM, Phillips WR, Gerber MA, Schwartz B. Otitis media—principles of judicious use of antimicrobial agents. Pediatrics 1998; 101:165–171.
37. Gonzales R, Steiner JF, Sande MA. Antibiotic prescribing for adults with colds, upper respiratory tract infection, and bronchitis by ambulatory care physicians. JAMA 1997; 278:901–904.
38. Bisno AL, Gerber MA, Gwaltney JM, Kaplan EL, Schwartz RH. Practice guidelines for the diagnosis and management of group A streptococcal pharyngitis. CID 2002; 35:113–125.
39. Red Book 2000. Report of the committee on infectious diseases. 25th ed. Elk Grove Village, IL: American Academy Pediatrics, 2000.
40. Sinus and Allergy Health Partnership. Antimicrobial treatment guidelines for acute bacterial rhinosinusitis. Otolaryngology-Head and Neck Surgery 2000; 123:S1–S32.
41. Sethis S. Infectious exacerbation of chronic bronchitis: diagnosis and management. J Antimicrob Chemother 1999; 43(suppl A):97–105.
42. American Thoracic Society. Standards for the diagnosis and care of patients with chronic obstructive pulmonary disease (COPD) and asthma. Am Rev Resp Dis 1987;138:225–244.
43. Gwaltney JM Jr. Acute bronchitis. In: Mandell GL Bennett JE, Dolin R, eds. Principles and Practice of Infectious Diseases. 4th ed. New York, NY: Churchill Livingstone, 1995:606–608.
44. Anthonisen NR, Manfreda J, Warren CPW, Hershfield ES, Harding GKM, Nelson NA. Antibiotic therapy in exacerbation of chronic obstructive pulmonary disease. Ann Intern Med 1987; 106:196–204.
45. Saint S, Bent S, Vittinghoff E, Grady D. Antibiotics in chronic obstructive pulmonary disease exacerbation: a meta-analysis. JAMA 1995; 273:957–960.
46. Snow V, Lascher S, Mottur-Pilson C, for the Joint Expert Panel on Chronic Obstructive Pulmonary Disease of the American College of Chest Physicians and the American College of Physicians-American Society of Internal Medicine. Evidence base for management of acute exacerbation of chronic obstructive pulmonary disease. Ann Intern Med 2001;134:595–599.
47. Adams SG, Anzueto A. Antibiotic therapy in acute exacerbation of chronic bronchitis. Semin Respir Infect 2000; 15:234–247.
48. Sethi S. Etiology and management of infections in chronic obstructive pulmonary disease. Clin Pulm Med 1999; 6:327–332.
49. File TM Jr. Treating CAP caused by penicillin-resistant *S pneumoniae*. J Respir Dis 1999; 20:833–842.
50. Bartlett JG, Dowell SF, Mandell LA, File TM Jr, Musher DM, Fine MJ. Community-acquired pneumonia in adults. Clin Infect Dis 2000; 31:347–382.
51. Metlay JP, Kapoor WN, Fine MJ. Does this patient have community-acquired pneumonia? Diagnosing pneumonia by history and physical examination. JAMA 1997; 278:1440–1445.
52. Doern GV, Heilman KP, Huynh HK, Rhomberg PR, Coffman SL, Brueg-

gemann AB. Antimicrobial resistance among clinical isolates of *Streptococcus pneumoniae* in the United States during 1999–2000, including a comparison of resistance rates since 1994–1995. Antimicrob Agents Chemother 2001; 45:1721–1729.

53. Thornsberry C, Ogilvie PT, Holley HP Jr, et al. Survey of susceptibilities of Streptococcus pneumoniae, Haemophilus influenzae, and Moraxella catarrhalis isolates to 26 antimicrobial agents: a prospective U.S. study. Antimicrob Agents Chemo 1999; 43(11):2612–2623.
54. Doern GV, Heilmann KP, Huynh HK, et al. Antimicrobial resistance among clinical isolates of Streptococcus pneumoniae in the United States during 1999–2000, including a comparison of resistance rates since 1994–1995. Antimicrob Agents Chemo 2001; 45(6):1721–1729.
55. Whitney CG, Farley MM, Hadler J, et al. Increasing prevalence of multidrug-resistant streptococcus pneumoniae in the United States. N Engl J Med 2000; 343:1917–1924.
56. Hoban DJ, Doern GV, Fluit AC, Roussel-Delvallez M, Jones RN. Worldwide prevalence of antimicrobial resistance in *Streptococcus pneumoniae*, *Haemophilus influenzae* and *Moraxella catarrhalis* in the SENTRY Antimicrobial Surveillance Program, 1997–1999. Clinical Infectious Diseases 2001; 32(suppl 2): S81–S93.
57. Felmingham D. Evolving resistance patterns in community-acquired respiratory tract pathogens: first results from the PROTEKT global surveillance study. J Infection 2002; 44(suppl A):3–10.
58. Felmingham D, Gruneberg RN, Appelbaum PC, Jacobs MR, & The Alexander Project Group. The Alexander Project 1998–2000: susceptibility of pathogens isolated from community-acquired lower respiratory tract infection to commonly used antimicrobial agents (to be submitted).
59. Richter SS, Heilmann KP, Coffman SL, et al. The molecular epidemiology of penicillin-resistant Streptococcus pneumoniae in the United States, 1994–2000. Clin Infect Dis 2002; 34:330–339.
60. Heffelfinger JD, Dowell SF, Jorgensen JH, et al, and Drug-Resistant Streptococcus pneumoniae Therapeutic Working Group. Management of community-acquired pneumonia in the era of pneumococcal resistance: a report from the Drug-Resistant *Streptococcus pneumoniae* Therapeutic Working Group. Arch Intern Med 2000; 160:1399–1408.
61. File TM Jr. Appropriate use of antimicrobials for drug-resistant pneumonia: focus on the significance of β-lactam-resistant Streptococcus pneumoniae. CID 2002; 34(suppl 1):S17–S26.
62. File TM Jr, Jacobs M, Poole M, Richard M, Wynne B. Clinical efficacy of pharmacokinetically enhanced amoxicillin/clavulanate (AMX/CA) vs comparators against *Streptococcus pneumoniae* (Sp) in respiratory tract infections (RTIs). Intern J Antimicrob Agents 2002; 20:235–247.
63. Feikin DR, Schuchat A, Kolczak M, et al. Mortality from invasive penumococcal pneumonia in the era of antibiotic resistance, 1995–1997. Am J Public Health 2000; 90:223–229.
64. Metlay JP, Hofmann J, Cetron MS, et al. Impact of penicillin susceptibility on

medical outcomes for adult patients with bacteremic pneumococcal pneumonia. Clin Infect Dis 2000; 30:520–528.
65. Campbell GD Jr, Silberman R. Drug-resistant Streptococcus pneumoniae. Clin Infect Dis 1998; 26:1188–1195.
66. Leclercq R, Courvalin P. Resistance to macrolides and related antibiotics in Streptococcus pneumoniae. Antimicrob Agents Chemother 2002; 46:2727–2734.
67. Amsden GW. Pneumococcal macrolide resistance – myth or reality? J Antimicrob Chemother 1999; 44:1–6.
68. Bishai W. The in vivo-in vitro paradox in pneumococcal respiratory tract infections. J Antimicrob Chemother 2002; 49:433–436.
69. Lynch JP III, Martinez FJ. Clinical relevance of macrolide-resistant Streptococcus pneumoniae for community-acquired pneumonia. Clin Infect Dis 2002; 34(suppl 1):S27–S46.
70. Siegel RE. The significance of serum vs tissue levels of antibiotics in the treatment of penicillin-resistant Streptococcus pneumoniae and community-acquired pneumonia. Are we looking in the wrong place? Chest 1999; 116: 535–538.
71. Rodvold KA, Gotfried MH, Danziger LH, et al. Intrapulmonary steady-state concentrations of clarithromycin and azithromycin in healthy adult volunteers. Antimicrob Agents Chemother 1997; 41(6):1399–1402.
72. Hyde TB, Gay K, Stephens DS, et al. Macrolide resistance among invasive Streptococcus pneumoniae isolates. JAMA 2001; 286:1857–1862.
73. Fogarty C, Goldschmidt R, Bush K. Bacteremic pneumonia due to multidrug-resistant pneumococci in 3 patients treated unsuccessfully with azithromycin and successfully with levofloxacin. Clin Infect Dis 2000; 31:613–615.
74. Kelley MA, Weber DJ, Gilligan P, et al. Breakthrough pneumococcal bacteremia in patients being treated with azithromycin and clarithromycin. Clin Infect Dis 2000; 31:1008–1011.
75. Musher DM, Dowell ME, Shortridge VD, et al. Emergence of macrolide resistance during treatment of pneumococcal pneumonia. N Engl J Med 2002; 346(8):630–631.
76. Lonks JR, Garau J, Gomez L, et al. Failure of macrolide antibiotic treatment in patients with bacteremia due to erythromycin-resistant Streptococcus pneumoniae. Clin Infect Dis 2002; 35:556–559.
77. Chen D, McGeer A, de Azavedo JC, Low DE, & The Canadian Bacterial Surveillance Network. Decreased susceptibility of *Streptococcus pneumoniae* to fluoroquinolones in Canada. N Engl J Med 1999; 341:233–239.
78. Ho PL, Yung RWH, Tsang DNC, et al. Increasing resistance of Streptococcus pneumoniae to fluoroquinolones: results of a Hong Kong multicentre study in 2000. J Antimicrob Chemother 2001; 48:659–665.
79. McGee L, Goldsmith CE, Klugman KP. Fluoroquinolone resistance among clinical isolates of *Streptococcus pneumoniae* belonging to international multiresistant clones. J Antimicrob Chemother 2002; 49:173–176.
80. Davidson R, Cavalcanti R, Brunton JL, et al. Levofloxacin treatment failures of pneumococcal pneumonia in association with resistance. N Engl J Med 2002; 346:747–750.

81. Kays NB, Smith DW. Levofloxacin treatment failure in a patient with fluoroquinolone resistant *Streptococcus pneumoniae* pneumonia. Pharmacotherapy 2002; 22:395–399.
82. Ho PL, Tse WS, Tsang KW, et al. Risk factors for acquisition of levofloxacin-resistant Streptococcus pneumoniae: a case-control study. Clin Infect Dis 2001; 32:701–707.
83. File TM Jr. Telithromycin: the first ketolide. Pharmacy & Therapeutics. 2002; 27:14–23.
84. Ball P, Baquero F, Cars O, File T, Garau J, Klugman K, Low DE, Rubinstein E, Wise R. The Consensus Group on Resistance and Prescribing in Respiratory Tract Infection. Antibiotic therapy of community respiratory tract infections: strategies for optimal outcomes and minimized resistance emergence. J Antimicrob Chemother 2002; 49:31–40.
85. Hamm RM, Hicks RJ, Bemben DA. Antibiotics and respiratory infections: Are patients more satisfied when expectations are met? J Fam Pract 1996; 43:56–62.
86. Pihlajamaki M, Kotilainen P, Teemu K, Klaukka T, Palva E, Huovinen P. Macrolide resistant *Streptococcus pneumoniae* and use of antimicrobial agents. The Finnish Study Group for Antimicrobial Resistance. Clin Infect Dis 2001; 33:483–488.
87. Rahal JJ, Urban Horn D, Freeman K, Segal-Maurer S, Maurer J, et al. Class restriction of cephalosporin use to control total cephalosporin resistance in nosocomial Klebsiella. JAMA 1998; 280:1233–1237.
88. Gonzales R, Steiner JF, Lum A, Barrett PHJ. Decreasing antibiotic use in ambulatory practice: impact of a multidimensional intervention on the treatment of uncomplicated acute bronchitis in adults. JAMA 1999; 281: 1512–1519.
89. Dagan R, Klugman KP, Craig WA, et al. Evidence to support the rationale that bacterial eradication in respiratory tract infection provides guidance for antimicrobial therapy. J Antimicrob Chemother 2001; 47:129–140.
90. Marchant CD, Carlin SA, Johnson CE, et al. Measuring the comparative efficacy of antibacterial agents for acute otitis media: the 'Pollyanna phenomenon'. J Ped 1992; 120:72–77.
91. Craig WA. Pharmacokinetic/pharmacodynamic parameters: rationale for antibacterial dosing of mice and men. Clin Infect Dis 1998; 26:1–12.
92. Boles M, Harbarth S, Chinn C, et al. Assessing the cost implications of microbiological sensitivity results of antibiotic treatment in lower respiratory tract infections. In program and abstracts of the fortieth Interscience Conference on Antimicrobial Agents and Chemotherapy, Toronto, Canada. Abstract 2129, pl 509. American Society for Microbiology, Washington, DC, 2000.
93. Grimshaw JM, Russell IT. Effect of clinical guidelines on medical practice: A systematic review of rigorous evaluations. Lancet 1993; 342(8883):1317–1322.
94. Beilby J, Marley J, Walker D, et al. The impact of changes in antibiotic prescribing on patient outcomes in a community setting: a natural experiment in Australia. Presented at: 37th Annual Meeting of the Infectious Diseases Society of America (IDSA); November 18–21, 1999; Philadelphia PA. Abstract 534.

95. Cabana MD, Rand CS, Powe NR, et al. Why don't physicians follow clinical practice guidelines? A framework for improvement. JAMA 1999; 282(15):1458–1465.
96. Hoberman A, Paradise JL, Block S, Burch DJ, Jacobs MR, Balanescu MI. Efficacy of amoxicillin/clavulanate for acute otitis media. Relation to *Streptococcus pneumoniae* susceptibility. Pediatr Infect Dis J 1996; 15(10):955–962.
97. Christenson B, Lunbergh P, Hedlund J, et al. Effects of a large scale intervention with influenza and 23-valent pneumococcal vaccines in adults aged 65 years or older: a prospective study. Lancet 2001; 357:1008–1011.
98. Centers for Disease Control and Prevention. General recommendations on immunization. Recommendations of the Advisory Committee on Immunization Practices (ACIP) and the American Academy of Family Practice Physicians. MMWR Morb Mortal Wkly Rep 2002; 51:No. RR-2.
99. Gardner P, Pickering LK, Orenstein WA, Gershon AA, Nichol K. Guidelines for quality standards for immunization. Clin Infect Dis 2002; 35:503–511.
100. Cornu C, Yzebe D, Leophonte P, Gaillt J, Boissel JP, Cucherat M. Efficacy of pneumococcal polysaccharide vaccine in immunocompetent adults: a meta-analysis of randomized trials. Vaccine 2001; 19:4780–4790.

2

Current Issues Involved in the Treatment of Community-Acquired Pneumonia

Richard Quintiliani
Hartford Hospital, Hartford
and University of Connecticut School of Medicine
Farmington, Connecticut, U.S.A.

Naomi R. Florea
Hartford Hospital, Hartford
Connecticut, U.S.A.

Charles H. Nightingale
Hartford Hospital, Hartford
and University of Connecticut School of Pharmacy
Storrs, Connecticut, U.S.A.

INTRODUCTION

Community-acquired pneumonia is a common and serious illness, with an estimated 5.6 million cases a year in the United States. Of these, approximately 1.1 million patients require hospitalization [1,2]. Community-acquired pneumonia ranks sixth among the leading causes of death in the United States and first among causes of death from an infectious disease, with 50,000 to 60,000 deaths attributed to the infection each year [1,2]. The mortality rate among outpatients with community-acquired pneumonia is low (< 1–5%), but increases to 8–12% among those requiring hospitalization, and to 40% among those patients in the intensive care unit [3,4]. Moreover, the economic cost of community-acquired respiratory tract infections is high, with approximately 150 million workdays lost each year and medical costs exceeding $10 billion annually [5].

Of growing concern is the increase in resistance to traditionally potent antimicrobials among common organisms associated with community-acquired pneumonia. Ubiquitous organisms such as *Streptococcus pneumoniae* are becoming widely resistant to penicillins, cephalosporins, macrolides, tetracyclines, and trimethoprim/sulfamethoxazole. Resistance is even more of an issue with pathogens responsible for chronic care– and hospital-acquired pneumonia, such as *Psuedomonas aeruginosa*, *Acinetobacter baumannii*, *Klebsiella pneumoniae*, and *Enterobacter cloacae*. As a result, lower respiratory tract infections now often require treatment with expanded-spectrum antimicrobial agents.

As a result of this "arms race" between bacteria and antibiotics, the need for optimal treatment strategies, as well as the use of newer antibiotics such as the antipneumococcal fluoroquinolones, to treat respiratory tract infections is becoming increasingly urgent. This chapter reviews the current issues, guidelines, and pharmacodynamic optimization of antimicrobials in the treatment of community acquired respiratory tract infections.

COMMUNITY-ACQUIRED PNEUMONIA

Community-acquired pneumonia (CAP) remains one of the more serious medical problems, being associated with considerable morbidity and mortality. It is estimated that 5.6 million American adults suffer from CAP each year, imposing a significant economic burden on society, with annual expenditures approaching $10 billion [1,2,5]. Although diagnostic techniques and antibiotic therapies have improved, the optimal management of this disease remains controversial.

Over the past decade, four principal guidelines have been published in North America by the following societies: the Infectious Diseases Society of America (IDSA) [6], the Centers for Disease Control and Prevention (CDC) [5], the American Thoracic Society (ATS) [7], and the Canadian Infectious Disease Society and the Canadian Thoracic Society [8]. The Canadian guideline recommendations are in agreement with those from the IDSA guideline except that it focuses on Canadian regional characteristics. Therefore, only the IDSA, CDC, and ATS will be discussed in this chapter, with an emphasis on empiric antibiotic management.

GENERAL CONCEPTS FOR THE UNDERSTANDING OF THE GUIDELINES FOR THE TREATMENT OF COMMUNITY-ACQUIRED PNEUMONIA

To understand the guidelines, one must be familiar with four important observations. First, the best outcomes in this infection occur with antibiotic regimens that provide reliable coverage against both the usual "typical" extracellular bacterial pathogens (e.g., *Haemophilus influenzae*, *Streptococcus pneumoniae*, *Moraxella catarrhalis*) and the "atypical" intracellular pathogens (e.g., *Chlamydia pneumoniae*, *Mycoplasma pneumoniae*, *Legionella pneumophila*). Although it was customary in the past to almost ignore the role of the atypicals, it is now recognized that at least 30% of serious pneumonia, especially in patients with various comorbidities, are caused by these organisms [9,10]. Furthermore, when a patient is first seen, it is basically impossible to determine whether the responsible pathogen belongs to the typical or atypical group. Unfortunately, there is too much overlap in the x-ray, physical, and laboratory findings to make this separation. This observation has had a major impact on the guidelines because neither penicillins (e.g., amoxacillin, ampicillin/sulbactam, piperacillin/tazobactam) nor cephalosporins (e.g., ceftriaxone, cefotaxime, cefuroxime) penetrate inside cells and, hence, do not exhibit activity against the intracellular organisms. As a result, to obtain coverage for the atypical pathogens, another antibiotic, like a macrolide, that displays both activity against these organisms and good intracellular penetration has to be combined with these β-lactam agents. As will be discussed later, this has become the basis for the recommendation to use a combination of a β-lactam antibiotic and a macrolide for the treatment of CAP.

Second, it has been shown that there is a significant increase in morbidity and mortality if appropriate therapy is not initiated within 8 hours of the diagnosis, particularly in the elderly patient with multiple medical comorbidities [7]. This observation negates much of the value of sputum cultures, because the growth of bacteria typically requires more than 48 hr. Moreover, even the Gram stain of sputum may not be helpful unless it is performed on an adequate specimen that has been stained and interpreted properly. The use of guidelines to determine initial empiric therapy not only provides coverage for the possibility of a mixed bacterial and intracellular pathogen infection, but also provides for appropriate rccommendations in a timely manner.

Finally, once easily cured with old narrow-spectrum antibiotics, lower respiratory tract infection now often requires treatment with expanded-spectrum agents, mainly due to the emergence of antibiotic-resistant strains of bacteria. Even ubiquitous organisms involved in CAP, such as S. *pneumoniae*, are becoming widely resistant to penicillins (~40%), cephalosporins, macrolides, tetracyclines, and trimethoprim/sulfamethoxazole [11]. Interestingly, this resistance is usually not a significant problem in otherwise healthy patients but may be one in those with comorbid conditions, such as chronic pulmonary, cardiac, or renal disease, or in the elderly. Antimicrobial agents such as the antipneumococcal fluoroquinolones, the ketolides, vancomycin, and linezolid maintain activity against drug-resistant *S. pneumoniae* (DRSP) and are viable treatment modalities in these circumstances.

CENTERS FOR DISEASE CONTROL AND PREVENTION (CDC) GUIDELINE

The CDC guideline (Fig. 1) was based on the draft of a meeting held in March 1998 that convened the Drug-Resistant *Streptococcus pneumoniae* Therapeutic Working Group (DRSP-TWG) [5].

For the outpatient management of CAP, the CDC guidelines strongly recommend monotherapy with a macrolide (clarithromycin or azithromycin) or doxycycline. For children under age five, an oral β-lactam (cefuroxime axetil, amoxicillin, or amoxicillin-clavulanate) alone is recommended for outpatient empiric treatment because atypical pneumonia is extremely uncommon in this age group and doxycycline and fluoroquinolones should be avoided.

For non–intensive care unit–hospitalized patients, combination therapy with a parenteral β-lactam (cefuroxime, cefotaxime, ceftriaxone, or ampicillin/sulbactam) plus a macrolide (clarithromycin or azithromycin) is recom-

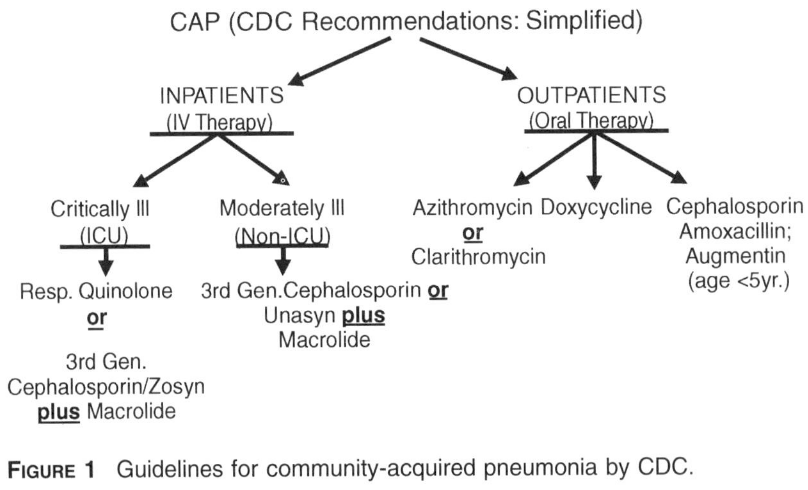

FIGURE 1 Guidelines for community-acquired pneumonia by CDC.

mended. For intubated or intensive care patients, the clinician has two suggested choices: combination intravenous therapy of a β-lactam antibiotic (ceftriaxone, cefotaxime, piperacillin/tazobactam) plus an intravenous macrolide or monotherapy with an antipneumococcal fluoroquinolone.

INFECTIOUS DISEASES SOCIETY OF AMERICA (IDSA) GUIDELINE

The IDSA guideline is summarized in Fig. 2 [6]. Like the CDC, the IDSA society also supports the use of monotherapy with macrolides or doxycycline for outpatients with CAP. However, they also recommend the use of antipneumococcal fluoroquinolone as a therapeutic option for outpatients, especially those with multiple comorbidities. Furthermore, although the IDSA guideline still supports the use of combination therapy with a third-generation cephalosporin or a β-lactamase inhibitor and a macrolide, it mainly recommends monotherapy with the use of antipneumococcal fluoroquinolones as first-line drug therapy for the hospitalized patient.

AMERICAN THORACIC SOCIETY (ATS) GUIDELINE

The ATS guidelines [7] (Fig. 3) are based on four patient stratification groups. Patients are stratified according to their need for hospitalization, underlying cardiopulmonary disease, and risk factors for DRSP, enteric gram-negative organisms, or *P. aeruginosa*. Risk factors for DRSP include age older than 65 years, β-lactam therapy within the past 3 months, immune-suppressive illness (including treatment with corticosteroids), multiple medical comorbidities, and exposure to a child in a day-care center. Those at risk for infection with an enteric gram-negative organism include nursing home residents, those with

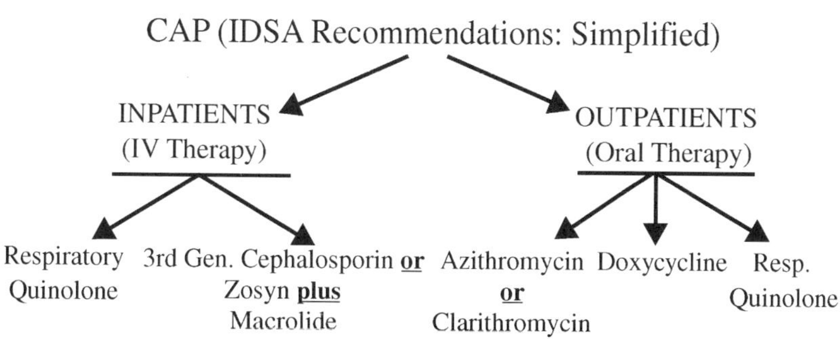

FIGURE 2 Guidelines for community-acquired pneumonia by IDSA.

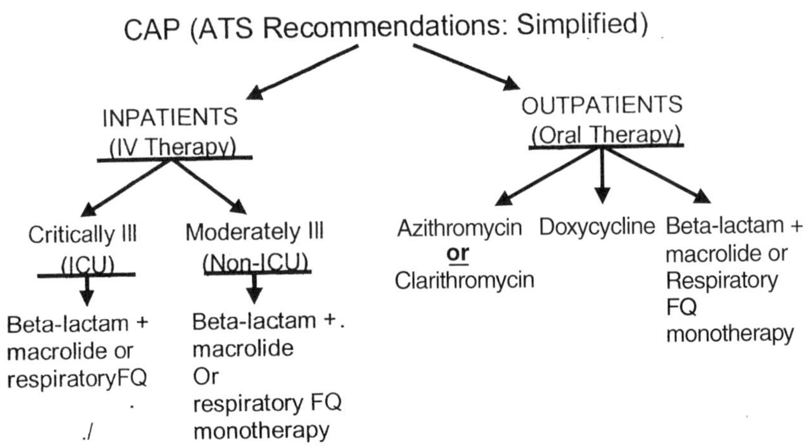

FIGURE 3 Guidelines for community-acquired pneumonia by ATS.

underlying cardiopulmonary disease, recent antibiotic therapy, and those with other medical comorbidities. Finally, patients at risk for infection with *P. aeruginosa* include those with structural lung disease, patients on corticosteroid therapy (>10 mg prednisone/day), use of broad-spectrum antibiotics for more than 7 days in the past month, malnutrition, and undiagnosed HIV infection [12–14].

Group one consists of outpatients that do not have cardiopulmonary disease and/or risk factors for DRSP or gram-negative organisms. Treatment of these patients is limited to an advanced-generation macrolide such as azithromycin or clarithromycin, with doxycycline as an alternative in those patients that are allergic to or intolerant of macrolides. Group 2 consists of outpatients that have cardiopulmonary disease and/or risk factors for DRSP or gram-negative organisms. Recommended therapy for these patients is an oral β-lactam (oral cefpodoxime, cefuroxime, high-dose amoxicillin, amoxicillin/clavulanic acid, or I.V. ceftriaxone followed by oral cefpodoxime) plus a macrolide or doxycycline. As with the IDSA guideline, the ATS guideline also recommends that an antipneumococcal fluoroquinolone can be used in these patients as monotherapy. Patients in Group 3 are those requiring hospitalization. The guidelines suggest that in those patients with no risk factors, a macrolide or an antipneumococcal fluoroquinolone used as monotherapy would suffice. However, in those patients with underlying risk factors, the addition of an intravenous β-lactam (cefotaxime, ceftriaxone, ampicillin/sulbactam, high-dose ampicillin) plus a macrolide or doxycycline should be employed. Once again, the use of a respiratory fluoroquinolone as monotherapy is recommended in these patients. Finally, group 4 consists of those patients that require admission to an intensive care unit. Treatment of these patients includes intravenous β-lactam therapy (cefotaxime, ceftriaxone) plus either intravenous azithromycin or an intravenous antipneumococcal fluoroquinolone. Patients in the ICU that have risk factors for *P. aeruginosa* should receive an intravenous antipseudomonal β-lactam (cefepime, imipenem, meropenem, piperacillin/tazobactam) plus an antipseudomonal fluoroquinolone (ciprofloxacin) or an antipseudomonal β-lactam plus an aminoglycoside plus either azithromycin or an antipneumococcal fluoroquinolone.

INCREASING POPULARITY OF THE FLUOROQUINOLONES IN THE TREATMENT OF RESPIRATORY TRACT INFECTIONS

A look at the current guidelines highlights the growing popularity of monotherapy with the antipneumococcal or third-generation fluoroquinolones, such as levofloxacin, gatifloxacin, and moxifloxacin. This popularity is due in most part to their almost uniform activity against the entire target organisms causing CAP, the ability to give them once-a-day, and their high degree of oral absorption (>90%), whereby allowing many patients to be treated without injectable antibiotics. These antimicrobials have sufficient pharmacokinetic properties to ensure delivery of active drug to the bacteria and thus are agents that are believed to be very effective in bacterial eradication. Since they are very active and have good pharmacokinetics, the probability of selecting or stimulating the emergence of resistant bacteria is considered to be low. This is one of the major reasons for their current popularity. Another is the reported resistance of *S. pneumoniae* to the macrolides. Most of these reports come from isolates collected in hospitalized patients and may not have relevance to the treatment of patients in the community. In addition the reports of resistance are based on breakpoints, which may or may not be set properly. Unfortunately the perception (not the reality) of clinically relevant resistance causes many physicians to use a quinolone in place of a macrolide.

PHARMACODYNAMIC CONCEPTS

A discussion of guidelines and optimal treatment modalities for CAP would not be complete without a brief focus on pharmacodynamic principles. In the past, dosing methods for antibiotics have been more a matter of style or habit than science. Recently, significant information has emerged from animal models, in vitro pharmacodynamic experiments, volunteer studies and clinical outcomes studies that now allow us to administer antibiotics in an optimal way. This means administering the antibiotic to attain the best clinical response, the least amount of toxicity, the lowest cost, and the lowest chance for the emergence of bacterial resistance.

The relationship between bacterial killing and microbiological activity is described by the area under the serum concentration-time curve (AUC) and minimum inhibitory concentration (MIC) of the antibiotic for the target organism(s) (i.e., the AUC:MIC ratio). Under certain conditions, the AUC can be simplified to either concentration or time of antibiotic exposure dependent activity against microorganisms.

β-Lactams, glycopeptides, clindamycin, and macrolide agents kill bacteria in a similar, time-dependent fashion, in which the time that the drug concentration exceeds the MIC (time > MIC) at the site of the infection drives the killing of the infecting microbes [15]. The time above MIC pharmacodynamic parameter can therefore be used to predict the efficacy of these drugs.

Aminoglycosides (e.g., tobramycin, gentamicin, amikacin), fluoroquinolones (e.g., ciprofloxacin, ofloxacin, levofloxacin, gatifloxacin), and amphotericin B eliminate microorganisms most rapidly when their concentrations are appreciably above the MIC of the targeted microorganism(s); hence, their type of killing is referred to as concentration-dependent or dose-dependent killing [17]. In animal models of infection, including neutropenic animals, many more animals survive a potentially lethal challenge of bacteria if aminoglycosides are given as a single daily dose than if the same dose is divided on a q8h basis [16]. In humans it has been shown that aminoglycosides eradicate organisms best when they achieve levels that are approximately 10 to 12 times above the microorganism's MIC [17].

Although fluoroquinolones also exhibit concentration-dependent killing, excessively high concentrations (>10 μg/mL) of these agents in serum can be associated with seizures and other potentially serious central nervous system (CNS) adverse reactions. When targeted against very sensitive organisms, a serum peak to MIC ratio of 10:1 can be obtained. For more moderately sensitive (or moderately resistant organisms), this ratio often cannot be reached without producing excessive toxicity. The goal in this situation is still, however, to maximize concentration-dependent killing for as long as possible without moving into toxic serum levels. Because the AUC is a measurement of both serum concentration and time of exposure of the organism to the antibiotic, the AUC:MIC relationship becomes the best predictor of the clinical response. Predictions from animal models of sepsis, in vitro pharmacodynamic experiments, and clinical outcomes studies indicate that the magnitude of the 24-hour AUC:MIC ratio can be utilized to predict clinical response. For instance, a 24-hour AUC:MIC ratio of 125 or greater has been associated with the best cure rates in the treatment of infections caused by gram-negative hospital-acquired aerobic enteric pathogens [18]. For gram-positive bacteria, like *S. pneumoniae*, it appears that the AUC:MIC ratio can be appreciably lower. Clinical failures or superinfections have not been associated with the respiratory fluoroquinolones when the AUC:MIC ratio for this bacterium is consistently 30 or greater [19]. Achieving AUC: MIC ratios greater than 30–40 against *S. pneumoniae*, however, has not been associated with better clinical responses or less likelihood of the emergence of bacterial resistance.

Regardless of the antibiotic chosen, the dose and dosing regimen must be such that a rapid response to the antibiotic is achieved. Unfortunately, most clinical trials do not report response rates as a function of time. Rather they use a somewhat arbitrary time called the test of cure (TOC). This is one time point where the patients are evaluated and the antibiotic is compared to the results of treating similar patients with the "gold standard." Unfortunately, this does not compare the speed of response of the patient to either drug regimen, and important information is lost.

TRANSITIONAL ANTIBIOTIC THERAPY

Clinical stability in CAP, as assessed by improvements in signs and symptoms as well as laboratory values, can usually be seen within the first 24–72 hours [7]. It is at this point that conversion from intravenous to oral therapy (I.V. to P.O.) should be initiated.

In 1987, we introduced the term antibiotic "streamlining" to refer to the process of converting patients from complicated, often expensive, intravenous therapy to equally efficacious, simple, and less expensive regimens [20]. When the conversion is from I.V. to P.O., the process is now often designated sequential, transitional, step-down, or switch therapy. The fluoroquinolones have gained considerable attention as excellent transitional choices because of their high degree of bioavailability, exceeding 90%.

There are many advantages to employing oral antibiotic therapy in the treatment of infections. Significant cost reductions result from the conversion from I.V. to P.O. therapy because of lower drug acquisition costs, a reduction in pharmacy time in the preparation and mixing of drugs, the ability to deliver a drug without the intervention of intravenous technicians, and a reduction in the length of hospital stay. Investigators at Hartford Hospital found that pharmacist-initiated I.V. to P.O. conversion programs of levofloxacin maximized the number of conversion candidates, led to a reduced length of stay, and resulted in a total provider savings of approximately $3,000 per eligible patient [21].

Perhaps the most important benefit derived from oral antibiotic therapy is the removal of intravenous catheters, which are the major source of nosocomial bacteremia, especially that caused by staphylococci. It has been established that there are more than 20 million vascular catheters inserted annually in patients admitted to hospitals in the United States, resulting in more than 50,000 episodes of bacteremia or line sepsis [22]. The frequency of these infections is directly correlated with the duration of catheter insertion [23]. In a recent cost analysis of 104 patients with line sepsis, it was noted that the average additional cost from each episode of line sepsis was $3,707, and even higher ($6,064) if it was caused by *Staphylococcus aureus*. A number of these episodes, particularly those due to staphylococci, were associated with significant morbidity and occasionally with mortality [24].

Criteria required for converting patients to oral therapy varies from hospital to hospital. The ATS guidelines recommend that patients should be switched to oral therapy if they meet four conditions: improvement in cough and dyspnea, afebrile ($< 100\,^{\circ}F$) on two occasions 8 hr apart, decreasing white blood cell count, and functioning gastrointestinal tract with adequate oral intake [7]. These guidelines can aid in formulating a set of criteria for one's individual institution in order to yield the benefits of conversion therapy.

CONCLUSIONS

At the present time, there are two popular ways to treat community-acquired pneumonia: one is to use monotherapy with a respiratory quinolone, doxycycline, or a macrolide, and the other approach is to employ the combination of a cephalosporin or β-lactamase inhibitor with a macrolide. Monotherapy with a macrolide or doxycycline is used for the otherwise healthy young adult, whereas monotherapy with a fluoroquinolone or combination therapy is usually given to older patients, those with comorbidities, or both. When administering antimicrobial therapy, it is of great importance that the pharmacodynamic parameters of each agent be optimized in order to achieve optimal concentrations for the defined dosing period. Finally, intravenous to oral conversion should be considered in order to reduce the length of hospitalization, risk of line sepsis, and additional labor and supply costs.

REFERENCES

1. Garibaldi RA. Epidemiology of community-acquired respiratory tract infections in adults: incidence, etiology, and impact. Am J Med 1985; 78:32S–37S.
2. Niederman MS, McCombs JI, Unger AN, et al. The cost of treating community-acquired pneumonia. Clin Ther. 1998; 20:820–837.
3. Marrie TJ, Durant H, Yates L. Community-acquired pneumonia requiring hospitalization: a 5 year prospective study. Rev Infect Dis 1989; 11:586–599.
4. Woodhead MA, MacFarlane JT, McCracken JS, et al. Prospective study of

the aetiology and outcome of pneumonia in the community. Lancet 1987; I:671–674.
5. Heffelfinger JD, Dowell SF, Jorgensen JH, et al. Management of community-acquired pneumonia in the era of pneumococcal resistance. Arch Intern Med 2000; 160:1399–1408.
6. Bartlett JG, Dowell SF, Mandell LA, File TM Jr, Musher DM, Fine MJ. Practice guidelines for the management of community-acquired pneumonia in adults. Clin Infect Dis 2000; 31:347–382.
7. Niederman MS, Mandell LA, Anzueto A, et al. American Thoracic Society guidelines for the management of adults with community-acquired pneumonia: diagnosis, assessment of severity, antimicrobial therapy, and prevention. Am J Respir Crit Care Med 2001; 163:1730–1754.
8. Mandell LA, Marrie TJ, Grossman RF, Chow AW, Hyland RH, the Canadian Community-Acquired Pneumonia Working Group. CID 2000; 31:383–421.
9. Marston BJ, Plouffe JF, File TM Jr, et al. Incidence of community-acquired pneumonia requiring hospitalization: results of a population-based active surveillance study in Ohio. The Community-Based Pneumonia Incidence Study Group. Arch Intern Med 1997; 157:1709–1718.
10. Lieberman D, Schlaeffer F, Boldur I, et al. Multiple pathogens in adult patients admitted with community-acquired pneumonia: a one year prospective study of 346 consecutive patients. Thorax 1996; 51:179–184.
11. Doern GV, Pfaller MA, Kugler K, Freeman J, Jones RN. Prevalence of antimicrobial resistance among respiratory tract isolates of Streptococcus pneumoniae in North America: 1997 results from the SENTRY antimicrobial Surveillance Program. Clin Infect Dis 1998; 27:764–770.
12. Ruiz M, Ewig S, Torres A, et al. Etiology of community-acquired pneumonia: impact of age, comorbidity, and severity. Am J Respir Crit Care Med 1999; 160:397–405.
13. Rello J, Rodriguez R, Jubert P, Alvarez B. Severe community-acquired pneumonia in the elderly: epidemiology and prognosis. Clin Infect Dis 1996; 23:723–728.
14. Porath A, Schlaeffer F, Lieberman D. The epidemiology of community acquired pneumonia among hospitalized adults. J Infect 1997; 34:41–48.
15. Craig WA. Interrelationship between pharmacokinetics and pharmacodynamics in determining dosage regimens for broad-spectrum cephalosporins. Diagn Microbiol Infect Dis 1995; 22:89–96.
16. Dudley MN. Pharmacodynamics and pharmacokinetics of antibiotics with special reference to fluoroquinolones. Am J Med 1991; Suppl 6A:45S–50S.
17. Moore RD, Lietman PS, Smith CR. Clinical response to aminoglycoside therapy: Importance of the ratio of peak concentration to minimal inhibitory concentration. J Infect Dis 1987; 155:93–99.
18. Schentag JJ, Nix DE, Adelman MH. Mathematical examination of dual individualization principles. I Relationships between AUC above MIC and area under the inhibitory curve for cefmenoxime, ciprofloxacin, and tobramycin. DICP Ann Pharmacother 1991; 25:1050–1057.

19. Quintiliani R, Nicolau DP, Nightingale CH. Pharmacokinetic and pharmacodynamic principles in antibiotic usage. In: Johnson J, Yu V, eds. Infectious Disease and Antimicrobial Therapy of the Ears, Nose and Throat. chap 5. Philadelphia, Pa: W.B. Saunders Co, 1997:48–55.
20. Quintilani R, Cooper BW, Briceland LL, et al. Economic impact of streamlining antibiotic administration. Am J Med 1987; 82(4A):391–394.
21. Kuti JL, Le TN, Nightingale CH, Nicolau DP, Quintiliani R. Pharmacoeconomics of a pharmacist-managed program for automatically converting levofloxacin route from i.v. to oral. Am J Health Syst Pharm 2002; 59:2209–2215.
22. Maki DG. Infection due to infusion therapy. In: Bennett JV, Brachman PA, eds. Hospital Infection. Boston, Mass: Little, Brown, 1986:561–580.
23. Read I, Body GP. Infectious complications of indwelling vascular catheters. Clin Infect Dis 1992; 15:197–210.
24. Arnow PM, Quimosing EM, Beach M. Consequences of intravascular catheter sepsis. Clin Infect Dis 1993; 16:778–784.

3

Cost Considerations in the Use of Antibiotics for the Treatment of Community-Acquired Respiratory Tract Infections

Joseph L. Kuti
Hartford Hospital
Hartford, Connecticut, U.S.A.

INTRODUCTION

Community-acquired respiratory tract infections (CRTIs) are among the most prevalent and serious infections in the United States, accounting for over 50 million physician visits, 5 million hospitalizations, and 100 thousand deaths annually [1–3]. As a result, the economic impact of CRTIs is substantial. In 1985, the cost of treating CRTIs was estimated to be over $15 billion (US, 1985) [4]. Not only are these costs significantly greater today due to inflation as well as more costly treatment options, they also tend to be considerably underestimated because of the intrinsic error introduced in cost-of-illness studies. Moreover, the implications of increasing resistance among commonly encountered bacterial pathogens, which in turn may lead to clinical failure when inappropriate therapy is initiated empirically, will significantly add to the total economic burden of CRTIs [5].

Infections of the lower respiratory tract, including community-acquired pneumonia (CAP) and acute exacerbations of chronic bronchitis (AECB), account for the majority of hospitalizations and deaths associated with CRTIs. CAP is the sixth leading cause of death in the United States, causing approximately 1.1 million hospitalizations and 45,000 deaths annually [3]. Furthermore, inpatient management of CAP, estimated at $7.5 billion (US, 1995) annually, accounts for over 90% of total treatment-associated costs. As mentioned in separate chapters in this book, *Streptococcus pneumoniae* is the predominant bacterial pathogen in the etiology of CAP; furthermore, resistance to commonly used antimicrobials in the community and hospital make appropriate empiric therapy vital to clinical as well as economic outcomes. Penicillin-nonsusceptibility in *S. pneumoniae* has been shown to increase hospital length-of-stay (LOS), thereby adversely affecting hospital room, nursing, and pharmacy costs [6,7].

AECB, a component of chronic obstructive pulmonary disease, accounts for approximately 280,000 hospitalizations and $1.6 billion in total costs. Similar to CAP, costs due to hospitalizations accounted for the majority of expenses at approximately $1.5 billion [2]. *S. pneumoniae*, along with *Haemophilus influenzae* and *Moraxella catarrhalis*, are the predominant pathogens in AECB. Likewise, antimicrobial resistance among these pathogens can greatly affect clinical and economic outcomes [8,9].

Conversely, upper respiratory tract infections such as sinusitis, pharyngitis, and acute otitis media (AOM), although associated with less mortality and hospitalization, occur more frequently in the community population and thus also incur significant health care resource consumption and cost. AOM, for example, is the most commonly diagnosed bacterial infection in children and costs an estimated $5 billion annually [10]. Unlike CAP and AECB, the majority of these costs are incurred by prescription costs, physician office visits, and indirect costs, specifically work time lost by the caregiver [11].

It is obvious that the improper treatment of CRTIs can have devastating outcomes on health care costs. Consequently, health care reform and technological advances are creating changes in how health care interventions are evaluated. In the past decade, cost containment has at times appeared to overshadow clinical assessments; however, the goal of understanding both the costs and consequences of interventions is ultimately being acknowledged. Clinical endpoints are still necessary, of course, but are no longer sufficient to make fully informed patient care decisions. Nor is it appropriate to make a decision based primarily on cost. In other words, the cheapest antibacterial is not always the most cost-effective, especially when the costs associated with resistance, treatment failures, and adverse events are considered. The purpose of this chapter is to highlight potential methods for reducing health care costs associated with the antibacterial treatment of CRTIs. Because hospitalization and treatment failure–associated costs appear to be most significant, the greater part of this discussion will focus on these concerns. Examples of cost-beneficial approaches to managing such infections in the institution will be provided.

METHODS OF REDUCING ANTIMICROBIAL COST IN THE HEALTH CARE SETTING

There are numerous methods described in the literature for reducing costs when treating patients with CRTIs. These include administering appropriate empiric antibacterial therapy based on pharmacodynamic principles (as covered in other chapters in this book) and providing therapy that encourages good patient compliance such as combination versus monotherapy, single daily dosing, and shorter treatment courses. Patient compliance to appropriate antibacterial therapy is cost-beneficial by reducing treatment failures and readmissions and delaying the emergence of resistance. Finally, promoting intravenous to oral transitional therapy may reduce hospital LOS and avoid costly intravenous complications. None of these methods, however, will be successful if not actually put into practice; therefore, guidelines or clinical pathways can be instituted to lead health care practitioners down the most efficient and cost-effective treatment path for a specific health care setting.

PATIENT COMPLIANCE

Combination Versus Monotherapy

Quintiliani and colleagues were the first to introduce the concept of antibiotic streamlining, which included, initially, transitioning antibiotic courses from combination to monotherapy [12,13]. This concept was tested by Briceland and colleagues when an infectious diseases physician and clinical pharmacist rounded on all patients who had received at least 3 days of parenteral combination antimicrobial therapy [14]. Streamlining recommendations were made in 54% of these patients, accepted in 82%, and resulted in an average cost savings of $138.51 (US, 1988) per patient. The majority of the recommendations suggested discontinuing the current combination therapy and substituting a different single agent, usually a broad-spectrum β-lactam. Monotherapy was more expensive in only 13 cases, usually when two inexpensive agents were replaced by a more costly single agent, such as converting from a gentamicin/cefazolin combination to ceftriaxone or cefotaxime. The increase in cost in these 13 cases was mainly due to the higher acquisition cost of the newer agent. However, comparisons of acquisition costs alone can be misleading if the two agents are not otherwise identical [15]. All costs incurred directly and indirectly by therapy must be considered in order to select the most cost-effective medication. These include drug costs, administration costs (labor and supplies), costs incurred by treatment failures, costs created by drug-induced side effects, drug interactions, and so forth [16].

Richerson and colleagues performed an economic evaluation of alternative antibiotic regimens in hospitalized patients with community-acquired pneumonia [17]. A decision-tree model was used to compare all associated costs from treatment of CAP with azithromycin, levofloxacin, or a combination of cefuroxime plus erythromycin. Probabilities for obtaining clinical success and adverse reactions were taken from the literature and added to the tree at all decision nodes, as denoted by a circle (Fig. 1). The costs for each arm were derived from actual Hartford Hospital costs (US, 1998) and included

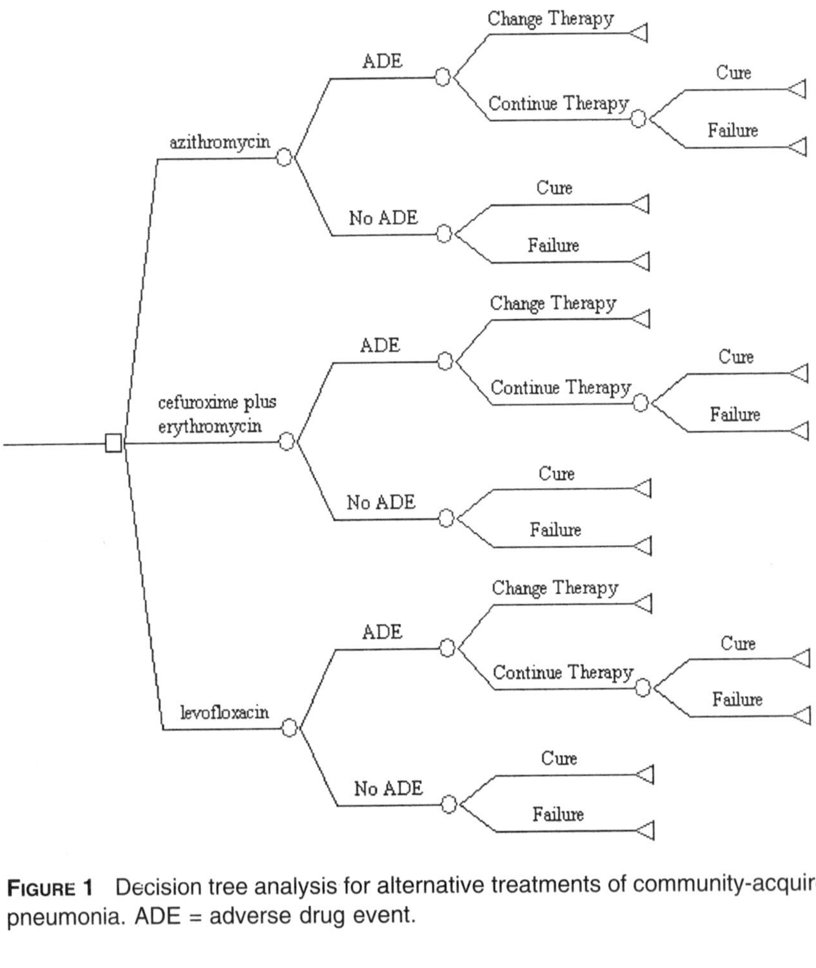

FIGURE 1 Decision tree analysis for alternative treatments of community-acquired pneumonia. ADE = adverse drug event.

expenses associated with drug acquisition, supplies, drug-related adverse events, discontinuation rates requiring alternative therapy, and treatment failure. After performing several analyses to determine the effect of significant component costs on the decision outcome, the authors found that when drug acquisition costs alone were considered, levofloxacin was the most expensive agent ($126), followed by the combination of cefuroxime/erythromycin ($83), and finally azithromycin ($80). However, as the authors added in other indirect costs, levofloxacin became the most cost-effective therapy ($208, 95% CI: 206–210), followed by azithromycin ($228, 95% CI: 224–232), and the combination regimen ($323, 95% CI: 320–326). Not until the effectiveness of levofloxacin was held below 70% did the decision change to favor azithromycin therapy; furthermore, under all reasonable estimates of effectiveness, the levofloxacin regimen was more cost-effective than the combination regimen.

Interestingly, this simulation may have actually underestimated the cost-effectiveness of levofloxacin therapy compared to other standards because the significant cost of hospital LOS was not included in the analysis. Due to its large economic impact, the ability to save even one day of hospitalization could sway the decision in any treatment direction. Using data from a large clinical trial of patients with CAP, Dresser and colleagues performed a cost-effectiveness analysis of another fluoroquinolone antibiotic, gatifloxacin, in comparison with the combination of ceftriaxone plus intravenous erythromycin [18]. Oral transitional therapy was encouraged after at least 2 days of intravenous therapy, and when clinically appropriate, patients could be converted to oral gatifloxacin or oral clarithromycin as per their randomized grouping. Costs were broken up into level 1, 2, and 3 costs. Level 1 costs considers only the acquisition price of the study medication. Gatifloxacin level 1 costs were significantly lower than the combination therapy by an average of $51 (US, 2000), $P < 0.0005$. Level 2 costs, which include all costs directly related to antibiotic use and infection treatment, excluding hospital per diem, were also significantly lower for gatifloxacin by an average of $94 (US, 2000), $P < 0.0005$. Finally, level 3 includes all hospital costs; on this level, gatifloxacin cost an average of $5,109 (US, 2000) per treatment course as compared with the combination therapy, which cost $6,164 (US, 2000), a difference of $1055 (US, 2000) in favor of the fluoroquinolone, $P = 0.0114$. The difference was primarily due to a slightly lower hospital LOS with the gatifloxacin regimen, 4.2 days versus 4.9. By including hospital LOS in the economic analysis, the difference in costs between these regimens was 21 times greater than if only acquisition pricing were considered. Furthermore, after performing sensitivity analysis by varying acquisition prices, hospital costs, and success rates, the economic decision could not be altered and remained in favor of once-daily monotherapy with gatifloxacin.

Once-Daily Dosing and Short-Duration Therapy

A survey of patients receiving antibiotics demonstrated that short-course therapy, once-daily dosing, good efficacy, and few side effects were the most important characteristics of an antibiotic regimen [19]. Administering antimicrobials with a long half-life that allows for once-daily dosing, especially during outpatient treatment, can also further reduce costs [20]. In most cases, total treatment acquisition costs will be similar between newer once-daily antimicrobials compared with older drugs that require more frequent dosing. However, this relationship can vary in either direction depending on the length of treatment and the availability of generic products, which significantly reduce cost. For example, penicillin VK administered at 250 mg four times a day for 10 days would cost an institution approximately $4.80 (US, 1997). Meanwhile, an azithromycin Z-Pak®, which lasts 5 days, would cost $36.24 (US, 1997) [21]. Although the penicillin must be administered four times a day and given for twice as long, it is one-seventh the price of the Z-Pak®. Of course, when failure rates and adverse reactions are considered, the economic decision might favor the azithromycin therapy. Part of that failure rate involves patient compliance with the prescribed medication. Studies have demonstrated improved compliance leading to improved outcomes with once daily dosing versus multiple doses [22,23]. Older, yet cheaper antimicrobials that require administration three to four times a day do not coincide with the increasingly busy schedules of today's lifestyle. What good is the cheaper agent if the patient does not take all the doses? More important, poor compliance to antibiotic therapy can lead to clinical failure, hospital readmission, and the emergence of bacterial resistance. For this reason, many older antibiotics have been remanufactured in extended-release formulations that allow for increased dosing intervals. Such is the case with clarithromycin, which is now available in an ER formulation enabling once-daily dosing. Table 1 displays a list of intravenous and oral antimicrobial agents that can be dosed once daily in the treatment of CRTIs.

Shorter courses of antibacterial therapy will also increase patient compliance, potentially leading to increased success rates, lower resistance rates, and lower costs. The optimal duration of therapy for many CRTIs is controversial. Only recently have clinical trials evaluated the clinical response rates, and more important, relapse rates of antimicrobials when administered for shorter durations.

A 5-day course of telithromycin, the first of a new class of antibiotics called ketolides, was shown to be as effective as 10-day courses of amoxicillin/clavulanic acid, cefuroxime axetil, penicillin VK, and clarithromycin in the treatment of AECB, acute maxillary sinusitis, group A β-hemolytic streptococcus tonsillopharyngitis, and CAP, respectively [24–27]. Other potent

TABLE 1 Intravenous and Oral Antimicrobials That Allow Once-Daily Dosing in the Treatment of CRTIs

Antibacterial	Once-Daily Dose
Intravenous	
Ceftriaxone	1 g
Ertapenem	1 g
Azithromycin	500 mg
Levofloxacin	500 mg
Gatifloxacin	400 mg
Moxifloxacin	400 mg
Oral	
Clarithromycin ER	2 × 500 mg tablets
Azithromycin	2 × 250 mg tablets
Telithromycin	1 × 800 mg tablet
Levofloxacin	1 × 500 mg tablet
Gatifloxacin	1 × 400 mg tablet
Moxifloxacin	1 × 400 mg tablet
Cefixime	1 × 400 mg tablet
Ceftibuten	1 × 400 mg tablet

antimicrobials such as gatifloxacin and moxifloxacin have also been studied for shorter 5-day courses in AECB and acute maxillary sinusitis and demonstrated good outcomes [28,29]. The macrolide, azithromycin, when administered for only 3 days, was shown to be as effective as a 10-day course of amoxicillin/clavulanate in children with acute lower respiratory tract infections (i.e., community-acquired pneumonia) [30]. Of importance is the fact that the majority of isolated pathogens in this study were highly susceptible intracellular bacteria (i.e., *Mycoplasma pneumoniae* and *Chlamydia pneumoniae*) and viruses. More resistant pathogens such as *S. pneumoniae* and *H. influenzae* were not isolated; therefore, the effect of a shorter course is not known for these bacteria. Azithromycin has also been approved as a single 30 mg/kg dose for the treatment of AOM in children [31].

The ability of many of the newer antimicrobials to be effective over a shorter course is associated primarily with their increased microbiologic potency and improved pharmacokinetics. However, as resistant isolates become more prevalent, lengthier treatment regimens as well as higher doses of these agents will likely be needed to maintain efficacy. Furthermore, although presumed to be less costly compared with longer course therapy due to increased patient compliance and equal efficacy, pharmacoeconomic studies of these short-duration regimens are still needed to fully elucidate their economic impact.

Transitional Therapy

An important phase of Quintiliani and colleagues' streamlining concept involved converting the treatment of a stable patient from an intravenous antibiotic to an active oral formulation in order to complete therapy at home. This usually took place around day seven [12]. Since the introduction of this concept in the late 1980s, it has been suggested that this intravenous to oral conversion can occur earlier, perhaps on day 3 or 4, or when certain clinical requirements are met [32–35]. Conversion from intravenous to oral antibiotics can result in important clinical and economic gains. Significant cost reductions occur because of lower drug acquisition costs, a reduction in pharmacy and nursing time for preparation and administration of intravenous formulations, and most important, a potential reduction in the length of hospital stay. Additionally, an important benefit derived from oral therapy is the elimination of the use of intravenous catheters, which are a significant source of nosocomial bacteremias, especially those caused by staphylococci. It has been estimated that there are more than 20 million vascular catheters inserted annually in patients admitted to hospitals in the United States, resulting in more than 50,000 episodes of bacteremia or line sepsis. The frequency of these infections is directly correlated with the duration of their use. In a cost analysis of 104 patients with line sepsis, it was noted that the average additional cost from each episode of line sepsis was $3,707 (US, 1993) and even higher ($6,064) if it was caused by *Staphylococcus aureus* [36].

Intravenous to oral conversion of antimicrobials is known as transitional therapy and can further be identified by the type of conversion made: step-down therapy, switch therapy, or sequential therapy [16]. Step-down therapy involves conversion to an oral agent of the same or different class but with less potency. An example of this is conversion from any parenteral β-lactam to an oral one. Switch therapy refers to the conversion of an intravenous antimicrobial to a different oral agent without reducing potency, such as the transition from intravenous ceftriaxone to oral ciprofloxacin to treat an *Escherichia coli* infection. Finally, conversion from a parenteral agent to its own oral formulation, without losing potency, is termed sequential therapy. Such is the case with the respiratory fluoroquinolones, levofloxacin, gatifloxacin, and moxifloxacin. Because of their high oral bioavailability, these agents would be expected to achieve similar serum concentrations regardless of the mode of administration [37,38].

Numerous studies have demonstrated cost savings when switch therapy is applied, specifically in the treatment of community-acquired pneumonia [33,35,39]. Despite strong clinical support, physician hesitancy still exists when converting patients to oral antibiotics, especially if a different drug or class of drugs has to be used. Therefore, sequential therapy would be expected to have an advantage over switch or step-down therapy; the two formulations of a specific drug have similar adverse effect profiles and the same susceptibility profiles, plus the oral formulation will often be significantly less costly than its parenteral form. This was evaluated in a cost-effectiveness analysis using results from a randomized, open-label, controlled trial comparing sequential ofloxacin versus standard switch therapy in patients hospitalized with complicated urinary tract infections, lower respiratory tract infections, or skin and soft tissue infections [40]. Success rates were similar between regimens; however, sequential ofloxacin therapy resulted in a one-day reduction in antibiotic-related hospitalization (a savings of $399 per patient, US, 1997). The investigators concluded that sequential therapy would lead to earlier oral conversion compared with switch therapy mainly because of an increased physician comfort level with using the same drug, only now in its oral formulation.

Still, the greatest cost savings in the treatment of hospitalized patients occurs in the presence of a reduction in LOS. Even if treatment is switched to oral antibiotics for community-acquired pneumonia, this doesn't automatically assure patient discharge from the hospital. It has been common practice to observe a patient for at least 24 hours after transitional therapy, usually to confirm that the oral formulation is still effective and well tolerated. However, this practice is based more on tradition than scientific evidence. Recently, several studies have confirmed that this observational period is unnecessary and only increases hospital cost, including the risk of acquiring a nosocomial infection [41–43]. While applicable to many patients with moderate CAP, this observation may be significantly different when treating AECB or older patients with more severe CAP as many of these patients will have other comorbidities that may prolong their hospitalization course.

Rhew and colleagues performed a retrospective review of "low-risk" patients with community-acquired pneumonia to assess the clinical benefit of in-hospital observation after oral conversion. Low-risk patients were defined as those patients with pneumonia in the absence of a serious comorbid disease (cancer, HIV, immunosuppression, organ transplantation, cystic fibrosis, empyema, or lung cavity), infection with a high-risk pathogen, an obvious reason for continued hospitalization, or a life-threatening complication during hospitalization. Of 142 patients identified, 102 were observed and 40 were discharged as soon as oral antibiotics were initiated. No patient required medical intervention within 24 hours after hospital discharge and no patient from either group died within the 30-day follow-up period. The LOS for the observed and nonobserved groups was 98 $\pm$ 33 hr and 83 $\pm$ 49 hr, respectively. The difference in LOS was 15 hr (95%

CI, 3 to 27 hr) and could translate into a cost savings of $550 per patient (US, 1993) [41].

A more recent observational study also found similar findings. Forty-eight percent of 266 patients with CAP were observed in-hospital for 24 hr or longer after switching from I.V. to oral antibiotic therapy, resulting in an unnecessary cost of approximately $119,370 (US, 2000). No underlying problem or comorbidity to justify continued hospitalization could be found. If these results were applied to all patients who were admitted to the hospital with CAP, 384,000 hospital days per year could be eliminated, resulting in savings of $265 million dollars [42].

It has been demonstrated that patients hospitalized with CAP generally become clinically stable on the third day of antimicrobial treatment, as indicated by an improvement in vital signs and ability to eat. More severe cases, such as in the elderly, patients with comorbidities, or those requiring ICU admission, can take longer to reach clinical stability (i.e., closer to 7 days) [34]. Initially, these time frames are useful to predict when patients should respond to therapy and would be candidates for transitional therapy. More specifically, vital signs, such as body temperature, systolic blood pressure, heart rate, and respiratory rate, plus the ability to tolerate oral intake would be the best markers to identify stable patients for conversion. Therefore, if a patient becomes stable as indicated by his or her vital signs on day one of treatment, there is no reason why oral therapy shouldn't be initiated and the patient discharged home, provided no other comorbidities require hospitalization and close monitoring.

Many institutions recommend that a pharmacist contact the physician with a recommendation for I.V. to oral conversion when such a patient is identified. Although usually effective, this practice is time consuming and doesn't assure that a candidate for transitional therapy will always be converted. Most studies that employ this technique have demonstrated acceptance in 80% of recommendations [33,35,44–47]. A more efficient method would be to allow pharmacists to automatically convert candidates to an oral formulation of the same drug precisely when clinical stability is identified. This practice would assure conversion in all identified patients because the pharmacist enters the order on the spot. Pharmacist-managed automatic conversion programs have been developed at several institutions with positive outcomes [48,49].

Kuti and colleagues performed an economic evaluation of the intravenous to oral conversion program for levofloxacin at their institution and compared this with a prospective observational period before implementation [49]. The majority of patients evaluated had a diagnosis of CAP or AECB. Of patients who met conversion criteria (temperature, HR, RR, BP, oral intake), 92% were converted when the pharmacists managed the program as compared with 37% beforehand, $P = 0.009$ (Fig. 2). Moreover, patients were converted earlier during the pharmacist-managed program, 3.65 days versus 7.09 days, $P = 0.010$. As a result, level 1, 2, and 3 costs were significantly reduced by the program. The average cost of a hospital stay for a patient meeting criteria was $3,267 (US, 2000) less after the pharmacist-managed program was implemented. This was predominantly due to a reduction in hospital LOS, 6 days versus 9.5 days, $P = 0.031$.

Pharmacoeconomics of Clinical Pathways

Despite all these methods for reducing the cost associated with antimicrobial treatment of CRTIs, little savings will be seen if they are not in turn applied to patient care. This can best be accomplished with implementation of guidelines, otherwise known as clinical pathways, for the treatment of these infections in a specific institution or outpatient setting. Originally developed by industry, clinical pathways are frequently used by health care systems to ensure optimum delivery of high-quality care and control costs. These pathways can include guidelines for ranking patient severity, recommendations whether or not to admit the patient, appropriate diagnostic tests to be ordered, and recommended treatment options. For CRTIs, clinical pathways can also include cost-effective recommendations such as the proper dose, most effective method of administration, and even criteria for oral conversion and hospital discharge. All of these recommendations should provide for the highest quality and most cost-effective treatment of patients.

Clinical pathways may also have positive effects on the time to first antibiotic dose and hospital LOS [50,51]. Marrie and colleagues evaluated

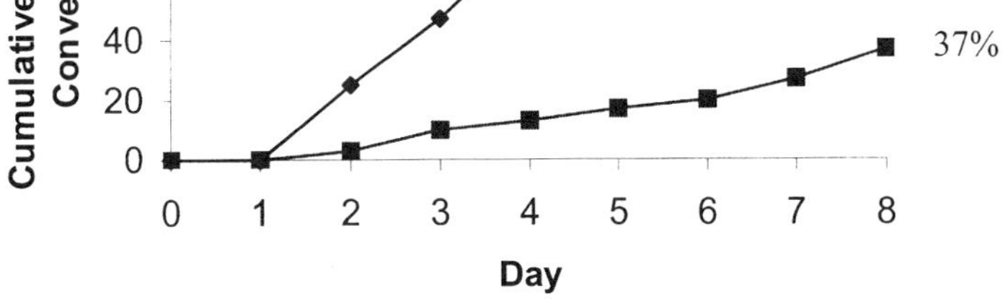

FIGURE 2 Cumulative percent of patients converted to oral levofloxacin over the first eight days of therapy. (From Ref. 49.)

the effect of a clinical pathway incorporating the Pneumonia Severity Index Scoring System [52] and intravenous or oral levofloxacin in 19 Canadian teaching or community hospitals. Hospitals were randomized to either introduce the developed clinical pathway or continue conventional management. No difference between quality of life, occurrence of complications, readmission, or mortality was observed between clinical pathway and conventional treatment sites. Pathway use was associated with a 1.7 day reduction in bed days per patient managed (BDPM), which is the product of the institutional average length of stay and the admission rate (4.4 versus 6.1 days, $P = 0.04$). Clinical pathway institutions also realized a reduction in median LOS (5.0 versus 6.7, $P = 0.01$) and 1.7 fewer days of intravenous antibiotic therapy (4.6 versus 6.3 days, $P = 0.01$). Although no formal economic analysis was included in this article, the investigators estimated that the reduction in use of hospital resources has the potential of saving approximately $1,700 (US, 2000) per patient treated [50].

Marrie and colleagues used levofloxacin as the antimicrobial agent of choice for their CAP clinical pathway. Certainly, any other respiratory fluoroquinolone, such as moxifloxacin and gatifloxacin, would be expected to have similar outcomes. Likewise, antibiotics in other classes such as β-lactams/macrolide combinations and telithromycin can also be equally included in a clinical pathway. The choice of antibiotic should depend on the types of patients being treated and the resistance rates specific to that area. Thus, if pneumococcal resistance to the β-lactam antibiotics were prevalent in an area, the most cost-effective agent would be a respiratory fluoroquinolone or telithromycin. These agents have activity against the most likely causative pathogens in CRTIs, including penicillin-resistant isolates as well as β-lactamase–producing *H. infuenzae* and *M. catarrhalis*, can be dosed once-daily to improve compliance, and are available in an oral formulation with excellent bioavailability. However, if resistance is not an issue in a specific institution, then a β-lactam, a macrolide, or both can be included on the clinical pathway. Recommendations can be based on numerous guidelines currently available for the treatment of CAP, AECB, and acute bacterial rhinosinusitis [3,53–56]. Combination therapy should be streamlined as soon as a pathogen is isolated, and parenteral agents, if used initially, should be transitioned to appropriate oral formulations when patients become stable. Finally, patient discharge immediately after oral conversion should be encouraged in order to reduce LOS, provided no other comorbidities require additional in-hospital monitoring.

CONCLUSION

Despite the advances in new therapies and approaches to diagnosis, the management of CRTIs remains a clinical and economic challenge. The concepts outlined within this discussion may be used as a guideline to create a strategic and economical approach to the management of these infections, specifically in the era of increasing antimicrobial resistance. As mentioned earlier in this chapter, acquisition costs alone do not accurately depict the total economic impact associated with the management of CRTIs. The most beneficial approach to therapy is one that produces a rapid, positive clinical outcome. Ultimately, rapid cure will also lead to positive economic outcomes, benefiting the patient, the institution, and society.

REFERENCES

1. Niederman MS, McCombs JS, Unger AN, Kumar A, Popovian R. The cost of treating community-acquired pneumonia. Clin Ther 1998; 20:820–837.
2. Niederman MS, McCombs JS, Unger AN, Kumar A, Popovian R. Treatment cost of acute exacerbations of chronic bronchitis. Clin Ther 1999; 21:576–591.
3. Bartlett JG, Dowell SF, Mandell LA, File TM, Musher DM, Fine MJ. Practice guidelines for the management of community-acquired pneumonia in adults. Clin Infect Dis 2000; 31:347–382.
4. Dixon RE. Economic costs of respiratory tract infections in the United States. Am J Med 1985; 78(suppl 6B):45–51.
5. Nicolau DP. Clinical and economic implications of antimicrobial resistance for the management of community-acquired respiratory tract infections. J Antimicrob Chemother 2002; 50(suppl S1):61–70.
6. Klepser M, Klepser D, Brooks J, Ernst E, Diekema D, Hoffman H, et al. Examination of healthcare resource utilization associated with the treatment of infections caused by susceptible and non-susceptible isolates of Streptococcus pneumoniae (abstract 2133). In Program and Abstracts of the 40th Interscience Conference on Antimicrobial Agents and Chemotherapy, Toronto, Canada, 2000. p 510. American Society for Microbiology, Washington, DC, USA.
7. Einarsson S, Kristjansson M, Kristinsson KG, Kjartansson G, Jonsson S. Pneumonia caused by penicillin-non-susceptible and penicillin-susceptible pneumococci in adults: a case-control study. Scand J Infect Dis 1998; 30:253–256.
8. Backhouse R, Shakespeare A, Hutton J. Economic evaluation of alternative antibiotic regimens in the management of acute exacerbations of chronic bronchitis. Br J Med Econ 1995; 8:11–25.
9. Pechere JC, Lacey L. Optimizing economic outcomes in antibiotic therapy of patients with acute exacerbations of chronic bronchitis. J Antimicrob Chemother 2000; 45:19–24.
10. Gates GA. Cost-effectiveness considerations in otitis media treatment. Otolaryng Head Neck Surg 1996; 114:525–530.
11. Alsarraf R, Jung CJ, Perkins J, Crowley C, Alsarraf NF, Gates GA. Measuring the indirect and direct costs of acute otitis media. Arch Otolaryng Head Neck Surg 1999; 125:12–18.
12. Quintiliani R, Cooper BW, Briceland LL, Nightingale CH. Economic impact

of streamlining antibiotic administration. Am J Med 1987; 82(suppl 4A):391–394.

13. Quintiliani R. Strategies for the cost-effective use of antibiotics. Infectious Diseases. 2d ed. Philadelphia, PA: W.B. Saunders, 1998:417–422.
14. Briceland LL, Nightingale CH, Quintiliani R, Cooper BW, Smith KS. Antibiotic streamlining from combination therapy to monotherapy utilizing an interdisciplinary approach. Arch Intern Med 1988; 148:2019–2022.
15. Klepser ME, Nightingale CH, Quintiliani R. Pharmacoeconomic analysis of piperacillin/tazobactam versus ticarcillin/clavulanate for the treatment of intra-abdominal infections. Pharm and Ther J 1994; 19:24–32.
16. Paladino JA. Pharmacoeconomics of antimicrobial therapy. Am J Health Syst Pharm 1999; 56(suppl 3):S25–S28.
17. Richerson MA, Ambrose PG, Quintiliani R, Bui KQ, Nightingale CH. Pharmacoeconomic evaluation of alternative antibiotic regimens in hospitalized patients with community-acquired pneumonia. Infect Dis Clin Pract 1998; 7: 227–233.
18. Dresser LA, Niederman MS, Paladino JA. Cost-effectiveness of gatifloxacin vs ceftriaxone with a macrolide for the treatment of community-acquired pneumonia. Chest 2001; 119:1439–1448.
19. Branthwaite A, Pechere JC. Pan-Europenam survey of patients' attitudes to antibiotics and antibiotic use. J Int Med Res 1996; 24:229–238.
20. Davey P, Parker S. Cost-effectiveness of once-daily oral antimicrobial therapy. J Clin Pharmacol 1992; 32:706–710.
21. Nightingale CH, Quintiliani R. Cost of oral antibiotic therapy. Pharmacother 1997; 17:302–307.
22. Jordan WC. Doxycycline versus tetracycline in the treatment of men with gonorrhea: the compliance factor. Sex Transm Dis 1981; 8(suppl 2):105–109.
23. Cockburn J, Gibberd RW, Reid AL, Sanson-Fischer RW. Determinants of noncompliance with short term antibiotic regimens. Br Med J 1987; 295:814–818.
24. Zervos M, Aubier M, Rangaraju M, Leroy B. Five-day telithromycin, a new ketolide, is as effective as standard 10-day comparators in the treatment of acute exacerbation of chronic bronchitis [abstract L-916]. 41st Interscience Conference on Antimicrobial Agents and Chemotherapy, Chicago, Illinois, December 2001.
25. Roos K, Tellier G, Baz M, Rangaraju M, Leroy B. Five-day therapy with the new ketolide telithromycin is as effective as standard 10-day comparators in the treatment of acute maxillary sinusitis [abstract L-909]. 41st Interscience Conference on Antimicrobial Agents and Chemotherapy, Chicago, Illinois, December 2001.
26. Norrby SR, Quinn J, Rangaraju M, Leroy B. Five-day therapy with telithromycin, a new ketolide, is as effective as standard 10-day comparators in the treatment of tonsillopharyngitis [abstract L-915]. 41st Interscience Conference on Antimicrobial Agents and Chemotherapy, Chicago, Illinois, December 2001.
27. Tellier G, Isakov T, Petermann W, Patel M, Lavin B. Efficacy and safety of telithromycin (800 mg once daily) for 5 or 7 days vs clarithromycin (500 mg twice daily) for 10 days in the treatment of patients with community-acquired

pneumonia [abstract L-373]. 42nd Interscience Conference on Antimicrobial Agents and Chemotherapy, San Diego, California, September 2002.

28. Sher LD, Sokol WN, McAdoo MA, Bettis RB, Turner M, Li NF, et al. Short-course, 5-day gatifloxacin is comparable to a standard 10-day course of amoxicillin/clavulanate in patients with acute maxillary sinusitis [abstract L-907]. 41st Interscience Conference on Antimicrobial Agents and Chemotherapy, Chicago, Illinois, December 2001.
29. Lorenz J, Busch W, Thate-Waschke IM. Moxifloxacin in acute exacerbations of chronic bronchitis: clinical evaluation and assessment by patients. J Intern Med Res 2001; 29:61–73.
30. Ferwerda A, Moll HA, Hop WCJ, Kouwenberg JM, Tjon Pian Gi CV, Robben SGF, et al. Efficacy, safety and tolerability of 3 day azithromycin versus 10 day co-amoxiclav in the treatment of children with acute lower respiratory tract infections. J Antimicrob Chemother 2001; 47:441–446.
31. Zithromax [package insert]. New York: Pfizer Inc., 2002.
32. Weingarten SR, Riedinger MS, Varis G, Noah MS, Belman MJ, Meyer RD, et al. Identification of low-risk hospitalized patients with pneumonia: implications for early conversion to oral antimicrobial therapy. Chest 1994; 105:1109–1115.
33. Ramirez JA, Srinath L, Ahkee S, Huang A, Raff MJ. Early switch from intravenous to oral cephalosporins in the treatment of hospitalized patients with community-acquired pneumonia. Arch Intern Med 1995; 155:1273–1276.
34. Halm EA, Fine MJ, Marrie TJ, Coley CM, Kapoor WN, Obrosky S, et al. Time to clinical stability in patients hospitalized with community-acquired pneumonia. JAMA 1998; 279:1452–1457.
35. Ramirez JA, Vargas S, Ritter GW, Brier ME, Wright A, Smith S, et al. Early switch from intravenous to oral antibiotics and early hospital discharge. Arch Intern Med 1999; 159:2449–2454.
36. Arnow PM, Quimosing EM, Beach M. Consequences of intravascular catheter sepsis. Clin Infect Dis 1993; 16:778.
37. Quintiliani R, Owens RC, Grant EM. Clinical role of fluoroquinolones in patients with respiratory tract infections. Infect Dis Clin 1999; 8(suppl 1):S28–S41.
38. Stein GE. The methoxyfluoroquinolones: gatifloxacin and moxifloxacin. Infect Med 2000; 17:564–570.
39. Siegel RE, Halpern NA, Almenoff PL, Lee A, Cashin R, Greene JG. A prospective randomized study of inpatient IV antibiotics for community-acquired pneumonia: the optimal duration of therapy. Chest 1996; 110:965–971.
40. Partsch DJ, Paladino JA. Cost-effectiveness comparison of sequential ofloxacin versus standard switch therapy. Ann Pharmacother 1997; 31:1137–1145.
41. Rhew DC, Hackner D, Henderson L, Ellrodt AG, Weingarten SR. The clinical benefit of in-hospital observation in 'low-risk' pneumonia patients after conversion from parenteral to oral antimicrobial therapy. Chest 1998; 113:142–146.
42. Andaya MRP, Raab TA. Is one day of in-hospital observation after switching from intravenous to oral antibiotic therapy in the treatment of community acquired pneumonia necessary? Infect Dis Clin Pract 2000; 9:372–375.

43. Beaumont M, Schuster M. Is an observation period necessary after intravenous antibiotics are changed to oral administration? Am J Med 1999; 106:114–116.
44. Prybylski KG, Rybak MJ, Martin PR, Weingarten CM, Zaran FK, Stevenson JG, et al. A pharmacist-initiated program of intravenous to oral antibiotic conversion. Pharmacotherapy 1997; 17:271–276.
45. Ahkee S, Smith S, Newman D, Ritter W, Burke J, Ramirez JA. Early switch from intravenous to oral antibiotics in hospitalized patients with infections: a 6-month prospective study. Pharmacotherapy 1997; 17:569–575.
46. Gums JG, Yancey RW, Hamilton CA, Kubilis PS. A randomized, prospective study measuring outcomes after antibiotic therapy intervention by a multidisciplinary consult team. Pharmacotherapy 1999; 19:1369–1377.
47. Sevine F, Prins JM, Koopmans RP, Langendijk PNJ, Bossuyt PMM, Dankert J, et al. Early switch from intravenous to oral antibiotics: guidelines and implementation in a large teaching hospital. J Antimicrob Chemother 1999; 43:601–606.
48. Wong-Beringer A, Nguyen KH, Razeghi J. Implementing a program for switching from i.v. to oral antimicrobial therapy. Am J Health Syst Pharm 2001; 58: 1139–1142.
49. Kuti JL, Le TN, Nightingale CH, Nicolau DP, Quintiliani R. Pharmacoeconomics of a pharmacist-managed program for automatically converting levofloxacin route from i.v. to oral. Am J Health Syst Pharm 2002; 59:2209–2215.
50. Marrie TJ, Lau CY, Wheeler SL, Wong CJ, Vandervoort MK, Feagan BG. A controlled trial of a critical pathway for treatment of community-acquired pneumonia. JAMA 2000; 283:749–755.
51. Benenson R, Magalski A, Cavanaugh S, Williams E. Effects of a pneumonia clinical pathway on time to antibiotic treatment, length of stay, and mortality. Acad Emerg Med 1999; 6:1243–1248.
52. Fine MJ, Auble TE, Yealy DM, Donald M, Hanusa BH, Weissfeld LA, et al. A prediction rule to identify low-risk patients with community-acquired pneumonia. N Engl J Med 1997; 336:243–250.
53. Niederman MS, Mandell LA, Anzueto A, Bass JB, Broughton WA, Campbell GD, et al. Guidelines for the management of adults with community-acquired pneumonia: diagnosis, assessment of severity, antimicrobial therapy, and prevention. Am J Respir Crit Care Med 2001; 163:1730–1754.
54. Mandell LA, Marrie TJ, Grossman RF, Chow AW, Hyland RH. Canadian guidelines for the initial management of community-acquired pneumonia: an evidence based update by the Canadian Infectious Diseases Society and the Canadian Thoracic Society. Clin Infect Dis 2000; 31:383–421.
55. Heffelfinger JD, Dowell SF, Jorgensen JH, Klugman KP, Mabry LR, Musher DM, et al. Management of community-acquired pneumonia in the era of pneumococcal resistance: a report from the Drug-Resistant *Streptococcus pneumoniae* Therapeutic Working Group. Arch Intern Med 2000; 160:1399–1408.
56. Sinus and Allergy Health Partnership. Antimicrobial treatment guidelines for acute bacterial rhinosinusitis. Otolaryng Head Neck Surg 2000; 123:S4–S32.

4

The Role of Macrolides in the Treatment of Community-Acquired Pneumonia

William R. Bishai
Johns Hopkins School of Medicine
Baltimore, Maryland, U.S.A.

Charles H. Nightingale
Hartford Hospital, Hartford
and University of Connecticut School of Pharmacy
Storrs, Connecticut, U.S.A.

Erythromycin, the first member of the macrolide class to enter clinical use, was introduced in 1952. Erythromycin remained a mainstay antibiotic for several decades both as an inpatient, infusible agent and as an outpatient, orally administered drug until the introduction of the newer macrolide and azalide agents, clarithromycin and azithromycin, in the early 1990s. The macrolide antibiotic class has activity against each of the major pyogenic pathogens playing etiologic roles in respiratory tract infections: *Streptococcus pneumoniae*, *Haemophilus influenzae*, and *Moraxella catarrhalis*. Moreover, they are potent against atypical respiratory tract pathogens: *Legionella pneumophila*, *Mycoplasma pneumoniae*, and *Chlamydia pneumoniae*. As such they comprise a class of agents with focused activity against respiratory pathogens. It is important to note that they have little role in the treatment of skin and soft tissue infections for which staphylococci are common causes, enteric infections caused by gram-negative bacilli, or opportunistic gram-negative infections such as *Pseudomonas aeruginosa*. Hence, macrolides are considered excellent focused therapy agents for use against respiratory tract infections.

MACROLIDE PK/PD RELATIONSHIPS

Despite being related structurally and by mechanism of action, the pharmacodynamic parameters most predictive of success are different for the major drugs in the macrolide/azalide family. For clarithromycin and erythromycin (as with the β-lactams), time above MIC seems to be the critical parameter; for azithromycin the AUC/MIC ratio seems to be most predictive. For optimal efficacy against *S. pneumoniae*, clarithromycin and erythromycin should achieve concentrations above the MIC for greater than 40% of the dosing interval [1]; and for azithromycin an AUC/MIC ratio above 25 is optimal [2]. Beyond pharmacodynamics, clarithromycin and azithromycin have dramatically different human pharmacokinetics (Fig.1). The C_{max} achieved with a 500 mg oral dose of clarithromycin is approximately 2.5 μg/mL with a half-life of 6 hr [3]. Thus, this agent achieves a concentration above 1 μg/mL, which is the current NCCLS breakpoint between intermediate and high level clarithromycin resistance, for greater than 50% of a 12-hr treatment cycle. Likewise, extended-release clarithromycin achieves a C_{max} of 2.5 μg/mL with a half-life of 12–16 hr, also providing drug concentrations well above the MIC of intermediately resistant organisms for greater than half of its 24-hr treatment cycle. In contrast, the C_{max} of azithromycin is only 0.4 μg/mL with an AUC of 4.5 mg-h/mL following administration of a 500 mg dose [3]. Thus, for isolates with an MIC of less than 0.25 μg/mL, azithromycin achieves the target AUC/MIC ratio needed for optimal efficacy in the serum; however, for isolates with higher MICs, effectiveness may be less.

Beyond serum concentration, however, macrolides may exert their potency through a high degree of tissue penetration in the respiratory tract. This phenomenon is combined with the fact that pyogenic respiratory tract pathogens such as *S. pneumoniae*, *H. influenzae*, and *M. catarrhalis* are extracellular agents that induce disease by infection in the alveolar spaces or on mucosal surfaces. Appreciation of this fact has prompted an investigation of macrolide drug levels in key compartments such as the epithelial surface and the intracellular space of leukocytes and macrophages, which are recruited to the site of infection [4,5]. As seen in Figure 2, concentrations of clarithromycin and azithromycin in the epithelial lining fluid (ELF) are typically approximately 10 times higher than the achievable serum levels

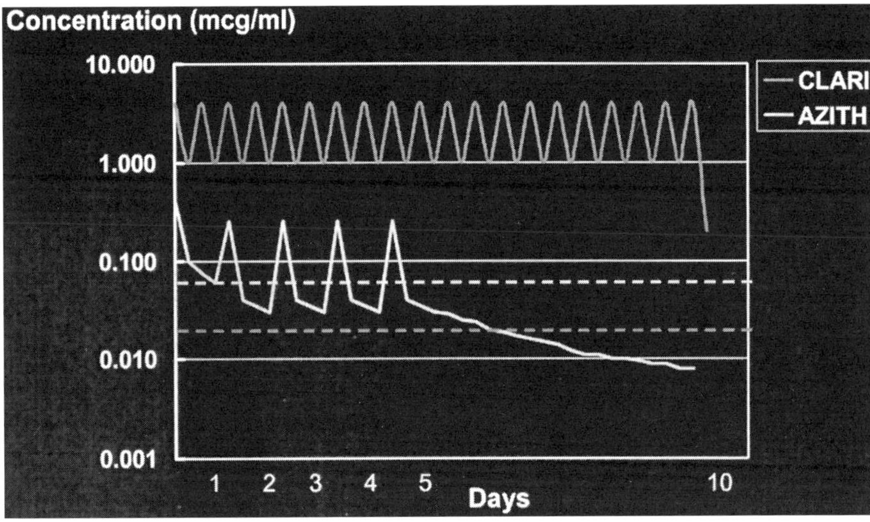

FIGURE 1 Plasma concentrations of clarithromycin and azithromycin during the treatment cycle with standard U.S. dosing of 500 mg twice daily and 250 mg once daily, respectively. For comparison, the NCCLS MIC_{90} breakpoints between susceptible and nonsusceptible strains of *Streptococcus pneumoniae* are shown for the two agents in dotted lines. (From Ref. 43.)

[6,7]. Clarithromycin, after standard dosage, achieves ELF levels of approximately 35 μg/mL and alveolar macrophage intracellular concentrations of approximately 350–500 μg/mL 6 hr after oral dosage in humans [6]. Twenty-four hours after oral dosing, the ELF concentration is approximately 4.5 μg/mL and the alveolar macrophage concentration 100 μg/mL. Azithromycin achieves ELF levels of 1–2 μg/mL but much higher levels in the alveolar macrophage intracellular compartment [6]. A number of investigators have emphasized that the presence of inflammation, which recruits leukocytes to the site of infection, enhances the bioavailability of macrolides, in particular that of azithromycin [8–10]. Levels of azithromycin inside neutrophils and monocytes have been measured at 10 μg/mL or higher, suggesting that these cells may be an important source of macrolide drug during inflammation [4].

By taking into account macrolide concentrations in the epithelial lining fluid, it is apparent that sustained concentrations of greater than 25 to 35 μg/mL may be achieved in the ELF with clarithromycin for a greater than 50% of the treatment cycle. Because more than 90% of the *S. pneumoniae* isolates in the United States have MICs to clarithromycin of 16 μg/mL or less, the

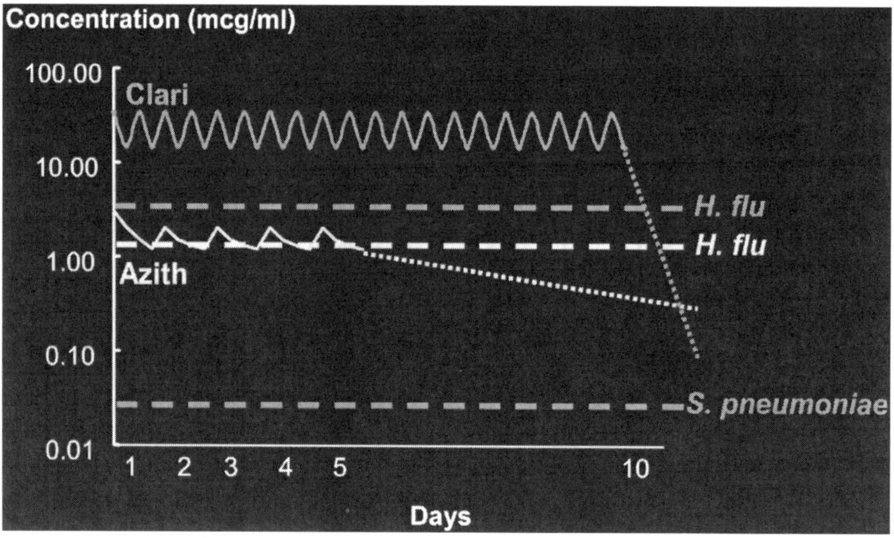

FIGURE 2 Lung epithelial lining fluid (ELF) concentrations of clarithromycin and azithromycin during the treatment cycle with standard U.S. dosing of 500 mg twice daily and 250 mg once daily, respectively. For comparison, the NCCLS MIC_{90} breakpoints between susceptible and nonsusceptible strains of *Haemophilus influenzae* are shown for the two agents in dotted color-coded lines for the two drugs, and the clarithromycin NCCLS MIC_{90} breakpoints between susceptible and nonsusceptible strains of *Streptococcus pneumoniae* are also shown. (From Ref. 43.)

pulmonary concentration effect of macrolides may well explain their continued treatment efficacy despite the emergence of strains that are defined as resistant by current NCCLS breakpoints.

BACTERIAL RESISTANCE TO THE MACROLIDES

S. pneumoniae Resistance Mechanisms to Macrolides

Macrolide resistance in the United States is currently approximately 20–26% in recent surveillance studies [11–13]. Among *S. pneumoniae* isolates resistant to penicillin, macrolide coresistance is approximately 75% [11]. In parts of southern Europe and in the Far East, macrolide resistance rates of 75% or greater have been reported [14].

Pneumococcal resistance to the macrolides falls into two categories. Relatively low level resistance with MICs from 1 to 32 μg/mL are observed with pneumococcal isolates harboring macrolide efflux pump genes (*mef* genes). These pump genes show inducible activity and are capable of pumping macrolides drugs out of the bacterial cell in a concentration-dependent manner. Newer ketolide drugs, such as telithromycin, are not substrates of the *mef* efflux pumps currently present in pneumococci, and hence they remain active in pneumococci expressing *mef* genes.

The second mechanism of resistance occurs via target modification. Erythromycin ribosomal methylase (*erm*) genes of several different types are capable of methylating key residues in the ribosomal RNA of the 50S ribosome, rendering the ribosomal binding pocket of macrolides nonsusceptible to macrolide inhibition. This form of resistance is concentration-independent and confers MICs of greater than 64 μg/mL to pneumococci. Many of the *erm* genes identified in pneumococci are also inducible following the administration of macrolide drugs.

In addition to the genotypic categorization of pneumococcal resistance to macrolides, there is a phenotypic resistance system. MLS_B phenotypic resistance indicates coresistance to macrolides, lincosamides, and streptogramins, and is generally synonymous with target modification mechanisms with the *erm* genotype. The M phenotype of pneumococcal macrolide resistance represents resistance to macrolides only, without lincosamide and streptogramin resistance. Such isolates are susceptible to the lincosamide drug clindamycin, while resistant to erythromycin and other macrolides. Usually, M-type resistance correlates with the presence of an efflux pump–based mechanism with a *mef* genotype.

In the United States, approximately 60 to 75% of macrolide-resistant strains are the M phenotype with an efflux-based mechanism of resistance and MICs between 1 and 32 μg/mL. Only about 25% of isolates are of the high level resistance, MLS_B phenotype with MICs of greater than 64 μg/mL [15]. There is some evidence that while the rate of MLS_B resistance is remaining relatively stable, there has been a gradual shift toward higher MIC levels of resistance within the M-phenotype strains, with an increasing proportion of strains with MICs of 8 or 16 μg/mL observed in recent surveys [15]. In contrast to the situation in the United States, in southern Europe and in other parts of the world there appears to be a higher rate of MLS_B macrolide resistance. In fact, some studies have identified 75 to 80% MLS_B (or *erm*-based) resistance to the macrolides [14].

The new ketolide agent, telithromycin, which is a 14-membered ring macrolide derivative, is active against the majority of MLS_B and M-phenotype pneumococcal isolates. In addition telithromycin is not an inducer of the *mef* and *erm* genes [16]. However, there have been reports of in vitro–derived resistance [17], and some clinical isolates have been identified with telithromycin resistance of 1 to 8 μg/mL, which may be due to a mutation in the ribosomal L4 protein [18].

Macrolide Immunomodulatory Effects

An interesting drug-host interaction has been demonstrated for some macrolides, showing that the drug may have an immune-enhancing effect in addition to its direct antibacterial effect [5]. It has been shown that macrolides enhance ciliary clearance and reduce levels of proinflammatory cytokines, which may reduce the recruitment of tissue-damaging mononuclear cells to the site of resolving infection and accelerate recovery. Such immunomodulatory abilities may significantly augment the activity of an antibiotic and may account for high treatment success rates even when there is relative antimicrobial resistance.

IN VIVO–IN VITRO PARADOX WITH PNEUMOCOCCAL RESPIRATORY TRACT INFECTIONS

Despite rising rates of pneumococcal resistance to β-lactam and macrolide antibiotics, there remains little evidence that this microbiologic phenomenon is correlated with increased rates of treatment failure. The controversy brings into focus the question of whether microbiologic resistance determinations in vitro, in fact, predict treatment outcomes in vivo. A number of large-scale clinical studies in community-acquired pneumonia due to *S. pneumoniae* have looked for inferior treatment outcomes with drug-resistant *S. pneumoniae* (DRSP) infections compared with drug susceptible.

The In Vivo–In Vitro Paradox with Penicillin-Resistant *S. Pneumoniae* (PRSP)

The first study to evaluate this question was conducted in Barcelona in a series of 504 patients with culture-proven pneumococcal pneumonia [19]. Although this study contained a high proportion of penicillin-resistant isolates, there was no increase in mortality in patients who had DRSP compared with those who had drug-susceptible isolates. Moreover, the use of discordant therapy in the study during the first 48 hours was not associated with an increase in mortality compared with concordant therapy. More recently Feikin et al. evaluated the clinical impact of resistance in the United States and Canada from 1995 to 1997, identifying a series of 5837 cases of community-acquired invasive pneumococcal pneumonia. The study did not identify a statistically significant difference in the mortality rate between penicillin-susceptible infection and penicillin-resistant infection [20].

Numerous other such studies have been conducted, and several have looked at nonmortality measures of outcome (Table 1). In general, there has been no consistent effect on either morbidity or mortality in pneumonia due to

TABLE 1 Studies Comparing Mortality Outcomes of Invasive Pneumococcal Pneumonia Caused by Penicillin-Susceptible (Pen-S) and Penicillin-NonSusceptible (Pen-NS) Strains

Location	Year	Fraction of patients with DRSP	Mortality		*P* value	Reference
			Pen-S	Pen-NS		
Barcelona, Spain	1984–93	145/504 (29%)	24%	38%	NS	Pallares et al. (Ref. 19)
Israel	1987–92	67/293 (23%)	11%	16%	NS	Rahav et al. (Ref. 38)
Ohio	1991–94	39/499 (8%)	19%	21%	NS	Plouffe et al. (Ref. 39)
New York[a]	1992–96	30/421—Pen IR (7%)	14%	27%	NS	Turett et al. (Ref. 21)
		19/421—Pen R (5%)	16%	42%	<0.01	
S. Africa (children)	1993–94	35/108 (32%)	16%	24%	NS	Friedland et al. (Ref. 40)
Atlanta	1994	44/192 (23%)	11%	23%	NS	Metlay et al. (Ref. 41)
North America	1995–97	741/4193 (18%)	11%	14%	NS	Feikin et al. (Ref. 20)
Barcelona	1996–98	49/101—Pen (49%)	6%	16%	NS	Ewig et al. (Ref. 42)
		12/101—Mac (12%)	14%[b]	7%[c]	NS	

[a] 70% of patients with the Pen-NS strains were HIV-infected.
[b] Mac-S.
[c] Mac-NS
Source: Ref. 22.

β-lactam–resistant *S. pneumoniae*, although one study with small numbers of patients with a high rate of HIV infection did identify a mortality difference [21]. These findings have been recently summarized [22].

The In Vivo–In Vitro Paradox with Macrolide-Resistant *S. Pneumoniae* (MRSP)

Similar scrutiny has been applied to the outcome of pneumonia due to macrolide-resistant *S. pneumoniae* (MRSP). Ewig et al. evaluated 101 consecutive patients in Barcelona between 1996 and 1998, 47% of whom had bacteremic pneumococcal pneumonia. In the study there was no statistically significant difference in mortality comparing pneumonia due to penicillin-susceptible *S. pneumoniae* (mortality 6%) and penicillin-nonsusceptible *S.*

pneumoniae (mortality 16%). The investigators looked at the impact of macrolide resistance in the study. The mortality rate among patients with macrolide-susceptible isolates was 14% (10 deaths among 74 patients evaluated), whereas the mortality among patients with macrolide nonsusceptible isolates was 7% (2 deaths among 27 patients with MRSP), a result that was a trend in the counterintuitive direction but did not achieve statistical significance. Thus, as with β-lactam resistance, to date there has been no demonstration of statistically worse outcomes for mortality or morbidity with macrolide-resistant pneumococcal pneumonia.

Descriptive Reports of Macrolide Failures Associated with Bacteremic Pneumococcal Pneumonia

Pharmacodynamic considerations would predict that while the macrolides should have excellent efficacy for tissue-based pneumonia, they might have less activity in bacteremic pneumonia because of their relatively lower serum drug levels compared with tissue levels. Several recent case reports and small case series have documented pneumococcal bacteremia due to resistant isolates associated with macrolide therapy [23–29]. Typically such failures occur in outpatients receiving oral macrolides, and the failures have been identified with isolates having MICs of 8 μg/mL or higher [25,28], although in one case, failure with breakthrough bacteremia was seen during parenteral macrolide therapy with azithromycin [29].

A recent case-control report by Lonks and colleagues evaluated patients treated with macrolides over a 13-year period in four study sites in Boston, Providence, and Barcelona. The study found that concurrent exposure to macrolides increased the likelihood of having macrolide intermediate-resistant *S. pneumoniae* (MISP) or fully macrolide resistant *S. pneumoniae* (MRSP) compared with age- and sex-matched controls [25]. The study suggested that macrolide resistance resulting from efflux strains of the M phenotype (low-level resistance with MICs of 1 to 16 μg/mL) was clinically relevant. However, evaluation of the data identified that only five instances of non-meningeal breakthrough bacteremia due to M-phenotype strains were observed. For two of these, no MIC data were included, two had MICs of 16 μg/mL, and only one had an MIC of 4 μg/mL (which is in the range commonly observed with efflux strains in the United States). Moreover, the patient for whom the latter isolate was obtained had been treated with his first macrolide dose within hours of the positive blood culture. Hence, these data do not conclusively link macrolide treatment failure with pneumonia caused by pneumococci with M-type (low level resistance) phenotypic resistance. Unfortunately, these anecdotal and small series reports lack incidence information because they do not include a denominator to suggest how common these occurrences are. Clearly more information and prospective studies will be needed to assess this important question.

COMMUNITY-ACQUIRED PNEUMONIA GUIDELINES AND MACROLIDES

Three Sets of Community-Acquired Pneumonia Guidelines in the United States

Although ATS was the first to write CAP guidelines in 1993, that document has been sorely out of date since it predated the introduction of respiratory fluoroquinolones. The IDSA introduced its CAP guidelines 5 years later in 1998. However, as resistance rates in respiratory tract infections have risen and more drugs have become available, there has been increasing pressure to generate new or updated practice recommendations. In 2000, CDC guidelines appeared in May [30], and updated IDSA Guidelines were published in September [31]. Updated ATS guidelines, which appeared in June 2001, are now the third major set of CAP guidelines to appear in the span of 13 months [32].

The market for respiratory tract antibiotics is estimated to approach $10 billion annually. Within this pie, the greatest fraction of antibiotic use and expenditure lies within outpatient management of respiratory tract infections. It is in this same arena that empiric management plays an important role, because in routine clinical practice, cultures and antimicrobial susceptibility testing, if performed, usually have a minimal impact on the clinical course. CAP guidelines, such as the new ATS statement, have their greatest influence in directing empiric management—particularly in outpatient practice.

The rising rates of resistance among respiratory tract pathogens, particularly the pneumococcus, are a major concern addressed by each of the guidelines. Although rates of microbiologic resistance have increased, all three guidelines specifically point out that there has not been a proven correlation between microbiologic resistance and loss of clinical efficacy among older drug classes such as the β-lactams, macrolides, and doxycycline. The paradox between increasing rates of microbiologic resistance but stable rates of therapeutic success has prompted a number of experts to question the current trend towards using new drug categories, such as the fluoroquinolones, when treatment failure is not being seen with older agents.

There has been a steady trend toward greater stratification of patient categories in respiratory tract infections. The Fine criteria [33,34] gave methodologic criteria for stratifying patients with pneumonia to four categories depending on severity. Both the IDSA and the ATS guidelines are based on categories developed by Fine risk stratification with pneumonia. The IDSA

TABLE 2 Recommendations for Outpatient Management of CAP

Guideline body	Date	Antibiotic Category Recommended	Reference
CDC	5/00	Macrolide[a] or Doxycycline or β-lactam[b]	30
IDSA	9/00	Macrolide or Doxycycline or Fluoroquinolone[c]	31
ATS	6/01	*Uncomplicated*: Macrolide or Doxycycline *Complicated*: Fluoroquinolone alone or a β-lactam[d] plus either a Macrolide or Doxycycline	32

[a] Recommended macrolides: clarithromycin, erythromycin, or azithromycin.
[b] Recommended β-lactams: amoxicillin, amoxicillin/clavulanate, cefuroxime axetil, cefpodoxime, or cefprozil. Cefdinir, a new agent, also acceptable.
[c] Recommended fluoroquinolones: levofloxacin, gatifloxacin, or moxifloxacin.
[d] Recommended β-lactams: cefpodoxime, cefuroxime, amoxicillin (3 g/day), or amoxicillin/clavulanate. Cefdinir, a new agent, also acceptable.

guidelines used three severity categories, whereas the new ATS guidelines have six: two for outpatients and four for inpatients. Significantly, the ATS guidelines are the first to subdivide the all-important category of outpatient CAP.

As may be seen in Table 2, the four categories of drugs recommended for outpatient CAP management are: (1) macrolides, (2) fluoroquinolones, (3) certain β-lactams, and (4) doxycycline. Comparison of the guidelines reveals several areas of discrepancy in managing outpatients with CAP. Significantly, all three guideline bodies recommend macrolides (clarithromycin, erythromycin, or azithromycin) or doxycycline for managing outpatient CAP. The drugs for which there is disagreement are the β-lactams and fluoroquinolones.

ROLE FOR β-LACTAM MONOTHERAPY IN CAP GUIDELINES?

The CDC guidelines have suggested that certain β-lactam drugs are effective in outpatient CAP, but there is considerable concern over their lack of activity against the causative agents of atypical pneumonia such as *Legionella* and *Mycoplasma pneumoniae*. Some studies of CAP suggest that mycoplasma may be more prevalent in older individuals than reported earlier [35]. Among the β-lactam agents with relatively high activity against *S. pneumoniae*, *H. influenzae*, and *M. catarrhalis* that are deemed appropriate under the CDC guidelines are amoxicillin, amoxicillin/clavulanate, cefuroxime axetil, cefpodoxime, or cefprozil. The new agent, cefdinir, has potency and pharmacokinetic properties which make it acceptable as well. Monotherapy with a β-lactam in CAP is not recommended by ATS or IDSA.

Macrolides Versus Fluoroquinolones as First-Line Agents for the Empiric Management of Outpatient CAP

One of the most pressing issues in the outpatient management of community-acquired pneumonia is the appropriate use of fluoroquinolones. While all three guideline groups—CDC, IDSA and ATS—have recommended fluoroquinolones for inpatient management of community-acquired pneumonia, they have disagreed over the appropriate role for these drugs on the outpatient side. The respiratory fluoroquinolones levofloxacin, gatifloxacin, and moxifloxacin have gained popularity because of their broad spectrum of action, their convenience of dosing, and the convenience of dual I.V. and P.O. dosing routes.

The IDSA guidelines, which endorsed the outpatient use of fluoroquinolones in CAP, emphasized the rising rates of pneumococcal resistance to macrolides and doxycycline. Concern over the possibility of treatment failure due to resistance has fueled the popularity of fluoroquinolones for respiratory tract infections. Current rates of resistance to the fluoroquinolones among respiratory tract pathogens are low. For *Streptococcus pneumoniae*, U.S. rates of fluoroquinolone resistance remain under 5%. This contrasts with higher rates of microbiologic resistance to the macrolides among pneumococci of approximately 25%.

Despite the relatively high rate of microbiologic resistance to the macrolides, the ATS guidelines point out that treatment failure has not been observed at an appreciable rate in spite of the growing rate of resistance. The ATS and the CDC have been concerned that expanded use of the fluoroquinolones for outpatient management of respiratory tract infection may be unnecessary and could accelerate the emergence of resistance to this class, thereby damaging the future usefulness of the fluoroquinolone category. Out of concern over the emergence of new resistance, the CDC guidelines took a conservative approach, recommending strict restrictions on the use of fluoroquinolones for empiric management of outpatient CAP. The CDC has recommended that outpatient use of fluoroquinolones be restricted to patients known (1) to be allergic to all other agents, (2) to have a high-level drug resistant strain, or (3) to have had previous treatment failure. On the other hand, the IDSA guidelines took the opposite stand, recommending use of fluoroquinolones for empiric management of outpatient pneumonia with no restriction.

The ATS guidelines recommend an intermediate approach by restricting fluoroquinolones for uncomplicated outpatient CAP, but endorsing their use in high-risk patients with CAP being managed as outpatients. The ATS defines high-risk patients as those with preexisting COPD, immunosuppression, recent hospitalization, or residence in a chronic care facility. For such complicated CAP patients, the ATS recommends one of two regimens: (1) a β-lactam plus either a macrolide or doxycycline, or (2) a respiratory fluoroquinolone. For uncomplicated CAP, the ATS guidelines recommend that a macrolide or doxycycline be used in the interest of restricting fluoroquinolones to prevent the emergence of resistance.

Issues in Appropriate Use of Antibiotics

Underlying the differences in these guidelines is a controversy among infectious diseases and pulmonary experts on just when resistance may be expected to emerge in respiratory tract pathogens. Leading the list of pathogens in this arena is *Streptococcus pneumoniae*, in which we have witnessed the emergence of alarming levels of resistance (35% to penicillin, 25% to macrolides) over the past decade. Looking back, historically, few pathogen-drug combinations have escaped the inexorable emergence of resistance. (Notable exceptions to the generalization that increased use produces increased resistance are *Streptococcus pyogenes* and *Treponema pallidum*, which have remained uniquely susceptible to penicillin for over 50 years.) Thus, we have learned that increased use eventually leads to resistance.

With regard to penicillin resistance in the pneumococcus, it is perhaps a more intriguing question to consider why it took 40 years for this resistance to occur beginning in the early 1990s despite high-level use of β-lactam drugs. Here an important observation has been made from the molecular epidemiologic studies of pneumococcal spread in the United States. The majority of drug-resistant *S. pneumoniae* (DRSP) strains in North America belong to one of six serotypes [36]. Hence, the increased prevalence of DRSP is due to clonal spread. The fact that additional pneumococcal serotypes have not acquired mutations conferring β-lactam resistance suggests a significant genetic barrier to achieving resistance.

Unlike β-lactam resistance, pneumococcal fluoroquinolone resistance in North America has been polyclonal and associated with multiple strains independently acquiring, or mutating to, the resistance phenotype. In Canada, where ciprofloxacin was used extensively for the treatment of respiratory tract infections beginning in the late 1980s and throughout the 1990s, multiple DNA fingerprint types and multiple serotypes of fluoroquinolone-resistant pneumococci have been observed [37]. These data suggest that the barrier to resistance development in the pneumococcus is substantially lower for the fluoroquinolones than it is for the β-lactam drugs. With lower genetic barriers to developing resistance, the emergence of quinolone resistance in pneumococci may occur more rapidly under conditions of expanded use than was witnessed with β-lactams.

Guidelines have emerged as an influential part of clinical practice during the past decade. The CDC, IDSA, and ATS guidelines for the management of community-acquired pneumonia represent scholarly contributions and offer rational approaches on the empiric management of outpatient community acquired pneumonia. One lingering concern is the number of different guidelines on the same topic and the lack of complete consensus on the topic of fluoroquinolone use in CAP. There has been a considerable interest in combining the expert societies in future years to publish a single set of guidelines rather than multiple independent, and sometimes conflicting, documents. Indeed, plans are currently in progress to achieve such a consensus statement, which will be endorsed by the ATS, CDC, and IDSA.

REFERENCES

1. Craig WA. Pharmacokinetic/pharmacodynamic parameters: rationale for antibacterial dosing of mice and men. Clin Infect Dis 1998; 26:1–10.
2. Craig WA. The hidden impact of antibacterial resistance in respiratory tract infection. Re-evaluating current antibiotic therapy. Respir Med 2001; 95(suppl A):S12–S19.
3. Carbon C. Pharmacodynamics of macrolides, azalides, and streptogramins: effect on extracellular pathogens. Clin Infect Dis 1998; 27:28–32.
4. Amsden GW. Pneumococcal macrolide resistance—myth or reality? J Antimicrob Chemother 1999; 44:1–6.
5. Baldwin DR, Honeybourne D, Wise R. Pulmonary disposition of antimicrobial agents: methodological considerations. Antimicrob Agents Chemother 1992; 36:1171–1175.
6. Rodvold KA, Gotfried MH, Danziger LH, Servi RJ. Intrapulmonary steady-state concentrations of clarithromycin and azithromycin in healthy adult volunteers. Antimicrob Agents Chemother 1997; 41:1399–1402.
7. Patel KB, Xuan D, Tessier PR, Russomanno JH, Quintiliani R, Nightingale CH. Comparison of bronchopulmonary pharmacokinetics of clarithromycin and azithromycin. Antimicrob Agents Chemother 1996; 40:2375–2379.
8. Girard AE, Cimochowski CR, Faiella JA. Correlation of increased azithromycin concentrations with phagocyte infiltration into sites of localized infection. J Antimicrob Chemother 1996; 37(suppl C):9–19.
9. Ballow C, Amsden GW, Highet VS. Healthy volunteer pharmacokinetics of oral azithromycin in serum, urine, polymorphonuclear leukocytes and inflammatory vs. non-inflammatory skin blisters. Clinical Drug Investigation 1998; 15: 159–167.
10. Freeman CD, Nightingale CH, Nicolau DP, Belliveau PP, Banevicius MA, Quintiliani R. Intracellular and extracellular penetration of azithromycin into

inflammatory and noninflammatory blister fluid. Antimicrob Agents Chemother 1994; 38:2449–2451.
11. Doern GV, Heilmann KP, Huynh HK, Rhomberg PR, Coffman SL, Brueggemann AB. Antimicrobial resistance among clinical isolates of *Streptococcus pneumoniae* in the United States during 1999–2000, including a comparison of resistance rates since 1994–1995. Antimicrob Agents Chemother 2001; 45:1721–1729.
12. Thornsberry C, Sahm DF, Kelly LJ, et al. Regional trends in antimicrobial resistance among clinical isolates of *Streptococcus pneumoniae*, *Haemophilus influenzae*, and *Moraxella catarrhalis* in the United States: results from the TRUST Surveillance Program, 1999–2000. Clin Infect Dis 2002; 34(suppl 1):S4–S16.
13. Hyde TB, Gay K, Stephens DS, et al. Macrolide resistance among invasive *Streptococcus pneumoniae* isolates. JAMA 2001; 286:1857–1862.
14. Lynch J, Martinez FJ. Clinical relevance of macrolide-resistant *Streptococcus pneumoniae* for community-acquired pneumonia. Clin Infect Dis 2002; 34 (suppl 1):S27–S46.
15. Gay K, Baughman W, Miller Y, et al. The emergence of *Streptococcus pneumoniae* resistant to macrolide antimicrobial agents: a 6-year population-based assessment. J Infect Dis 2000; 182:1417–1424.
16. Leclercq R, Courvalin P. Resistance to macrolides and related antibiotics in *Streptococcus pneumoniae*. Antimicrob Agents Chemother 2002; 46:2727–2734.
17. Davies TA, Dewasse BE, Jacobs MR, Appelbaum PC. In vitro development of resistance to telithromycin (HMR 3647), four macrolides, clindamycin, and pristinamycin in *Streptococcus pneumoniae*. Antimicrob Agents Chemother 2000; 44:414–417.
18. Tait-Kamradt A, Davies T, Appelbaum PC, et al. Two new mechanisms of macrolide resistance in clinical strains of *Streptococcus pneumoniae* from Eastern Europe and North America. Antimicrob Agents Chemother 2000; 44:3395–3401.
19. Pallares R, Linares J, Vadillo M, et al. Resistance to penicillin and cephalosporin and mortality from severe pneumococcal pneumonia in Barcelona, Spain. N Engl J Med 1995; 333:474–480.
20. Feikin DR, Schuchat A, Kolczak M, et al. Mortality from invasive pneumococcal pneumonia in the era of antibiotic resistance, 1995–1997. Am J Public Health 2000; 90:223–229.
21. Turett GS, Blum S, Fazal BA, Justman JE, Telzak EE. Penicillin resistance and other predictors of mortality in pneumococcal bacteremia in a population with high human immunodeficiency virus seroprevalence. Clin Infect Dis 1999; 29: 321–327.
22. Bishai W. The in vivo-in vitro paradox in pneumococcal respiratory tract infections. J Antimicrob Chemother 2002; 49:433–436.
23. Sanchez C, Armengol R, Lite J, Mir I, Garau J. Penicillin-resistant pneumococci and community-acquired pneumonia. Lancet 1992; 339:988.
24. Lonks J, Medeiros AA. High Rate of erythromycin and clarithromycin

resistance among *Streptococcus pneumoniae* isolates from blood cultures from Providence, R.I. Antimicrob Agents Chemother 1993; 37:1742–1745.
25. Lonks JR, Garau J, Gomez L, et al. Failure of macrolide antibiotic treatment in patients with bacteremia due to erythromycin-resistant *Streptococcus pneumoniae*. Clin Infect Dis 2002; 35:556–564.
26. Fogarty C, Goldschmidt R, Bush K. Bacteremic pneumonia due to multidrug-resistant pneumococci in 3 patients treated unsuccessfully with azithromycin and successfully with levofloxacin. Clin Infect Dis 2000; 31:613–615.
27. Kelley MA, Weber DJ, Gilligan P, Cohen MS. Breakthrough pneumococcal bacteremia in patients being treated with azithromycin and clarithromycin. Clin Infect Dis 2000; 31:1008–1011.
28. Waterer GW, Wunderink RG, Jones CB. Fatal pneumococcal pneumonia attributed to macrolide resistance and azithromycin monotherapy. Chest 2000; 118:1839–1840.
29. Musher DM, Dowell ME, Shortridge VD, et al. Emergence of macrolide resistance during treatment of pneumococcal pneumonia. N Engl J Med 2002; 346:630–631.
30. Heffelfinger JD, Dowell SF, Jorgensen JH, et al. Management of community-acquired pneumonia in the era of pneumococcal resistance: a report from the Drug-Resistant *Streptococcus pneumoniae* Therapeutic Working Group. Arch Intern Med 2000; 160:1399–1408.
31. Bartlett JG, Dowell SF, Mandell LA, File TM Jr, Musher DM, Fine MJ. Practice guidelines for the management of community-acquired pneumonia in adults. Infectious Diseases Society of America. Clin Infect Dis 2000; 31:347–382.
32. Niederman MS, Mandell LA, Anzueto A, et al. Guidelines for the management of adults with community-acquired pneumonia. Diagnosis, assessment of severity, antimicrobial therapy, and prevention. Am J Respir Crit Care Med 2001; 163:1730–1754.
33. Fine MJ, Auble TE, Yealy DM, et al. A prediction rule to identify low-risk patients with community-acquired pneumonia. N Engl J Med 1997; 336:243–250.
34. Fine MJ, Stone RA, Singer DE, et al. Processes and outcomes of care for patients with community-acquired pneumonia: results from the Pneumonia Patient Outcomes Research Team (PORT) cohort study. Arch Intern Med 1999; 159:970–980.
35. Marston BJ, Plouffe JF, File TMJr., et al. Incidence of community-acquired pneumonia requiring hospitalization. Results of a population-based active surveillance Study in Ohio. The Community-Based Pneumonia Incidence Study Group. Arch Intern Med 1997; 157:1709–1718.
36. Doern GV, Brueggemann AB, Blocker M, et al. Clonal relationships among high-level penicillin-resistant *Streptococcus pneumoniae* in the United States. Clin Infect Dis 1998; 27:757–761.
37. Chen DK, McGeer A, de Azavedo JC, Low DE. Decreased susceptibility of *Streptococcus pneumoniae* to fluoroquinolones in Canada. Canadian Bacterial Surveillance Network. N Engl J Med 1999; 341:233–239.

38. Rahav G, Toledano Y, Engelhard D, Simhon A, Moses A, Sacks T, Shapiro M. Invasive pneumococcal infections. A comparison between adults and children. Medicine (Baltimore) 1997; 76(4):295–303.
39. Plouffe JF, Breiman RF, Facklam RR. Bacteremia with *Streptococcus pneumoniae*. Implications for therapy and prevention. JAMA 1996; 275(3):194–198.
40. Friedland IR. Comparison of the response to antimicrobial therapy of penicillin-resistant and penicillin-susceptible pneumococcal disease. Pediatr Infect Dis J 1995; 14(10):885–890.
41. Metlay JP, Hofmann J, Cetron MS, et al. Impact of penicillin susceptibility on medical outcomes for adult patients with bacteremic pneumococcal pneumonia. Clin Infec Dis 2000; 30:520–528.
42. Ewig S, Ruiz M, Torres A, et al. Pneumonia acquired in the community through drug-resistant *Streptococcus pneumoniae*. Am J Respir Crit Care Med 1999; 159:1835–1842.
43. Nightingale CH, Mattoes HM. Macrolide, azelide and ketolide pharmacodynamics. In: Nightingale CH, Murakawa T, Ambrose PG, eds. Antimicrobial Pharmacodynamics in Theory and Clinical Practice. New York: Marcel Dekker, 1999:205–220.

5

Treatment of Community-Acquired Respiratory Tract Infections with Ketolides

Paul B. Iannini
Danbury Hospital, Danbury
and Yale University School of Medicine
New Haven, Connecticut, U.S.A.

INTRODUCTION

The ketolides are a new class of antibacterial agents derived from the 14-membered macrolactone ring that characterizes the macrolides. Novel structural modifications result in enhanced binding to bacterial ribosomes through tighter binding at domain V of bacterial rRNA relative to erythromycin A and direct binding at a second site in domain II of bacterial rRNA. The result of this improved ribosomal binding is increased potency against respiratory tract pathogens, including macrolide-resistant strains. Ketolides do not induce expression of macrolide-lincosamide-streptogramin$_B$ (MLS$_B$) resistance. They have an optimum spectrum of activity for the treatment of respiratory tract infections (RTIs), being highly active against common, atypical, and intracellular respiratory pathogens such as *Streptococcus pneumoniae* (including penicillin-, macrolide-, and azalide-resistant strains), *Haemophilus influenzae* and *Moraxella catarrhalis* (including β-lactamase–producing strains), *Staphylococcus aureus, Streptococcus pyogenes* (including many macrolide- and azalide-resistant strains), respiratory anaerobes, *Legionella pneumophila, Chlamydophila pneumoniae,* and *Mycoplasma pneumoniae.* Ketolides also possess good activity against *Coxiella burnetii, Francisella tularensis, Corynebacterium diphtheriae, Bordetella pertussis,* and *Bordetella parapertussis.* The ketolides display concentration-dependent bactericidal activity. They achieve high concentrations in plasma, respiratory tissues, alveolar macrophages, and neutrophils. Their targeted spectrum of antibacterial activity and favorable pharmacokinetic/pharmacodynamic (PK/PD) profile make this class of agents ideal for the treatment of lower and upper RTIs, including community-acquired pneumonia (CAP), acute exacerbations of chronic bronchitis (AECB), acute maxillary sinusitis (AMS), and tonsillitis/pharyngitis. Telithromycin—the first ketolide antibacterial to be approved for clinical use—has been both effective and well tolerated in over 1 million patients since its commercial introduction. Telithromycin retains clinical efficacy in the therapy of patients with resistant pathogens, and has been efficacious even in the setting of bacteremic pneumococcal disease caused by penicillin- and macrolide-resistant strains. Side effects, when they do occur, are mild and consistent in incidence and severity with other approved antibacterial agents, particularly the macrolides. Drug-drug interactions are few and are similar to those of the macrolides.

KETOLIDE STRUCTURE

The ketolides are structurally related to the 14-membered ring macrolides but a keto group replaces the L-cladinose at position 3 of the macrolactone ring [1] (Fig. 1). Replacement of the α L-cladinose sugar with a keto function avoids the induction of MLS_B resistance [2]. Ketolides also contain a methoxy group at position 6 of the macrolactone ring that, in conjunction with the 3-keto group, improves stability in acidic environments by preventing internal hemiketalization. The L-cladinose moiety at position 3 of the macrolactone ring was previously thought to be essential for the antibacterial activity of macrolides, but it is now known that derivatizing other positions of the macrolactone ring can provide the same activity. In most developmental ketolides, a C11, C12-carbamate group is present and more than compensates for the removal of the L-cladinose group (Fig. 2). Telithromycin also possesses an aryl alkyl side chain extension to the C11, C12-carbamate (Fig. 2) [3].

The mode of action of the ketolides is similar to that of the macrolides. Both antibacterial classes bind to the 50S subunit of bacterial ribosomes and prevent bacterial protein synthesis by preventing mRNA translation and ribosomal assembly. Both macrolides and ketolides bind to domain V of the 23S rRNA. Due to the C11, C12-carbamate group, ketolides, unlike the macrolides, bind directly to a second site in domain II of the 23S rRNA of the 50S ribosomal subunit [4,5]. The secondary structure of bacterial 23S rRNA

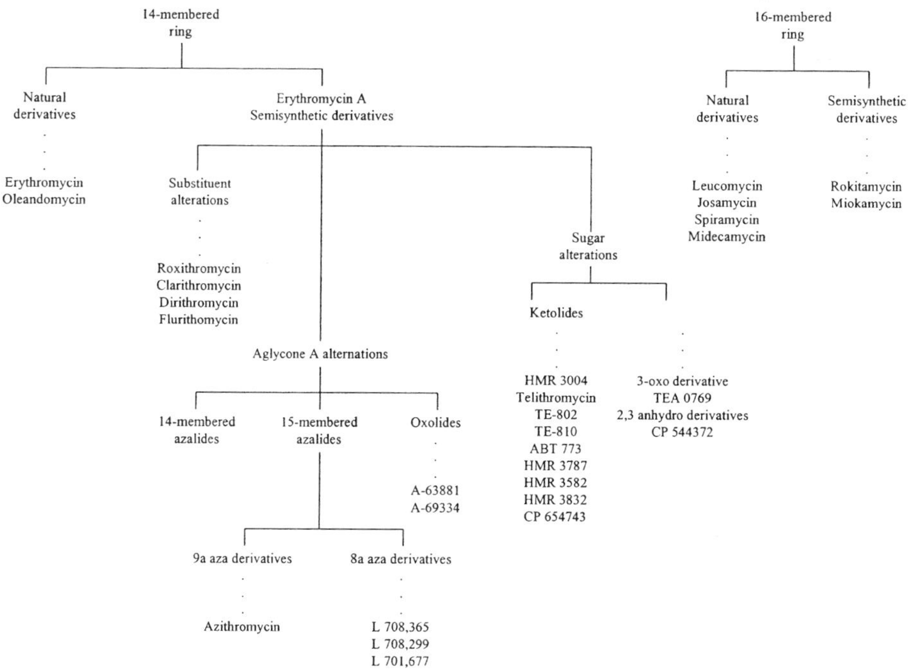

FIGURE 1 Macrolides and their derivatives. (From Ref. 2.)

showing the sites of interaction of the macrolides and ketolides is shown in Figure 3.

There are two main mechanisms by which streptococci become resistant to macrolide antibacterials: target-site modification (encoded by the *erm* genes) and drug efflux (encoded by the *mef* genes). Methylation of the adenine 2058 residue in domain V of bacterial rRNA causes MLS_B phenotypic resistance to macrolides such as erythromycin A and clarithromycin, azalides such as azithromycin, lincosamides such as clindamycin, and Group B streptogramins such as quinupristin. Folding of the 23S ribosomal subunit brings domains II and V very near to each other at the junction of the peptide exit channel and adjacent to the petidyl transferase center. Ketolides retain activity against strains that have become MLS_B resistant through methylation of adenine residue 2058 in domain V through their second interaction with adenine residue 752 in domain II of bacterial rRNA [6]. Ketolides do not elicit MLS_B phenotypic expression of inducible *erm* genes and, thus far, have not caused selection of resistant strains [7]. Telithromycin is a poor substrate for

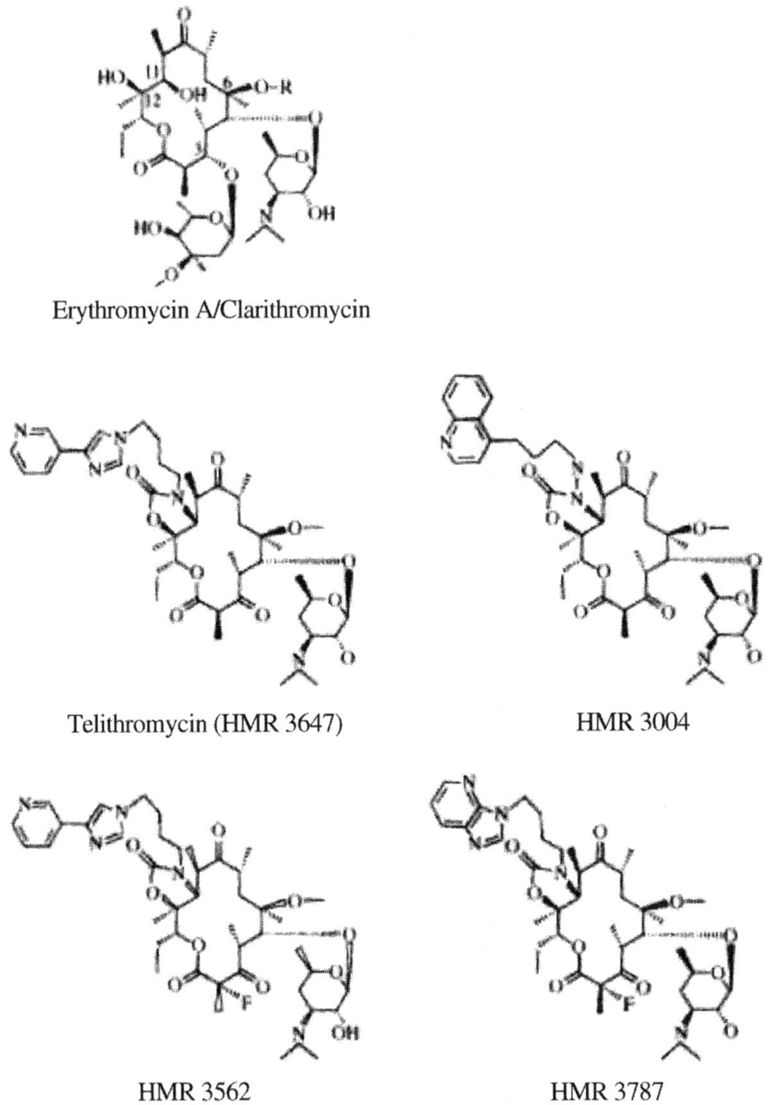

FIGURE 2 Macrolide/ketolide structure. (From Ref. 3.)

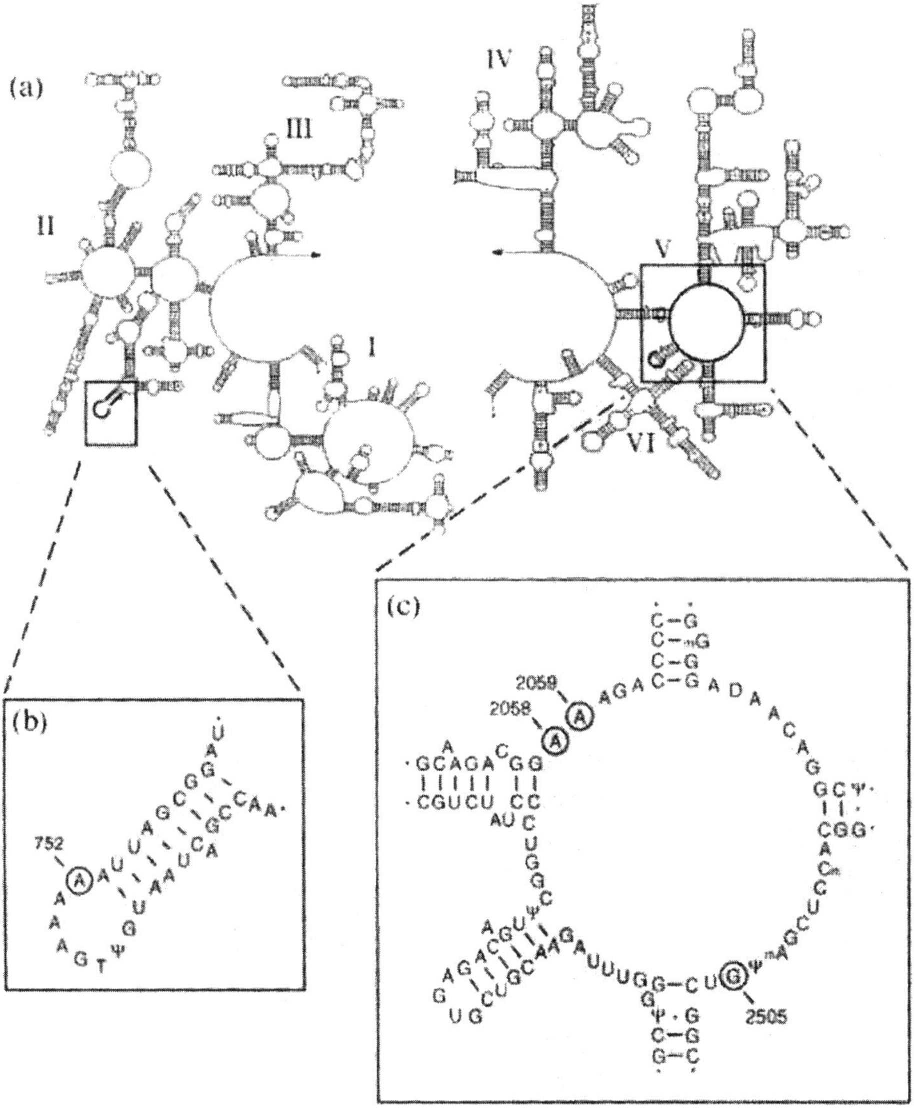

FIGURE 3 Bacterial 23S rRNA secondary structure showing the sites of interaction of the macrolides and ketolides. (From Ref. 3.)

the *mef* efflux pump of *S. pneumoniae* and so is not affected by this resistance mechanism. Telithromycin is also active against ribosomal protein L4 mutations in *S. pneumoniae* that confer resistance to macrolides and azalides [8]. Telithromycin binds wild-type ribosomes with 10-fold greater affinity than erythromycin A and six-fold greater affinity than clarithromycin, but its affinity for MLS_B-resistant ribosomes is more than 20 times greater than either macrolide [1]. Two fluoroketolides (HMR 3562 and HMR 3787) that have a fluoride atom in position 2 of the lactam ring are also under evaluation and may have increased potency against respiratory pathogens compared with their nonfluorinated ketolide derivatives [9].

GENERAL CLASS ASPECTS

The ketolides have an optimal spectrum of antibacterial activity for the treatment of community-acquired RTIs. All of the common bacterial species involved in these infections are susceptible to ketolides, including strains of *S. pneumoniae* resistant to macrolides and azalides (including both *mef* and *erm* genotypes), β-lactams, and fluoroquinolones. Ketolides are active against *H. influenzae* and *M. catarrhalis* (including β-lactamase–producing strains), *S. aureus*, oral anaerobes, atypical pathogens such as *M. pneumoniae*, and intracellular pathogens such as *L. pneumophila* and *C. pneumoniae*. β-Hemolytic group A streptococci (GABHS; *S. pyogenes*) are also susceptible, including many macrolide-resistant strains, particularly those with *mef*(A) or *erm*(A) subclass *erm*(TR) genotypes. Ketolides demonstrate concentration-dependent bactericidal activity against *S. pneumoniae*, and achieve high concentrations in respiratory tissues and serum. There is moderate cytochrome P450 metabolism and active drug is excreted by the kidneys and, to some extent, the liver. Drug-drug interactions are few and are similar to those of the macrolides. The targeted spectrum of activity of the ketolides makes these compounds attractive candidates for the treatment of community-acquired RTIs including CAP, AECB, AMS, and tonsillitis/pharyngitis, particularly in the current era of increasing bacterial resistance.

TELITHROMYCIN

Antibacterial Activity

Telithromycin has potent activity against common, atypical, and intracellular respiratory pathogens, including strains that are resistant to β-lactam, MLS_B, and fluoroquinolone antibacterial agents (Table 1) [10, 11]. Telithromycin is more potent *in vitro* and *in vivo* against gram-positive cocci than clarithromycin or azithromycin. It is also highly active against inducible *erm*- (MLS_B)

TABLE 1 In vitro Susceptibility of Respiratory Tract Pathogens to Telithromycin

Organism	Minimum inhibitory concentration (MIC; mg/L)	
	MIC_{50}	MIC_{90}
Streptococcus pneumoniae		
All	0.015	0.125
Penicillin resistant	0.06	0.125
Macrolide resistant	0.06	0.5
Fluoroquinolone resistant	0.03	0.125
Streptococcus pyogenes		
All	0.015	0.015
Macrolide resistant	0.25	8
Haemophilus influenzae		
All	1	2
β-lactamase producing	1	2
Moraxella catarrhalis		
All	0.06	0.06
β-lactamase producing	0.06	0.125
Chlamydophila pneumoniae	0.03	0.06
Legionella pneumophila	0.015	0.03
Mycoplasma pneumoniae	≤0.015	≤0.015

Penicillin (penicillin G resistant; intermediate plus resistant), minimum inhibitory concentration (MIC) ≥0.12 mg/L; macrolide (erythromycin A) resistant, MIC ≥1 mg/L; fluoroquinolone (levofloxacin) resistant, MIC ≥8 mg/L.
Source: Refs. 10 and 11.

or *mef*-mediated macrolide-resistant strains of *S. pneumoniae, S. pyogenes*, and *S. aureus*, and constitutive *erm* (MLS_B)-resistant strains of *S. pneumoniae* [12]. The activity of telithromycin against isolates of *S. pneumoniae* and *S. pyogenes* is superior to that of the respiratory quinolones such as levofloxacin. The mode minimum inhibitory concentration (MIC) for *S. pneumoniae* is 0.008 mg/L, with an MIC_{90} of 0.125 mg/L. The MIC_{90} is essentially unchanged in penicillin-intermediate (MIC = 0.12 mg/L) or resistant (MIC ≥2 mg/L) strains (Table 1) [12, 13]. The MIC_{90} for erythromycin A-resistant strains of *S. pneumoniae* is moderately higher than that for susceptible strains (0.5 mg/L vs 0.015 mg/L, respectively) [14]. Telithromycin provides uniform bactericidal activity, with 99.9% killing after 24 hours and 99.0% killing at 12 hours at two times the MIC against both erythromycin A–sensitive and –resistant strains. Comparable activity for erythromycin A, clarithromycin, and azithromycin is achieved only in erythromycin A-susceptible strains [14].

Similar results for telithromycin were obtained by the same investigators with time-kill curves for penicillin-susceptible and -resistant strains of *S. pneumoniae*. Telithromycin is also active against fluoroquinolone-resistant strains of *S. pneumoniae*, with an MIC_{90} of 0.125 mg/L, regardless of the mechanism of resistance (either efflux or topoisomerase target mutation) [15]. Postantibiotic effects of telithromycin for erythromycin A–susceptible gram-positive cocci are optimal: *S. pneumoniae*, 9.7 hr; *S. pyogenes*, 8.9 hr; *S. aureus*, 3.7 hr; only slightly shorter in erythromycin A-resistant strains [16].

The MIC_{90} for GABHS is 0.015 mg/L, compared with 0.12 mg/L for clarithromycin and 0.5 mg/L for azithromycin [15]. A large proportion of erythromycin A–resistant strains remains susceptible to telithromycin, with 98.5% of strains being inhibited at less than 0.5 mg/L [17].

Telithromycin's activity against *H. influenzae* is significantly greater than erythromycin A and clarithromycin, and similar to that of azithromycin, with an MIC range of 0.12–8.0 mg/L and an MIC_{90} of 2–4 mg/L (Table 1) [10,11,13]. The MIC_{90} of telithromycin for *H. influenzae* is unaffected by β-lactamase production [18]. Telithromycin has concentration-dependent bactericidal activity against *H. influenzae* over the initial 4 hr at concentrations equal to or above its MIC [18]. Telithromycin levels attained in pulmonary tissues and epithelial lining fluid exceed these MICs. Telithromycin also possesses potent activity against isolates of *M. catarrhalis*, with an MIC_{90} of 0.06 mg/L, which is essentially unaffected by β-lactamase production (Table 1) [13].

Telithromycin possesses excellent activity against atypical/intracellular respiratory pathogens (Table 1). Telithromycin is highly active against *C. pneumoniae* with an MIC range of 0.015–0.0625 mg/L [19]; others have found an MIC range of 0.031–0.25 mg/L [18]. Telithromycin has bactericidal activity and significant sub-MIC effects against this intracellular pathogen [20,21]. Telithromycin is also highly active against *L. pneumophila in vitro* and in a guinea pig infection model [22], being more potent than erythromycin A against this pathogen [23]. *M. pneumoniae* is also extremely susceptible to telithromycin [24].

Telithromycin's activity against gram-positive and -negative anaerobes is excellent and superior to that of macrolides and azalides [25]. Telithromycin is also more potent than macrolides against *B. pertussis* and has equal potency against *B. parapertussis* [26]. Telithromycin is bactericidal against intracellular *F. tularensis* [27], is more active against *C. diphtheriae* than macrolides and azalides [28], and is more active than erythromycin A against *C. burnetii* [29].

The activity of telithromycin has been compared with various macrolides, azithromycin, and pristinamycin using in vivo mouse infection models (including systemic infection and thigh muscle infection models). Telithromycin was found to be one of the most potent agents tested, being particularly effective in protecting against systemic infection caused by macrolide-resistant pathogens and the most effective compound against *H. influenzae* [30].

Pharmacokinetics and Pharmacodynamics

The PK parameters of telithromycin in healthy volunteers following single and repeated once-daily oral doses of 800 mg are shown in Table 2. Steady-state plasma concentrations are achieved after 2–3 days with repeated dosing and slight accumulation occurs at 7–10 days, with an accumulation ratio of 1.2–1.5. The C_{max} is dose proportional; the $AUC_{0\text{-}24h}$ increases threefold with a twofold increase in dose [31,32]. Telithromycin is 57% bioavailable and this is not affected by food [33]. In clinical studies involving patients with RTIs, the C_{max} was moderately higher than in healthy volunteers at 2.89 mg/L [34]. In the elderly, C_{max} is 3.0–3.6 mg/L with an $AUC_{0\text{-}24h}$ of 11.56–17.17 mg.h/L and T_{max} is shortened to < 1 hr [35]. The terminal elimination half-life ($t_{1/2,\ \lambda z}$) is 9.81 hr in healthy volunteers following multiple doses and renal clearance is 12.5 L/hr [35]. Renal clearance is moderately lower in the elderly, with an accumulation ratio of 1.45. At 800 mg, there are no differences between those with mild or moderate renal impairment and healthy volunteers [5]. In persons with severe renal impairment, there is a 1.4-fold increase in C_{max} and a 1.9-fold increase in $AUC_{0\text{-}24h}$ [35]. Hepatic impairment of a moderate to severe degree reduces C_{max} by 20% but AUC is not affected [36]. Elimination of telithromycin is reduced in patients with hepatic impairment but does not lead to significant accumulation due to an increase in renal excretion [36]. A large study of the PK profile of more than 200 patients with CAP showed no significant differences due to age, sex, body size, or renal function [37].

TABLE 2 Pharmacokinetic Parameters of Telithromycin in Healthy Volunteers after Single and Multiple 800 mg Doses

	Mean (%CV)	
Parameter	Single dose	Multiple dose[a]
C_{max} (mg/L)	1.90 (42)	2.27 (31)
t_{max} (h)	1.0 (0.5-4.0)[b]	1.0 (0.5–3.0)[b]
$AUC_{0\text{-}24h}$	8.25 (31)	12.5 (43)
$t_{1/2,\ \lambda z}$ (h)	7.16 (19)	9.81 (20)

[a] Once daily dosing for 7 days.
[b] Median (range).
Source: Refs. 31 and 32.

TABLE 3 Site to Serum Concentrations of Telithromycin after 800 mg Once-Daily Oral Dosing for 5–10 days

Site	Healthy volunteers	Patients
Alveolar macrophages[a]	55.0–540.0	40.9–2159.6
Bronchial mucosa[a]	ND	2.1–12.1
Epithelial lining fluid[a]	4.8–14.3	8.6–14.4
Tonsillar tissue[a]	ND	3.4–13.1
White blood cells[b]	101.0–2201.0	ND

Abbreviation: ND, not determined.
[a] 5-day telithromycin.
[b] 10-day telithromycin.
Source: Refs. 38 through 42.

Telithromycin concentrations in oropharyngeal and bronchopulmonary tissues are above the MICs for most key respiratory pathogens for a full 24 hr (38–41). Tissue-to-plasma ratios for respiratory and inflammatory cells and tissues are high [38–41] (Tables 3 and 4). Saliva to plasma ratios at C_{max} are 1.2–1.5 and at C_{min} are 3–5, with an $AUC_{0\text{-}24\ h}$ of 1.7 mg.h/L. Telithromycin is avidly taken up by neutrophils and is concentrated 300-fold in azurophilic granules compared with plasma [42]. Fusion of telithromycin-laden azurophilic granules with bacteria contained in phagosomes ensures high local intracellular drug levels [43]. In human volunteer studies with cantharidin-induced skin blisters, the blister fluid concentration of telithromycin is 0.44 mg/L 9 hr after a single oral dose of 600 mg, with a plasma $AUC_{0\text{-}24h}$ ratio of 1.38 [44].

After oral administration of telithromycin, approximately 90% of the dose is absorbed. Prior to entering the systemic circulation, telithromycin undergoes a first-pass effect (33% of dose) due to presystemic metabolism mainly by the liver, but to some extent by the intestine. After reaching sys-

TABLE 4 AUC/MIC_{90} Ratios for Common Pathogens in CAP and AECB

	AUC/MIC_{90}	
Pathogen	CAP	AECB
S. pneumoniae	12.5/0.03 = 416.7	12.5/0.03 = 416.7
H. influenzae	12.5/4 = 3.1	12.5/4 = 3.1
M. catarrhalis	12.5/0.12 = 104.2	12.5/0.12 = 104.2
S. aureus	12.5/0.12 = 104.2	12.5/0.5 = 25.0

temic circulation (absolute bioavailability = 57%), telithromycin is eliminated via multiple pathways with 7% excreted unchanged in the feces by biliary and/or intestinal excretion, 13% excreted unchanged by the kidney and 37% metabolized by the liver. The metabolism is mediated by both the hepatic cytochrome P450 (CYP) system (mainly 3A4) and the non-CYP system [35,45]. Telithromycin exists in five forms in the circulating plasma, the majority (57%) of which is an unchanged form. Lesser amounts exist as *N*-desmethyl-desosamine, *N*-oxide-pyridine derivatives, an alcohol, and an acid [45].

Therapeutic Uses

Telithromycin at a dosage of 800 mg once daily is approved for clinical use in the treatment of RTIs, based on clinical studies of CAP, AECB, and AMS in patients 18 years and older, and for tonsillitis/pharyngitis in patients 12 years and older.

Community-Acquired Pneumonia

Telithromycin 800 mg once daily for the recommended treatment duration of 7–10 days was evaluated in patients with CAP across six Phase III clinical studies (three open-label and three comparator-controlled studies vs clarithromycin 500 mg twice daily for 10 days, amoxicillin 1000 mg three-times daily for 10 days, or trovafloxacin 200 mg twice daily for 7–10 days). Telithromycin was clinically effective in 92.4% (1046/1132) and 91.0% (356/391) of patients in pooled and comparator-controlled studies, respectively, and clinical cure rates for telithromycin were equivalent to those of pooled comparators (90.4% [356/394]) [46,47]. Clinical cure rates were high for the major causative pathogens of CAP: 94.8% for *S. pneumoniae*, 90.5% for *H. influenzae*, and 86.7% for *M. catarrhalis* (Table 5) [35,48,49]. The clinical cure rate for patients with CAP caused by penicillin G– and/or erythromycin A–resistant *S. pneumoniae* (single- and mixed-pathogen infections) was 87.0% (Table 5) [48]. Clinical cure rates remained high in patients with risk factors for morbidity and mortality, including elderly patients (65 years and over; 90.3% [139/154]); patients with pneumococcal bacteremia (91.5% [43/47]); patients with a Fine score of III or over (92.0% [161/175]); and patients with infections caused by the atypical/intracellular pathogens *C. pneumoniae*, *M. pneumoniae*, and *L. pneumophila* (94.1% [32/34], 96.8% [30/31], and 100% [12/12], respectively) [50,51].

Acute Exacerbations of Chronic Bronchitis

Telithromycin 800 mg once daily for 5 days is the recommended dosing regimen for the treatment of AECB. Clinical cure rates following 5-day telithro-

TABLE 5 Clinical and Bacteriologic Cure Rates by Pathogen in Patients with Community-Acquired Pneumonia Who Were Treated with Telithromycin 800 mg Once Daily for 7–10 days

Pathogen	Clinical cure, n/N (%)	Bacteriologic cure, n/N (%)
S. pneumoniae		
All	165/174 (94.8)	165/174 (94.8)
PEN-R	13/16 (81.3)	13/16 (81.3)
ERY-R	13/16 (81.3)	13/16 (81.3)
PEN-R and/or ERY-R	20/23 (87.0)	20/23 (87.0)
H. influenzae	95/105 (90.5)	94/105 (89.5)
M. catarrhalis	26/30 (86.7)	27/30 (90.0)
S. aureus	15/19 (78.9)	15/19 (78.9)
Other	102/114 (89.5)	98/114 (86.0)
All pathogens	403/442 (91.2)	400/442 (90.5)

Abbreviations: PEN-R, penicillin G-resistant (minimum inhibitory concentration [MIC] ≥2 mg/L); ERY-R, erythromycin A-resistant (MIC ≥1 mg/L).
Source: Refs. 35, 48, and 49.

mycin therapy compared favorably with those of a 10-day course of comparator antibacterials (cefuroxime axetil 500 mg twice daily or amoxicillin-clavulanate 500/125 mg three-times daily). The overall clinical and bacteriologic cure rates for telithromycin were 86.3% [220/255] and 71.9% [46/64], respectively, and were similar to those of pooled comparators (82.7% [210/254] and 74.1% [43/58], respectively) [35,52]. Clinical cure rates for telithromycin remained high in elderly patients (87.8% [79/90]), in patients with one or more and two or more risk factors for morbidity (86.5% [128/148] and 84.3 [59/70], respectively), and in patients with severe bronchial obstruction (forced expiratory volume in 1 sec/forced vital capacity less than 60%; 82.4% [56/68]) [35,52]. Clinical and bacteriologic cure rates for telithromycin were similar to those of comparators at the late post-therapy visit (Table 6). The relapse rate at late post-therapy was low for telithromycin-treated patients and similar to the rates of comparator-treated patients (Table 6).

Acute Maxillary Sinusitis

Treatment with telithromycin 800 mg once daily for 5 or 10 days was compared with a 10-day course of comparator antibacterials (amoxicillin-clavulanate 500/125 mg three-times daily or cefuroxime axetil 250 mg twice daily) in patients with acute maxillary sinusitis. Clinical and bacteriologic cure rates following telithromycin therapy for 5 days (83.6% [383/458] and 87.6% [155/177]), respectively were equivalent to those of 10-day course of telithromycin (81.7% [223/273] and 89.5% [68/76], respectively) and a 10-day course of

TABLE 6 Late Post-Therapy Clinical and Bacteriologic Cure Rates and Relapse Rates in Patients with Acute Exacerbations of Chronic Bronchitis Who Were Treated with Telithromycin or a Comparator Antibacterial

Therapeutic regimen	Clinical cure, n/N (%)	Bacteriologic cure, n/N (%)	Relapse, n/N (%)
Telithromycin 800 mg once daily, 5 days	185/236 (78.4)	38/58 (65.5)	16/236 (6.8)
Amoxicillin/clavulanate 500/125 mg three-times daily, 10 days	81/108 (75.0)	16/26 (61.5)	7/108 (6.5)
Cefuroxime axetil 500 mg twice daily, 10 days	104/136 (76.5)	18/27 (66.7)	8/136 (5.9)

Source: Ref. 35.

comparator antibacterials (77.4% [175/226] and 78.9% [45/57], respectively) [35,53]. Clinical cure rates by pathogen for 5- and 10-day telithromycin are shown in Table 7. Five-day telithromycin therapy retained high clinical cure rates in at-risk patients including those with severe infection (86.3% [82/95]), those with total sinus opacity (88.4% [153/173]), and patients with allergic rhinitis (81.3% [61/75]) [35,53]. A 5-day course of telithromycin is currently recommended for the treatment of AMS.

TABLE 7 Clinical Cure Rates by Pathogen in Patients with Acute Maxillary Sinusitis Who Were Treated with Telithromycin 800 mg Once Daily for 5 or 10 Days

Pathogen	Clinical cure, n/N (%)	
	5-day telithromycin	10-day telithromycin
S. pneumoniae		
All	55/61 (90.2)	27/30 (90.0)
PEN-R and/or ERY-R	14/16 (87.5)	6/7 (85.7)
H. influenzae	42/48 (87.5)	15/16 (93.8)
M. catarrhalis	13/14 (92.9)	3/4 (75.0)
S. aureus	18/19 (94.7)	4/4 (100)
S. pyogenes	2/2 (100)	3/3 (100)
Other	62/81 (76.5)	38/42 (90.5)
All pathogens	192/225 (85.3)	90/99 (90.9)

Abbreviations: PEN-R, penicillin G-resistant (minimum inhibitory concentration [MIC] ≥2 mg/L); ERY-R, erythromycin A-resistant (MIC ≥1 mg/L).
Source: Refs. 35 and 53.

Tonsillitis/Pharyngitis

Telithromycin 800 mg once daily for 5 days has been evaluated in the therapy of tonsillitis/pharyngitis caused by GABHS (*S. pyogenes*) in adults and adolescents. Telithromycin achieved clinical and bacteriologic cure rates of 93.6% (248/265) and 88.3% (234/265), respectively, which were equivalent to the rates of 92.5% (235/254) and 88.6% (225/254), respectively, achieved with a 10-day course of comparator antibacterials (clarithromycin 250 mg twice daily or phenoxymethylpenicillin 500 mg three-times daily) [54–57]. *S. pyogenes* eradication rates were similar in telithromycin-, penicillin-, and clarithromycin-treated patients (Table 8) [54–56]. Five-day telithromycin therapy is currently recommended for the treatment of GABHS tonsillitis/pharyngitis.

Safety and Tolerability

The safety and tolerability of telithromycin have been investigated across nine comparator-controlled Phase III clinical studies (telithromycin, n = 2045; comparators, n = 1672). Telithromycin was consistently well tolerated. Adverse events, when they did occur, were of mild to moderate intensity, and less than 4% of telithromycin-treated patients discontinued therapy due to adverse events considered possibly related to treatment—a rate that was similar to that for comparator antibacterials (Table 9) [35]. Gastrointestinal adverse events such as diarrhea, nausea, and vomiting were the most frequently reported adverse events considered possibly related to treatment, although dizziness was also reported (Table 9) [35]. The majority of discontinuations in both the telithromycin and comparator treatment groups were due to possibly treatment-related adverse events of the gastrointestinal system (diarrhea, nausea, and vomiting). The safety profile of telithromycin was similar across patient age groups, with elderly (≥65 years) and adolescent patients (13–18 years) experiencing adverse events with a similar frequency and intensity to adult patients (> 13–< 65 years) [35].

TABLE 8 *Streptococcus pyogenes* Eradication Rates in Patients with GABHS Pharyngitis Tonsillitis Who Were Treated with Telithromycin or a Comparator Antibacterial

Therapeutic regimen	Eradication rate, n/N (%)
Telithromycin 800 mg once daily, 5 days	235/265 (88.7)
Penicillin V 500 mg three-times daily, 10 days	106/119 (89.1)
Clarithromycin 250 mg twice daily, 10 days	120/135 (88.9)

Source: Refs. 54 through 56.

TABLE 9 Incidence of Treatment-Related Adverse Events in Patients Receiving Telithromycin or a Comparator Antibacterial for the Treatment of Respiratory Tract Infections

	Patients, n (%)			
	Telithromycin (n=2045)		Pooled comparators (n=1672)	
	Adverse events	Discontinuations	Adverse events	Discontinuations
All adverse events	712 (34.8)	76 (3.7)	465 (27.8)	51 (3.1)
All GI events	495 (24.2)	56 (2.7)	246 (14.7)	28 (1.7)
Diarrhea	272 (13.3)	19 (0.9)	158 (9.5)	13 (0.8)
Nausea	166 (8.1)	18 (0.9)	64 (3.8)	9 (0.5)
Vomiting	57 (2.8)	19 (0.9)	24 (1.4)	6 (0.4)
Dizziness	73 (3.6)	5 (0.2)	26 (1.6)	1 (0.1)

Abbreviation: GI, gastrointestinal.
Source: Ref. 35.

The effect of telithromycin on QTc interval was very small (mean QTc increase of approximately 1 msec) and similar to that of clarithromycin [35]. The incidence of arrhythmia and cardiovascular adverse events was low for telithromycin and similar to that for comparator antibacterials (0.2% [3/1793] and 2.6% [47/1793], respectively, vs. 0.1% [2/1537] and 3.0% [46/1537], respectively) [35]. The incidence of clinically noteworthy abnormal laboratory values (abnormal hematology and clinical chemistry) was low and similar for telithromycin- and comparator-treated patients [36]. Telithromycin is a competitive inhibitor of CYP3A4 and, like the macrolides, may produce increases in plasma levels of drugs that are metabolized by this isoenzyme such as simvastatin, midazolam, and cisapride. Coadministration of potent CYP 3A4 inhibitors such as ketoconazole and itraconazole may lead to moderate increases in telithromycin exposure [35].

REFERENCES

1. Douthwaite S. Structure-activity relationships of ketolides vs macrolides. Clin Microbiol Infect 2001; 7(suppl 3):11–17.
2. Bryskier A, Denis A. Ketolides: novel antibacterial agents designed to overcome resistance to erythromycin A within Gram-positive cocci. In: Schonfeld W, Kirst HA, eds. Macrolide antibiotics. Basel, Switzerland: Birkhauser Verlag, 2002:97–140.
3. Douthwaite S, Champney S. Structures of ketolides and macrolides determine their mode of interaction with the ribosomal target site. J Antimicrob Chemother 2001; 48:1–8.

4. Novotny GW, Andersen NM, Poehlsgaard J, Douthwaite S. Telithromycin interacts directly with the base of A752 in domain II of 23S ribosomal RNA, in contrast to erythromycin and clarithromycin. Clin Microbiol Infect 2001; 7 (suppl 1):76.
5. Hansen LH, Mauvais P, Douthwaite S. The macrolide–ketolide antibiotic binding site is formed by structures of domain II and V of 23S ribosomal RNA. Mol Microbiol 1999; 31:623–631.
6. Douthwaite S, Hanse LH, Mauvais P. Macrolide–ketolide inhibition of MLS-resistance is improved by alternative drug interaction with domain II of 23S rRNA. Mol Microbiol 2000; 36:183–193.
7. Bonnefoy A, Girard A, Agouridas C, Chanot J. Ketolides lack inducibility properties of MLS(B) resistance phenotype. J Antimicrob Chemother 1997; 40: 85–90.
8. Nagai K, Appelbaum PC, Davies TA, Kelly LM, Hoellman DB, Andrasevic AT, et al. Susceptibilities to telithromycin and six other agents and prevalence of macrolide resistance due to L4 ribosomal protein mutation among 992 pneumococci from 10 central and Eastern European countries. Antimicrob Agents Chemother 2002; 46:371–377.
9. Denis A, Bretin F, Fromentin C, Bonnet A, Pittan G, Bonnefoy A, et al. Beta-keto-ester chemistry and ketolides. Synthesis and antibacterial activity of the 2-halogeno, 2-methyl and 2,3 enol-ether ketolides. Bioorg Med Chem Lett 2000; 10:2019–2022.
10. Jenkins S, Pluim J. Telithromycin has potent in vitro activity against common and atypical/intracellular and resistant respiratory tract pathogens: a review (Abstract 02.26). Program and Abstracts of the 6th International Conference on the Macrolides, Azalides, Streptogramins, Ketolides and Oxazolidinones. Atlanta, GA: ICMAS Inc. and the Sixth International Conference on the Macrolides, Azalides, Streptogramins, Ketolides and Oxazolidinones, 2002.
11. Felmingham D. Evolving resistance patterns in community-acquired respiratory tract pathogens: first results from the PROTEKT study. J Infect 2002; 22(suppl A):3–10.
12. Felmingham D. Microbiological profile of telithromycin, the first ketolide antimicrobial. Clin Microbiol Infect Dis 2001; 7(suppl 3):2–10.
13. Wootton M, Bowker KE, Janowska A, Holt HA, MacGowan AP. In-vitro activity of HMR 3647 against *Streptococcus pneumoniae, Haemophilus influenzae, Moraxella catarrhalis* and beta-hemolytic streptococci. J Antimicrob Chemother 1999; 44:445–453.
14. Pankuch G, Visalli M, Jacobs M, Appelbaum P. Susceptibilities of penicillin- and erythromycin-susceptible and -resistant pneumococci to HMR 36479 (RU6647), a new ketolide, compared with susceptibilities to 17 other agents. Antimicrob Agents Chemother 1998; 42:624–630.
15. Nagai K, Hoellman D, Davies T, Jacobs M, Appelbaum P. Activity of telithromycin against 26 quinolone-resistant pneumococci with known quinolone-resistance mechanisms. Clin Microbiol Infect 2001; 7:703–705.
16. Munckhof W, Borlace G, Turning J. Postantibiotic suppression of growth of

erythromycin A-susceptible and -resistant Gram-positive bacteria by the ketolides telithromycin (HMR 3647) and HMR 3004. Antimicrob Agents Chemother 2000; 44:1749–1753.

17. Nagai K, Appelbaum PC, Davies TA, Kelly LM, Hoellman DB, Andrasevic AT, et al. Susceptibility to telithromycin in 1,011 *Streptococcus pyogenes* isolates from 10 central and Eastern European countries. Antimicrob Agents Chemother 2002; 46:546–549.
18. Pankuch GA, Hoellman DB, Lin G, Bajaksouzian S, Jacobs MR, Appelbaum PC. Activity of HMR 3647 compared to those of five agents against *Haemophilus influenzae* and *Moraxella catarrhalis* by MIC determination and time-kill assay. Antimicrob Agents Chemother 1998; 42:3032–3034.
19. Roblin PM, Hammerschlag MR. In vitro activity of a new ketolide antibiotic, HMR 3647, against *Chlamydia pneumoniae*. Antimicrob Agents Chemother 1998; 42:1515–1516.
20. Miyashita N, Fukano H, Niki Y, Matsushima T. In vitro activity of telithromycin, a new ketolide against *Chlamydia pneumoniae*. J Antimicrob Chemother 2001; 48:403–405.
21. Gustafsson I, Hjelm E, Cars O. In vitro pharmacodynamics of the new ketolide HMR 3004 and HMR 3647 (Telithromycin) against *Chlamydia pneumoniae*. Antimicrob Agents Chemother 2000; 44:1846–1849.
22. Edelstein P, Edelstein M. In vitro activity of the ketolide HMR 3647 (RU6647) for *Legionella* spp., its pharmacokinetics in guinea pigs, and use of the drug to treat guinea pigs with *Legionella pneumophila* pneumonia. Antimicrob Agents Chemother 1999; 43:90–95.
23. Schulin T, Wennersten CB, Ferraro MJ, Moellering RC. Susceptibilities of *Legionella* spp. to newer antimicrobials in vitro. Antimicrob Agents Chemother 1998; 42:1520–1523.
24. Kenny G, Cartwright F. Susceptibilities of *Mycoplasma hominis, M. pneumoniae,* and *Ureoplasma urealyticum* to GAR-936, dalfopristin, dirithromycin, evernimicin, gatifloxacin, linezolid, moxifloxacin, quinupristin-dalfopristin, and telithromycin compared to their susceptibilities to reference macrolides, tetracyclines, and quinolones. Antimicrob Agents Chemother 2001; 45:2604–2608.
25. Credito KL, Ednie LM, Jacobs MR, Appelbaum PC. Activity of telithromycin (HMR 3647) against anaerobic bacteria compared to those of eight other agents by time-kill methodology. Antimicrob Agents Chemother 1999; 43:2027–2031.
26. Hoppe JE, Bryskier A. In vitro susceptibilities of *Bordetella pertussis* and *Bordetella parapertussis* to two new ketolides (HMR 3004 and HMR 3647), four macrolides (azithromycin, clarithromycin, erythromycin A, and roxithromycin), and two ansamycins (rifampin and rifapentine). Antimicrob Agents Chemother 1998; 42:965–966.
27. Maurin M, Mersali N, Raoult D. Bactericidal activities of antibiotics against intracellular *Francisella tularensis*. Antimicrob Agents Chemother 2000; 44: 3428–3431.
28. Engler K, Warner M, George R. In vitro activity of ketolides HMR 3004 and

HMR 3647 and seven other antimicrobial agents against *Corynebacterium diphtheriae*. J Antimicrob Chemother 2001; 47:27–31.
29. Rolain JM, Maurin M, Bryskier A, Raoult D. In vitro activities of telithromycin HMR3647) against *Rickettsia rickettsii, Rickettsia conorii, Rickettsia africae, Rickettsia typhi, Rickettsia prowazekii, Coxiella burnetii, Bartonella henselae, Bartonella quintana, Bartonella bacilliformis,* and *Ehrlichia chaffeensis*. Antimicrob Agents Chemother 2000; 44:1391–1393.
30. Bonnefoy A, Guitton M, Delachaume C, LePriol P, Girard A. In vivo efficacy of the new ketolide telithromycin (HMR 3647) in murine infection models. Antimicrob Agents Chemother 2001; 45:1688–1692.
31. Namour F, Wessels DH, Pascual MH, Reynolds D, Sultan E, Lenfant B. Pharmacokinetics of the new ketolide telithromycin (HMR 3647) administered in ascending single and multiple doses. Antimicrob Agents Chemother 2001; 45:170–175.
32. Lenfant B, Sultan E, Wable·C, Pascual MH, Meyer BH, Scholtz. Pharmacokinetics of 800 mg once-daily oral dosing of the ketolide, HMR 3647, in healthy young volunteers (Abstract A-49). Abstracts of the 38th Interscience Conference on Antimicrobial Agents and Chemotherapy. Washington DC: American Society for Microbiology, 1998.
33. Perret C, Wessels DH. Oral bioavailability of the ketolide telithromycin (HMR 3647) is similar in both elderly and young subjects. Clin Microbiol Infect 2000; 6(suppl 1):203–204.
34. Sultan E, Lenfant B, Wable C, Pascual M-H, Meyer B. Pharmacokinetic profile of HMR 3647 800mg once-daily in elderly volunteers. J Antimicrob Chemother 1999; 44(suppl A):54.
35. Briefing document for the FDA Anti-infective Drug Products Advisory Committee Meeting. Aventis, Bridgewater, NJ, USA, March 2001.
36. Sultan E, Cantalloube C, Patat A, Moirand R. Telithromycin (HMR 3647), the first ketolide antimicrobial, does not require dosage adjustment in individuals with hepatic impairment. Clin Microbiol Infect 2000; 6(suppl 1):203.
37. Pluim J. Population pharmacokinetics support the convenient once-daily 800 mg dosage of telithromycin in patients with upper and lower RTIs including special populations. Clin Microbiol Infect 2001; 7(suppl 1):266.
38. Gehanno P, Passot V, Nabet P, Sultan E. Telithromycin (HMR 3647) penetrates rapidly into tonsillar tissue achieving high and prolonged tonsillar concentrations. Clin Microbiol Infect 2000; 6(suppl 1):204.
39. Muller-Serieys C, Cantalloube C, Soler P, Ghia HP, Brunner F. HMR 3647 achieves high and sustained concentrations in broncho-pulmonary tissues. J Antimicrob Chemother 1999; 44(suppl A):57.
40. Kadota J, Ishimatsu Y, Iwashita T, Matsubara Y, Kohno S, Tateno M, et al. The ketolide antimicrobial telithromycin (HMR 3647) achieves high and sustained concentrations in alveolar macrophages and bronchoalveolar epithelial lining fluid in healthy Japanese volunteers (Abstract 2142). Abstracts of the 40th Interscience Conference on Antimicrobial agents and Chemotherapy. Washington DC: American Society for Microbiology, 2000.

41. Khair OA, Andrews JM, Honeybourne D, Jevons G, Vacheron F, Wise R. Lung concentrations of telithromycin after oral dosing. J Antimicrob Chemother 2001; 47:837–840.
42. Pham Gia H, Roeder V, Namour F, Sultan E, Lenfant B. HMR 3647 achieves high and sustained concentrations in white blood cells in man. J Antimicrob Chemother 1999; 44(suppl A):57–58.
43. Miossec-Bartoli C, Pilatre L, Peyron P, N'Diaye EN, Collart-Dutilleul V, Maridonneau-Parinin I, et al. The new ketolide HMR 3647 accumulates in the azurophilic granules of human polymorphonuclear cells. Antimicrob Agents Chemother 1999; 43:2457–2462.
44. Namour F, Sultan E, Pascual MH, Lenfant B. Penetration of telithromycin (HMR 3647), a new ketolide antimicrobial, into inflammatory blister fluid following oral administration. J Antimicrob Chemother 2002; 49:1035–1038.
45. Sultan E, Namour F, Mauriac C, Lenfant B, Scholtz H, et al. HMR 3647, a new ketolide antimicrobial, is metabolized and excreted mainly in feces in man. J Antimicrob Chemother 1999; 44(suppl A):54.
46. van Rensburg D, Rangaraju M, Jenkins S, Pluim J. Telithromycin provides high clinical and bacteriologic efficacy in patients with community-acquired pneumonia irrespective or gender or age (Abstract 62.013). In: Abstracts of the 10th International Congress on Infectious Diseases. Singapore: Society of Infectious Diseases (Singapore) and the Singapore Society for Microbiology and Biotechnology, 2002.
47. van Rensburg D, Moola S, Hagberg L, Rangaraju M, Leroy B. Oral telithromycin is as effective as standard comparators for the treatment of community-acquired pneumonia (Abstract 862). In: Abstracts of the 41st Interscience Conference on Antimicrobial Agents and Chemotherapy. Washington DC: American Society for Microbiology, 2001.
48. Hagberg L, Rangaraju M, Jenkins S. Efficacy of telithromycin in the treatment of community-acquired pneumonia caused by resistant pneumococci. Clin Microbiol Infect 2002; 8(suppl 1):318.
49. van Rensburg D, Rangaraju M, Jenkins S, Pluim J. Clinical and bacteriologic efficacy of telithromycin in patients with community-acquired pneumonia caused by Haemophilus influenzae (Abstract 62.014). In: Abstracts of the 10th International Congress on Infectious Diseases. Singapore: Society of Infectious Diseases (Singapore) and the Singapore Society for Microbiology and Biotechnology, 2002.
50. Rangaraju M, Leroy B, Pluim J. Telithromycin is effective in the treatment of high-risk patients with community-acquired pneumonia (Abstract 08.02). In: Program and Abstracts of the 6th International Conference on the Macrolides, Azalides, Streptogramins, Ketolides and Oxazolidinones. Atlanta, GA: ICMAS Inc. and the Sixth International Conference on the Macrolides, Azalides, Streptogramins, Ketolides and Oxazolidinones, 2002.
51. Dunbar L, Hagberg L, Rangaraju M, Leroy B. Seven to 10-day therapy with telithromycin, the first ketolide antimicrobial, is effective in community-acquired pneumonia caused by atypical and intracellular pathogens (Abstract 859). In:

Abstracts of the 41st Interscience Conference on Antimicrobial Agents and Chemotherapy. Washington DC: American Society for Microbiology, 2001.

52. Zervos M, Aubier M, Rangaraju M, Leroy B. Five-day telithromycin, a new ketolide, is as effective as standard 10-day comparators in the treatment of acute exacerbations of chronic bronchitis (Abstract 916). In: Abstracts of the 41st Interscience Conference on Antimicrobial Agents and Chemotherapy. Washington DC: American Society for Microbiology, 2001.
53. Roos K, Tellier G, Baz M, Rangaraju M, Leroy B. Five-day therapy with the new ketolide telithromycin is as effective as standard 10-day comparators in the treatment of acute maxillary sinusitis (Abstract 909). In: Abstracts of the 41st Interscience Conference on Antimicrobial Agents and Chemotherapy. Washington DC: American Society for Microbiology, 2001.
54. Norrby SR, Rabie W, Bacart P, Mueller O, Leroy B, Rangaraju M, Butticaz-Iroudayassamy E. Efficacy of 5 days' telithromycin (HMR 3647) vs 10 days' penicillin V in the treatment of pharyngitis in adults (Abstract 2242). In: Abstracts of the 40th Interscience Conference on Antimicrobial Agents and Chemotherapy. Washington DC: American Society for Microbiology, 2000.
55. Ziter P, Quinn J, Leroy B, Sidarous E, Belker M. Oral telithromycin (HMR 3647) 800 mg once daily for 5 days is well tolerated and as effective as oral clarithromycin 250 mg twice daily for 10 days in Group A-hemolytic streptococcal (GABHS) pharyngitis/tonsillitis (Abstract 2229). In: Abstracts of the 40th Interscience Conference on Antimicrobial Agents and Chemotherapy. Washington DC: American Society for Microbiology, 2000.
56. Norrby SR, Quinn J, Rangaraju M, Leroy B. Five-day therapy with telithromycin, a novel ketolide antimicrobial, is as effective as 10-day comparators for the treatment of tonsillopharyngitis (Abstract 915). In: Abstracts of the 41st Interscience Conference on Antimicrobial Agents and Chemotherapy. Washington DC: American Society for Microbiology, 2001.

6

Treatment of Community-Acquired Respiratory Tract Infections with Quinolone Antibacterial Agents

Vincent T. Andriole
Yale University School of Medicine
New Haven, Connecticut, U.S.A.

Paul G. Ambrose
Cognigen Corporation
Buffalo, New York, U.S.A.

Robert C. Owens, Jr.
Maine Medical Center
Portland, Maine, U.S.A.

QUINOLONES: A BRIEF HISTORY AND CHEMISTRY OVERVIEW

The dawn of modern antibacterial chemotherapy began in the 1930s when Germany's Gerhard Domagk identified sulfonamides as chemotherapeutic agents, for which he was awarded the Nobel prize in medicine in 1938 [1]. The development of penicillin G, by England's Sir William Dunn and Australia's Howard Florey, followed during the early 1940s [2]. Tetracycline (chlortetracycline, 1948), aminoglycoside (streptomycin, 1949), macrolide (erythromycin, 1952), and glycopeptide (vancomycin, 1956) antibacterial classes were introduced during the decade that followed the end of World War II [3].

The development of quinolone antibacterial agents began in the early 1960s. Nalidixic acid (Fig. 1B), chemically a naphthyridine, was serendipitously discovered during chloroquine synthesis in 1962 [4]. Due to its reliable activity against most Enterobactereaceae, for a time nalidixic acid became a popular choice for the treatment of uncomplicated urinary tract infections. In fact, early on it was often referred to as an oral therapeutic equivalent of kanamycin. Unfortunately, its serum and tissue concentrations were so low that it could not be employed for infections in other body sites. Moreover, its half-life was so short, nalidixic acid had to be given four times daily. Several other similar quinolones (e.g., oxolinic acid and cinoxacin) were developed

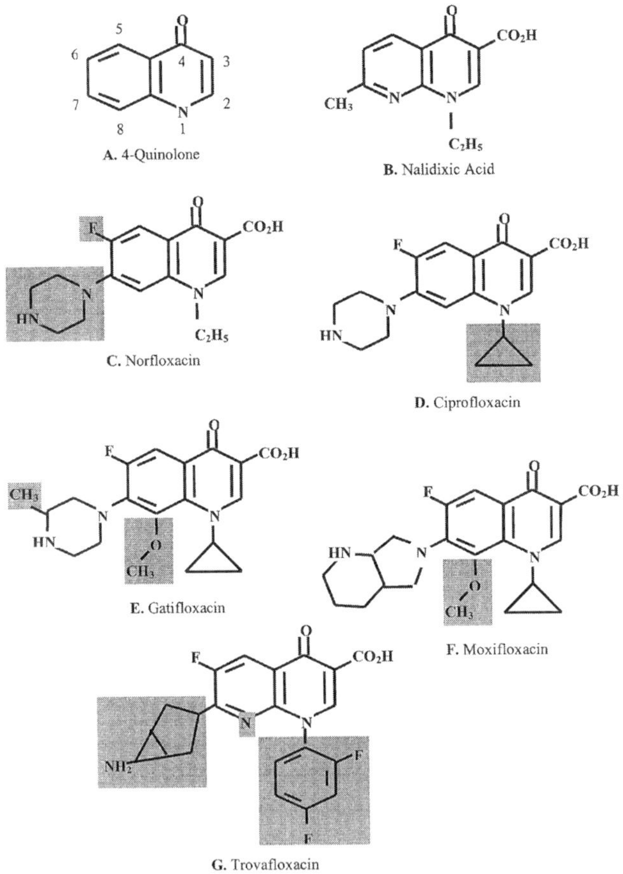

FIGURE 1 Structures of representative quinolones.

that were essentially identical with nalidixic acid but could be given less frequently. None of these first-generation quinolones exhibited any activity against *Pseudomonas aeruginosa*, anaerobes, or gram-positive bacteria.

Norfloxacin, the first second-generation quinolone, expanded quinolone bacterial coverage to include *P. aeruginosa* and staphylococci. This change was the result of the discovery that placement of a fluorine at the C-6 position of the 4-quinolone molecule and replacement of the C-7 methyl side chain of nalidixic acid with a piperazine group significantly enhanced microbiological activity (Fig. 1C) [5–7]. Generally, second-generation quinolones have a spectrum of microbiological activity similar to that of the aminoglycosides.

Replacement of norfloxacin's N-1 ethyl group with a cyclopropyl group resulted in compounds with greater bioavailability, such as ciprofloxacin (Fig. 1D) [5–7]. Due to the summation of the C-6, C-7, and N-1 structural changes, compounds such as ciprofloxacin and ofloxacin can be used in many sites of infection outside of the urinary tract. Moreover, these quinolones exhibit high intracellular penetration, allowing for the treatment of atypical organisms, such as *Chlamydia* spp., *Mycoplasma* spp., and *Legionella* spp. [8].

Norfloxacin is available as an oral formulation and is useful only for the treatment of urinary tract infections. Like norfloxacin, lomefloxacin and enoxacin are available only as oral formulations but may be used for a limited number of systemic infection sites. Ciprofloxacin and ofloxacin are available in both intravenous and oral formulations and are useful in treating many systemic sites of infection.

Unfortunately, none of the second-generation quinolones exhibit adequate pharmacokinetic/pharmacodynamic (PK-PD) profiles against *Streptococcus pneumoniae* and/or have sufficient clinical outcome data to be used reliably to treat serious infections caused by these organisms. Although, for a short time there was a quinolone, temafloxacin, with appreciable pneumococcal activity, it had to be withdrawn from the market due to the emergence of a syndrome of hemolysis and renal dysfunction [9]. This represented a serious problem for the clinician, because the leading cause of community-acquired pulmonary and sinus infection is *S. pneumoniae*, and the major cause of pharyngitis, soft tissue infections, and skin infections is *S. pyogenes*. This opened the door for the development of third-generation quinolones (sparfloxacin, grepafloxacin). These agents have moderate PK-PD profiles and in vitro microbiological activity against *S. pneumoniae*.

Forth-generation quinolones (garenoxacin, gatifloxacin, gemifloxacin, moxifloxacin, trovafloxacin, sitafloxacin) are characterized as having significantly improved PK-PD profiles against *S. pneumoniae* compared with levofloxacin. Moreover, these agents also have appreciable activity against anaerobes, such as *Bacteroides fragilus*. The enhanced streptococcal activity of these compounds results from modifications to the piperazine group at C-7 of the quinolone nucleus [7]. The addition of a sterically bulky group(s) on this substituent not only improved the PK-PD profile of these agents against gram-positive organisms but also diminished the potential for adverse CNS events and drug interactions (Fig. 1E,F).

The enhanced activity against anaerobes arise from either bulky substituents attached to the C-8 position of the 4-quinolone nucleus or N-8 substitutions of the 4-quinolone nucleus itself. While the C-8 methoxy group of moxifloxacin and gatifloxacin (Fig. 1E,F) and the sterically bulky group of garenoxacin confer moderate activity against many anaerobic species, an N-8 substitution (trovafloxacin) provides for superior anaerobic activity (Fig. 1G) [7,10,11].

PHARMACOKINETIC-PHARMACODYNAMIC PROPERTIES OF QUINOLONES

Pharmacokinetics-Pharmacodynamics: First Principles

Harry Eagle, a half-century ago, pioneered the first pharmacokinetic-pharmacodynamic (PK-PD) studies using penicillin in streptococcal and syphilitic animal models of infection [12–14]. It was at this time that dosing methods (e.g., continuous infusion vs. intermittent injection) as well as the dose of penicillin employed in relation to the minimum inhibitory concentration (MIC), were evaluated for its ability to impact in vivo outcome. Following a long respite, the science now known as PK-PD reemerged as Shah and colleagues classified antimicrobial agents based on their patterns of bactericidal activity [15]. Two patterns of bactericidal activity were described, time-dependent and concentration-dependent (Fig. 2).

The rate of bacterial killing exhibited by time-dependent agents is saturable over a narrow range of drug concentrations and usually reaches a plateau when drug concentrations are approximately 2–4 times the MIC of the pathogen to the drug [16]. (Fig. 2) β-Lactams (e.g., penicillins, cephalosporins, monobactams, carbapenems), lincosamides (e.g., clindamycin), macrolides (e.g., erythromycin, clarithromycin), and oxazolidinones (e.g., linezolid) best fit this pattern of bactericidal activity. Thus, the duration of time (T) that drug concentrations exceed some threshold (such as the MIC) would be predicted to be the PK parameter that determines in vivo efficacy [17].

On the other hand, the rate and extent of bacterial killing exhibited by concentration-dependent agents is saturable over a much broader range of drug concentrations, usually 10–20 times the MIC of the drug to the pathogen [16] (Fig. 2). In other words, as drug concentration increases, so does

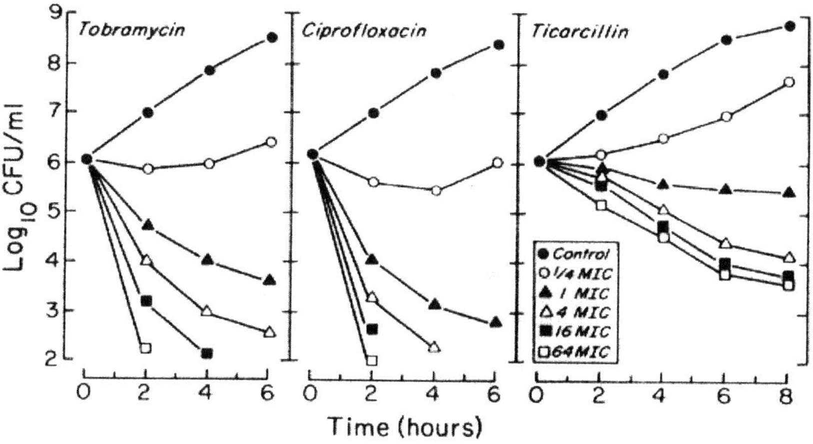

Figure 2 Time-kill curves of *Pseudomonas aeruginosa* with exposure to tobramycin, ciprofloxacin, and ticarcillin at concentrations ranging from one-fourth to 64 times the MIC. Tobramycin and ciprofloxacin exhibit a concentration-dependent pattern of bactericidal activity, whereas ticarcillin exhibits a concentration-independent pattern of bactericidal activity. (From Ref. 17.)

the rate of bacterial killing. Agents that demonstrate this pattern of bactericidal activity include the aminoglycosides, quinolones, daptomycin, vancomycin, teicoplanin, oritavancin, amphotericin B, and telithromycin. Thus, the peak drug concentration and the area under the serum concentration-time curve at 24 hours (AUC_{24}) would be predicted to be the PK parameters that determine in vivo efficacy [17].

Pharmacokinetic parameters determining efficacy may be transformed to PK-PD measures by indexing PK to a measure of drug potency, such as the MIC. More specifically, from a PK standpoint, bacterial killing can be characterized mathematically. Bacterial killing may be described by the integral of drug concentration (C) over time ($\int C dt$) or the AUC. Hence, from a PK-PD perspective, bacterial killing is a function of a drug's AUC when indexed to the MIC.

Under certain circumstances, changes in either concentration or time will make a small or negligible contribution to the killing process. In these instances, the PK-PD measure can be simplified to the peak concentration (peak):MIC ratio or time the serum concentration remains above the MIC ($T > MIC$). When one of these simplifying assumptions cannot be made, the efficacy of most antimicrobial agents can usually be linked to the AUC_{24}:MIC ratio [16].

TABLE 1 Quinolone Generations (PK-PD Classification)

First	Second		Third	Fourth
Nalidixic acid Oxolinic acid Cinoxacin	Norfloxacin (Noroxin) Enoxacin (Penetrex) Lomefloxacin (Maxaquin)	Ofloxacin (Floxin) Levofloxacin (Levaquin) Ciprofloxacin[a] (Cipro)	Sparfloxacin[a] (Zygam) Grepafloxacin[a] (Raxar)	Trovafloxacin[a] (Trovan) Gatifloxacin (Tequin) Moxifloxacin[a] (Avelox) Gemifloxacin[a] (Factive) Garenoxacin (BMS 284756) Sitafloxacin (DU 6859a)
Microbiological activity				
Enterobacteriaceae	Enterobacteriaceae + *P. aeruginosa*	Enterobacteriaceae + Atypicals *P. aeruginosa*	Enterobacteriaceae *P. aeruginosa* (+/−) Atypicals + *S. pneumoniae*	Enterobacteriaceae *P. aeruginosa* (+/−) Atypicals *S. pneumoniae* + Anaerobes
Site of infection				
Urine only	Urine +/− Systemic		Systemic +/− Urine	Systemic +/− Urine

[a] Dual elimination pathways exist.

Identification of the primary PK-PD measure that determines efficacy is complicated by the high degree of colinearity between measures. For instance, a larger dose of a given drug results not only in a larger peak:MIC ratio but also in a larger AUC_{24}:MIC ratio and a longer T > MIC. Because all three PK-PD measures increase with ascending dose, it can be difficult to determine which measure is most closely associated with any increase in efficacy. One way to overcome this colinearity is by comparng the effects of several total doses administered over various intervals (i.e., dose fractionation studies). In this way, one may identify the PK-PD measure that is most important to in vivo efficacy [17].

Pharmacokinetic-Pharmacodynamic Target Thresholds

For quinolones, like other agents that exhibit concentration-dependent bactericidal activity, bacterial killing is maximized when the free-drug (f) AUC_{24}:MIC ratio or the f peak:MIC ratio exceed a target threshold. It appears that the optimal PK-PD targets are pathogen- and patient population–specific. Generally, the PK-PD measure that best correlates with efficacy of quinolones is the $f\,AUC_{24}$:MIC ratio. Whereas the $f$peak:MIC ratio has been shown to be important in vitro and in vivo in the prevention of the emergence of quinolone-resistant mutants. In the following discussion we will explore quinolone PK-PD data derived from nonclinical models of infection (in vitro and animal) as well as that from clinical studies. Quinolones are classified based on their pharmacodynamic profile (Table 1).

PK-PD Target Thresholds and Gram-Negative Bacilli

Leggett et al. published the earliest study evaluating the PK-PD of quinolones against gram-negative bacilli in 1991. The study evaluated ciprofloxacin in neutropenic murine thigh and pulmonary infection models using strains of *P. aeruginosa* and *Klebsiella pneumoniae* [18]. Dose fractionation in these studies minimally impacted the extent of bacterial killing, suggesting that the $f\,AUC_{24}$:MIC ratio was the PK-PD measure most closely associated with efficacy. Since that time, it has become well established in animal models of infection involving gram-negative bacilli, where the change in bacterial density ($\Delta\ \log_{10}$ CFU) after 24 hours of therapy is used as the endpoint, $f\,AUC_{24}$:MIC ratios of approximately 50 are associated with a net bacteriostatic effect (i.e., no net change in $\log_{10}$ CFU), and ratios of 100 are associated with a 1 to 2 log-unit reduction (i.e., a 90–99% reduction in bacterial density). Similarly, in animal models of infection involving gram-negative bacilli, where mortality is used as the endpoint, about 50% and 90% animal survival is associated with $f\,AUC_{24}$:MIC ratios of approximately 50 and 100, respectively. The magnitude of the $f\,AUC_{24}$:MIC ratio associated with these endpoints have been consistent irrespective of dosing regimen, site of infection, or the quinolone studied [17].

Some of the first data to correlate PK-PD and response in humans were published by Peloquin and colleagues [19]. Intravenous ciprofloxacin was evaluated in the treatment of lower respiratory tract infections involving predominantly gram-negative bacilli in seriously ill patients hospitalized in the intensive care unit. A relationship between time of exposure and outcome was established. Interestingly, against *P. aeruginosa*, a low peak:MIC ratio (<10:1) was observed that resulted in the development of resistance in 10 of 13 pathogens. Although the authors concluded that the time of exposure was the important determinant of outcome against difficult-to-treat and less susceptible pathogens (e.g., *P. aeruginosa*), failure to obtain an optimal peak:MIC ratio resulted in the emergence of resistance. This is consistent with findings from the animal model of infection reported by Drusano, further emphasizing the importance of peak:MIC ratio when dealing with resistant subpopulations [20]. Eventually, after the addition of 24 new patients, Forrest and colleagues in 1993 published their reanalyzed data from the 1989 publication (Fig. 3) [21]. After the authors performed a multivariate analysis

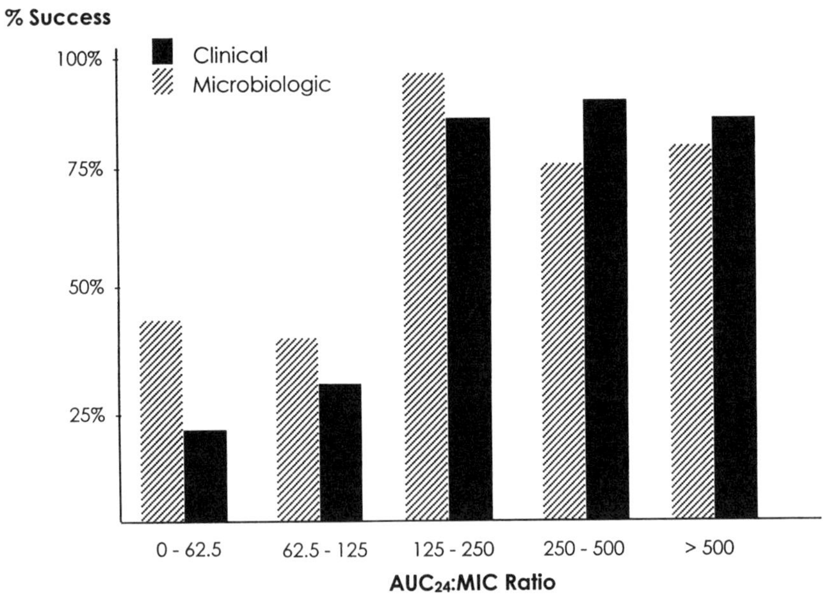

FIGURE 3 Relationship between the AUC_{24}:MIC ratio (total drug) and the probability (%) of clinical and microbiological response to therapy for ciprofloxacin against gram-negative bacilli in seriously ill patients. (From Ref. 21.)

and logistic regression, the AUC_{24}:MIC ratio predicted outcome best–not the time of exposure that was previously reported.

PK-PD Target Thresholds and Gram-Positive Cocci

As mentioned earlier, the optimal PK-PD targets are pathogen-and patient population–specific. Several recently published or presented studies have evaluated the PK-PD relationships of quinolones against gram-positive pathogens, particularly pneumococci. For *S. pneumoniae*, in vitro models of infection have demonstrated that for ciprofloxacin, garenoxacin, gatifloxacin, levofloxacin, moxifloxacin, and sparfloxacin, $f\,AUC_{24}$:MIC ratios of approximately 30 or greater are associated with a four log-unit reduction in bacterial density; lesser $f\,AUC_{24}$:MIC ratios are often associated with a significantly reduced extent of bacterial killing and in some instances bacterial regrowth (Fig. 4) [22–25].

Studies in animal models of infection identified a similar PK-PD target threshold. Onyeji and colleagues compared the efficacy of ciprofloxacin and levofloxacin in a murine model of peritoneal sepsis [26]. Clinical isolates of *S. pneumoniae* were used that displayed a range of susceptibilities to penicillin; MIC values for ciprofloxacin (1 and 2 μg/mL) and levofloxacin (1 and 2 μg/mL) were reflective of that seen clinically. Dosing regimens were varied in a

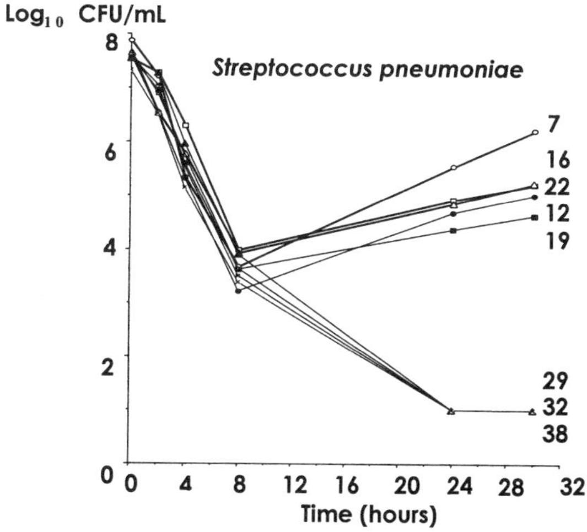

FIGURE 4 PK-PD time-kill curves of garenoxacin against *S. pneumoniae*. Each line represents changes in bacterial density over time for a single experiment; the numbers at the right side of each line represent the *f*AUC:MIC ratio for that experiment. *f*AUC:MIC ratios of 29 or greater resulted in the elimination of *S. pneumoniae* from the model, whereas lesser ratios did not. (Courtesy of Philip Lister.)

manner that resulted in drug exposures similar to those achieved in humans. Survival differences between ciprofloxacin and levofloxacin groups were negligible ($P > 0.05$), perhaps because the AUC_{24}:MIC ratios were not that different from those seen in humans. For ciprofloxacin, AUC_{24}:MIC ratios were between 17.5 and 35; and for levofloxacin, between 22 and 44. Neither ciprofloxacin nor levofloxacin achieved a desirable peak:MIC ratio of at least 10.

Further, Craig and Andes studied six quinolones in the mouse-thigh infection model in an effort to determine optimal $f\,AUC_{24}$:MIC ratios in terms of survival and change in bacterial density [27]. After being infected with *S. pneumoniae*, mice were treated with ciprofloxacin, gatifloxacin, gemifloxacin, levofloxacin, moxifloxacin, or sitafloxacin. The authors found that the fAUC:MIC ratio best predicted animal survival after 96 hr of therapy and the change in $\log_{10}$ CFU after 24 hr of therapy. $f\,AUC_{24}$:MIC ratios of 25 to 34 or greater were associated with approximately 90% animal survival and a 2 to 2.5 log-unit reduction in bacterial density (Fig. 5).

Preston and colleagues evaluated the association between different PK-PD measures for levofloxacin and both clinical and microbiological outcomes [28]. In this study, concentrations of levofloxacin in serum were obtained after administration of standard doses appropriate for site of infection in patients being treated for urinary tract, pulmonary, and skin/soft tissue infections. Of the initial 313 patients, 116 had sufficient pharmacokinetic, microbiological and clinical outcome data for evaluation. Patients in whom a peak:MIC ratio greater than 12.2 was achieved had a 100% chance of having the infecting organism eradicated from the site of infection. Conversely, if the peak:MIC ratio was less than 12.2, the likelihood of successful eradication was 80.8%. Although there was significant colinearity between the PK-PD measures of peak:MIC and AUC_{24}:MIC ratio on outcome predictability, the peak:MIC ratio reached a higher level of statistical significance for all pathogens and infection sites. A recent reanalysis of the infections caused by *S. pneumoniae*, however, revealed that $f\,AUC_{24}$:MIC ratios greater than 30 were associated with positive outcome [29]. These data are consistent with the previous work conducted by Drusano et al., which demonstrated that when a peak:MIC ratio of at least 10:1 could not be achieved, the PK-PD measure most closely associated with outcome is the AUC_{24}:MIC ratio.

Most recently, Ambrose et al. evaluated the relationship between the $f\,AUC_{24}$:MIC ratio of gatifloxacin and levofloxacin against *S. pneumoniae* and the microbiological response of patients enrolled in phase III, double-blinded, randomized trials conducted in North America [30]. Of the 778 patients enrolled in these studies involving either community-acquired pneumonia or acute bacterial exacerbation of chronic bronchitis, 376 patients had sufficient clinical and microbiological data for evaluation. Of these pa-

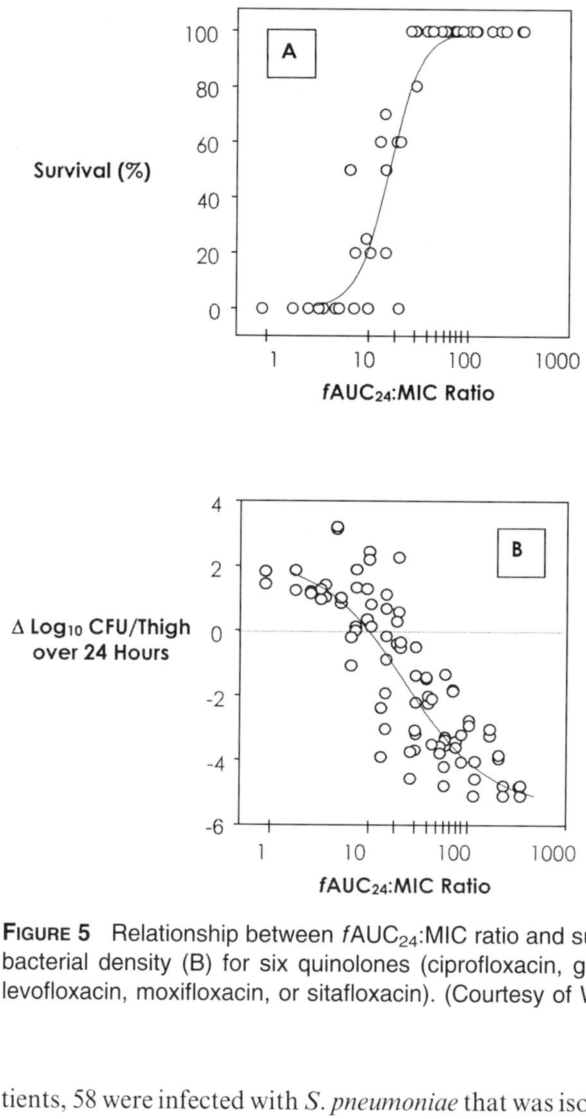

FIGURE 5 Relationship between $f\mathrm{AUC}_{24}$:MIC ratio and survival (A) and change in bacterial density (B) for six quinolones (ciprofloxacin, gatifloxacin, gemifloxacin, levofloxacin, moxifloxacin, or sitafloxacin). (Courtesy of William A. Craig.)

tients, 58 were infected with *S. pneumoniae* that was isolated from either blood or sputa. These data established that for gatifloxacin and levofloxacin, $f\mathrm{AUC}_{24}$:MIC ratio of at least 33.7 correlated with the eradication of *S. pneumoniae* in patients being treated for pneumococcal pulmonary infections (Fig. 6). $f\,\mathrm{AUC}_{24}$:MIC ratios greater than 33.7 were associated with patients having a 100% positive microbiological response to therapy, while those patients with $f\,\mathrm{AUC}_{24}$:MIC ratio less than 33.7 had only a 64% response to therapy.

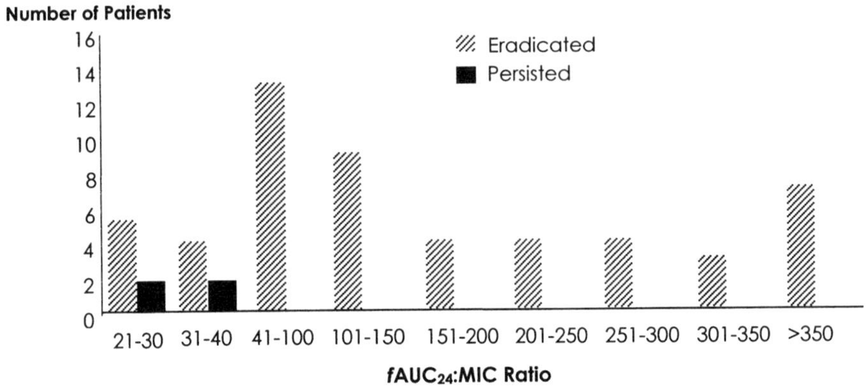

Figure 6 Relationship between the AUC_{24}:MIC ratio (free drug) and the probability (%) of microbiological response to therapy for gatifloxacin and levofloxacin against *Streptococcus pneumoniae* in patients with community-acquired respiratory tract infections. (From Ref. 27.)

PK-PD Target Thresholds and the Prevention of Resistance

Although there are considerably fewer data available, it is likely that a relationship also exists between the AUC_{24}:MIC and peak:MIC ratios and the development of resistance. Drusano and coworkers evaluated lomefloxacin in the neutropenic rat model of pseudomonas sepsis [20]. Doses were administered in a variety of regimens to study the effect of different PK-PD measures associated with outcome. The peak:MIC ratio was significantly associated with reduced mortality, compared with AUC_{24}:MIC ratio and the time over MIC. The doses used in this study provided peak:MIC ratios of approximately 20:1 and less than 10:1. The clear association between peak: MIC ratio and survival was postulated to be due to the increased inoculum size used (10^9) in the study. These findings demonstrated that with a higher burden of organisms, one is more likely to encounter resistant sub-populations, and in such settings the peak:MIC ratio becomes the more appropriate PK-PD measure that best predicts outcome.

Thomas and coworkers described this relationship in 107 hospitalized patients being treated for bacterial pneumonia [31]. Patients received a variety of dosing regimens of ciprofloxacin (200 mg q12h to 400 mg q8h) or a cephalosporin (cefmenoxime, 1–2 g q4–6hr or ceftazidime, 1–2 g q8–12hr), providing a wide range of exposures. Gram-negative pathogens predominated, as expected among patients with nosocomial pneumonia, accounting for over 90% of the organisms isolated. Gram-positive pathogens, such as *S. aureus* and *S. pneumoniae*, were isolated in less than 10% of cases. With the exception of Bush group 1 β-lactamase–elaborating organisms (e.g., *Enterobactor* spp.) treated with a β-lactam, PK-PD breakpoints were established. If a AUC_{24}:MIC ratio of at least 100 was achieved, the potential to develop resistance was less than 10%. In contrast, the probability of developing a resistant strain during therapy was greater than 80% if the AUC_{24}:MIC ratio was less than 100. Because the majority of pathogens encountered were gram-negative bacilli (most of which being *P. aeruginosa*), it is difficult to generalize these findings to gram-positive pathogens. Many more data are needed to further understand the relationship between PK-PD measures and the development of resistance.

Pharmacokinetics, Microbiology, and Toxicity

Pharmacokinetics

The pharmacokinetic profiles for the newer and some older quinolones are listed in Table 2. Due to intravenous-oral bioequivalence, quinolones have revolutionized the treatment of many infectious diseases. Whether quinolones are administered intravenously or orally, similar PK-PD relationships can be achieved with most quinolones because of their high degree of bioavailability that is consistent among the newer-generation agents.

Protein binding is one characteristic that is highly variable among the quinolones. The degree of protein binding not only influences penetration into tissues but also determines the amount of drug that is capable of interacting with bacteria at the site of infection [32]. The exact role of protein binding is often more controversial than not, but clearly, the pharmacokinetic parameter used in pharmacodynamic analyses should reflect free drug (active drug) rather than total drug concentrations.

Microbiology

The majority of community-acquired respiratory tract infections are most usually associated with one or more of six microbiologic etiologies. These include extracellular pathogens, such as *S. pneumoniae*, *H. influenzae*, and *M. catarrhalis* and intracellular pathogens such as *Legionella* spp. , *Mycoplasma pneumoniae*, and *Chlamydia pneumoniae*.

Quinolones, such as garenoxacin, gatifloxacin, levofloxacin, and moxifloxacin, have appreciable in vitro activity against both the extracellular and intracellular pathogens commonly associated with community-acquired respiratory tract infections. With regard to gram-positive microorganisms such as *S. pneumoniae*, garenoxacin and the 8-methoxy quinolones (gatifloxacin and moxifloxacin) are markedly more active than ciprofloxacin, ofloxacin, or levofloxacin. It is important to note that the activity of quinolones against *S. pneumoniae* is unrelated to penicillin resistance. The rank order of in vitro

TABLE 2 Overview of Pharmacokinetic Properties of Selected Quinolones

Parameter	Norfloxacin	Ciprofloxacin	Levofloxacin	Sparfloxacin	Gatifloxacin	Moxifloxacin	Trovafloxacin	Gemifloxacin
Dose (mg)	400	750	500	200	400	400	200	320
Bioavailability (%)	50	70	99	92	96	90	88	80
% Protein bound	15	25	30	40	20	55	75	59
Peak (μg/mL)	1.5	3.5	6	1.3	4.3	4.5	2.3	1.48
Free Peak (μg/mL)	1.3	2.6	4.2	0.8	3.4	2.0	0.6	0.6
$AUC_{(0-24)}$ (μg •h/mL)	13.6	64	47.5	17.7	51.3	48	31.2	9.3
Free $AUC_{(0-24)}$ (μg •h/mL)	11.6	48	33.3	10.6	41.0	21.6	7.8	3.8
$T_{1/2}$ (hr)	3.3	4	6	20	9	12	12	7.4
% Renal elim. (active drug)	40	60	95	10	85	20	6	30

activity of quinolones against *S. pneumoniae* is garenoxacin → moxifloxacin → gatifloxacin → levofloxacin → ciprofloxacin = ofloxacin. Against staphylococci, moxifloxacin = gatifloxacin → garenoxacin → levofloxacin → levofloxacin = ofloxacin.

Third- and fourth-generation quinolones have excellent in vitro activity against gram-negative respiratory pathogens such as *H. influenzae* and *M. catarrhalis*. Moreover, these agents have in vitro activity against most Enterobacteriaceae, such as *Citrobactor* spp., *Enterobactor* spp., *Escherichia coli*, and *Klebsiella pneumoniae*.

Finally, all third- and fourth-generation quinolones are highly active against *Legionella* spp. The newer agents (garenoxacin, gatifloxacin, and moxifloxacin), however, are more active against *M. pneumoniae* and *C. pneumoniae* than ciprofloxacin, levofloxacin, and ofloxacin.

Toxicities Associated with Quinolones

Phototoxicity. Phototoxicity is a dramatic dermatological complication of quinolone therapy that usually occurs within hours of exposure to ultraviolet (UV) light, with reactions ranging in severity from mild to severe. Phototoxicity has been observed with all known quinolones [33]. These reactions are most commonly associated with specific agents, particularly lomefloxacin, sparfloxacin, and clinafloxacin and are related to chemical structure. Compounds with a halogen (CL or F) at the 8-position of the quinolone nucleus have the most phototoxic potential [6]. Quinolones with an 8-methoxy group (gatifloxacin and moxifloxacin) have the least potential for phototoxicity [34]. The overall phototoxic potential of quinolones is lomefloxacin, fleroxacin → sparfloxacin, clinafloxacin → enoxacin → pefloxacin → grepafloxacin, ciprofloxacin → norfloxacin, ofloxacin, levofloxacin, trovafloxacin → gatifloxacin, moxifloxacin.

Central Nervous System. Seizures are rare and usually involve patients with central nervous system disorders such as epilepsy or patients who are also receiving NSAIDs or theophylline [33]. The exact mechanism by which quinolones induce seizures is controversial. There appears to be a strong association with similarities of structure for certain substituents at the 7-position of the quinolone nucleus and the structure of the gamma-aminobutyric acid (GABA) [35]. Some quinolones appear to displace or compete with GABA binding at receptor sites within the CNS, resulting in CNS stimulation. Several researchers have demonstrated associations between 7-piperazine–(ciprofloxacin, enoxacin, norfloxacin) and 7-pyrolidine–(tosufloxacin, clinafloxacin) containing quinolones and increased epileptic potential. Methyl-substituted 7-piperazinyl- or 7-pyrolidine- compounds (gatifloxacin, levofloxacin, and sparfloxacin) are associated with a reduction in epileptic potential. In general, quinolones should be used with caution in those patients who have a history of a seizure disorder or who are also receiving potentially epileptogenic medications.

Severe Idiosyncratic and Immune-Mediated Reactions. Trifluorinated quinolones (temafloxacin, tosufloxacin, fleroxacin, trovafloxacin) may pose greater risks of certain serious toxicities, the most serious being a hepato-renal syndrome (e.g., temafloxacin syndrome) characterized by serious hemolysis and often a new-onset renal and/or hepatic dysfunction (57% and 51% of cases, resepectively) [9]. The high frequency of adverse events associated with fleroxacin (84% with 48% being classified as severe, in a study of 79 patients), has been suggested to be related to triflourination [36,37]. Tosufloxacin was associated with eosinophilic pneumonitis in a study in Japan, where it is available for clinical use [38]. Trovafloxacin hepatic-related injury was also associated with eosinophilic infiltration.

Genotoxicity. Quinolones exert their activity by inhibiting bacterial DNA gyrase (topoisomerase II) and topoisomerase IV. Because mammalian cells also contain DNA gyrases, the possibility exists that quinolones may disrupt chromosomes in humans, a process known as clastogenicity. Position-1, -7, and -8 govern genotoxicity in humans. Groups associated with increased cytotoxicity potential include position-1 (cyclopropyl, tertiary butyl, 2,4 difluorophenyl) and position-8 (Cl, F, methoxy). The exact nature of such toxicities in humans has not been well elucidated.

Cardiotoxicity. Concerns about the cardiac safety of fluoroquinolones emerged after the withdrawal of grepafloxacin and sparfloxacin from the marketplace—owing, in part, to their potential to prolong the QTc interval, resulting in cardiac toxicity [39]. Fluoroquinolones were recently added to the growing list of antimicrobial agents that can cause delays in cardiac repolarization, leading to changes in the QTc interval manifested on the surface electrocardiogram (ECG). Macrolides, ketolides, azole antifungals, pentamidine, halofantrine, and very rarely trimethoprim/sulfamethoxazole are also associated with QTc prolongation [39].

The consequence of QTc prolongation is the establishment of an electrophysiological milieu that predisposes to the occurrence of cardiac arrhythmias, including torsades de pointes (TdP). The most common mechanism for drug-induced QTc prolongation is the blockade of the human ether-à-go-go related gene (HERG) that encodes the rapid delayed rectifier potassium current (lkr) [40]. This leads to QTc interval prolongation because it results in accumulation of potassium within the myocyte that delays cardiac repolarization. This delayed repolarization can lead to early after-depolarizations, which, if repetitive and self-sustaining, can lead to TdP.

The "multiple-hit hypothesis" suggests that multiple risk factors influence the development of TdP [41]. Risk factors include female gender; concurrent treatment with drugs also known to cause QTc interval prolongation, such as amiodarone and sotalol; metabolic drug interactions that result in significantly elevated levels of a drug known to prolong the QTc interval; organ impairment that results in larger than usual drug exposures; electrolyte derangements (e.g., hypokalemia, hypomagnesemia); underlying comorbid diseases (e.g., congestive heart failure, atrial fibrillation); bradycardia; and genetic polymorphisms (e.g., long QT syndrome) [39,42]. A case series of gatifloxacin-associated TdP and ventricular arrhythmias demonstrates the multiple-hit hypothesis, as multiple risk factors were present in all four patients [43]. Also, if drugs that prolong the QTc interval are concurrently administered, they may have an additive effect in blocking the lkr current, particularly if they are given with class Ia and class III antiarrhythmic agents (e.g., amiodarone, sotalol, dofetilide). Such combinations should be avoided.

Spontaneous reports to the Food and Drug Administration (FDA) Adverse Event Reporting System can be used to characterize risk factors for TdP in large populations once the drug has been approved for use [44,45]. These studies indicate that the overall risk associated with fluoroquinolones is very small. Levofloxacin had the most cases reported (n = 14), and moxifloxacin had the fewest (n = 3). Futhermore, large-scale post-marketing (phase IV) safety surveillance studies have been conducted for both gatifloxacin and moxifloxacin [46–48]. Results from a study of gatifloxacin in 15,625 patients, including 4906 who had underlying cardiovascular disease or were receiving cardiovascular drugs, indicated no cardiovascular events related to gatifloxacin [46]. Similarly, data from 7368 patients enrolled in clinical trials and 36,569 patients from safety surveillance studies indicated no significant arrhythmic potential associated with moxifloxacin [48]. In fact, in over 13 million patient exposures, four confirmed cases of TdP and one unconfirmed case have been reported [48]. The risk of TdP in patients receiving fluoroquinolones is very low. The concurrent use of gatifloxacin, moxifloxacin, or levofloxacin with class Ia or class III antiarrhythmic agents must be avoided in all patients.

Clinical Use of Quinolones

Food and Drug Administration Approved Indications

Ciprofloxacin. Ciprofloxacin is approved for use in pneumonia, acute exacerbation of chronic bronchitis, acute maxillary sinusitis, urinary tract infections including uncomplicated and complicated pyelonephritis, uncomplicated urogenital and rectal gonorrhea, chronic bacterial prostatitis, uncomplicated skin and soft tissue infections, bone and joint infections, infectious diarrhea, typhoid fever, intra-abdominal infection when used with metronidazole, Legionella infections, and febrile neutropenia.

Gatifloxacin. Gatifloxacin is approved for use in community-acquired pneumonia, acute exacerbation of chronic bronchitis, acute maxillary sinusitis, urinary tract infections including uncomplicated and complicated pyelonephritis, uncomplicated urogenital gonorrhea, and uncomplicated skin and soft tissue infections. Additionally, gatifloxacin is under FDA review for pediatric use for recurrent otitis media.

Levofloxacin. Levofloxacin is approved for the following indications: community-acquired pneumonia, acute exacerbation of chronic bronchitis, acute maxillary sinusitis, nosocomial pneumonia, urinary tract infections including uncomplicated and complicated pyelonephritis, and uncomplicated skin and soft tissue infections.

Moxifloxacin. Moxifloxacin is approved for use in community-acquired pneumonia, acute exacerbation of chronic bronchitis, acute maxillary sinusitis, and uncomplicated skin and soft tissue infections.

Trovafloxacin. Trovafloxacin is indicated for the treatment of patients whose therapy is initiated in inpatient health care facilities who have serious life- or limb-threatening infections, including nosocomial pneumonia, community-acquired pneumonia, complicated intra-abdominal infection, gynecologic and pelvic infecions, and complicated skin and skin structure infections.

Appropriate Use of Quinolones in Community-Acquired Respiratory Tract Infections

Community-Acquired Pneumonia. Recommendations for empirical therapy for inpatients with community-acquired pneumonia include the combination of a β-lactam and a macrolide or a fluoroquinolone alone [49]. Because fluoroquinolones are highly effective against the common extracellular (*S. pneumoniae*, *Haemophilus influenzae*, *Moraxella catarrhalis*) and atypical intracellular (*M. pneumoniae*, *C. pneumoniae*, *Legionella* spp.) respiratory pathogens, these agents offer an excellent approach to the treatment of community-acquired pneumonia.

Currently there are three quinolones available in the United States that are frequently used for the treatment of community-acquired pneumonia in both the in- and outpatient setting: gatifloxacin, levofloxacin, and moxifloxacin. Of the approved quinolones, moxifloxacin and gatifloxacin have superior pharmacokinetic-pharmacodynamic (PK-PD) profiles against *S. pneumoniae* compared with that of levofloxacin. A recent report for the

Antimicrobial Resistance Rate Epidemiology Team (ARREST Program) systematically compared the in vitro susceptibility patterns and estimated the probability of attainment of the PK-PD target ratios for gatifloxacin and levofloxacin against pneumococci worldwide [50]. Monte Carlo simulation was used to estimate the probability that gatifloxacin or levofloxacin would achieve a $fAUC_{24}$:MIC ratio of 30 or greater. The MIC at which 50% of isolates were inhibited (MIC_{50}) and the MIC_{90} for North American isolates were 0.25 and 0.5 mg/liter, respectively, for gatifloxacin, and 1 and 2 mg/liter, respectively, for levofloxacin. The probabilities of attaining a $fAUC_{24}$:MIC ratio greater than 30 for North American isolates were 97.6% for gatifloxacin and 78.9% for levofloxacin.

Moreover, there are similar data available comparing moxifloxacin or garenoxacin with levofloxacin with similar results [51,52]. The results of these types of analyses in combination with accumulating data on the development of levofloxacin resistance and subsequent treatment failure in pneumococcal pneumonia [53] suggest it may be the least attractive of the aforementioned quinolones for the treatment of community-acquired pneumonia.

Acute Exacerbation of Chronic Bronchitis. Patients with chronic bronchitis typically suffer from several acute exacerbations each year that adversely affect their quality of life and ability to function [54]. Acute exacerbations of chronic bronchitis are common and account for more than 10 million physician visits per year in the United States [55]. Approximately 50% of acute exacerbations of chronic bronchitis are bacterial in origin, and the predominant causative pathogens include *S. pneumoniae*, *H. influenzae*, and *M. catarrhalis* [56]. Routine treatment of acute exacerbations of chronic bronchitis is associated with failure or relapse rate of 17–32% [57]. Moreover, acute exacerbations of chronic bronchitis are a common cause of morbidity and mortality in sicker patients.

Quinolones such as gatifloxacin, levofloxacin, and moxifloxacin have proved to be safe and effective in treating patients with acute bacterial exacerbations of chronic bronchitis. Recent studies have shown that patients treated with moxifloxacin experience faster resolution of symptoms, fewer missed work hours, and higher work productivity than patients treated with early-generation quinolones, β-lactams, or macrolides [58]. Additionally, numerous studies have shown that bacteriological eradication rates are higher with quinolones compared with macrolide and β-lactam antimicrobial agents [59–62].

Acute Bacterial Maxillary Sinusitis. Diagnosis of patients with acute bacterial maxillary sinusitis involves the evaluation of various major and minor factors [63]. Major diagnostic factors include nasal congestion/obstruction, nasal purulence/drainage, facial pressure/pain, hyposmia/anos-

TABLE 3 FDA-Approved Dosing Regimens of Selected Quinolones for Community-Acquired Respiratory Tract Infections

						Dosage regimen for renal dysfunction	
Agent	Infection	Oral dose	Frequency	Length of therapy	Dose adjust for renal function	Creatinine clearance	Dose and frequency
Ciprofloxacin	CAP	500mg–750 mg	q12 hr	7–14 days	Yes	Cr_{cl} 30–50:	250–500 mg q12 hr
	ABECB	500 mg–750 mg	q12 hr	7–14 days		Cr_{cl} 5–29:	250–500 mg q18 hr
	Sinusitis	500 mg	q12 hr	10 days		Hemodialysis & peritoneal dialysis:	250–500 mg q24 hr (after dialysis)
Gatifloxacin	CAP	400 mg	q24 hr	7–14 days	Yes	Cr_{cl} < 40mL/min:	Initial dose: 400 mg Subsequent dose: 200 mg q24 hr
	ABECB	400 mg	q24 hr	5 days		Hemodialysis & CAPD:	Initial dose: 400 mg Subsequent dose: 200 mg q24 hr
	Sinusitis	400 mg	q24 hr	10 days			
Levofloxacin	CAP	500 mg	q24 hr	7–14 days	Yes	Cr_{cl} 20–49:	Initial dose: 500 mg Subsequent dose: 250 mg q24 hr
	ABECB	500 mg	q24 hr	7 days		Cr_{cl} 10–19:	Initial dose: 500 mg Subsequent dose: 250 mg q48 hr
	Sinusitis	500 mg	q24 hr	10–14 days		Hemodialysis & CAPD:	Initial dose: 500 mg Subsequent dose: 250 mg q48 hr
Moxifloxacin	CAP	400 mg	q24 hr	7–14 days	No		
	ABECB	400 mg	q24 hr	5 days			
	Sinusitis	400 mg	q24 hr	10 days			

CAP = community-acquired pneumonia; ABECB = acute bacterial exacerbation of chronic bronchitis; Cr_{cl} = Creatinine clearance.

mia, and fever; minor diagnostic factors include cough, ear pressure/fullness, fatigue, halitosis, headache, and dental pain. Diagnosis is based on the presence of two or more major factors, or one major and two minor factors and evidence of purulent nasal discharge on examination. The predominant causative pathogens include *S. pneumoniae* (20–43%), *H. influenzae* (22–35%), *M. catarrhalis* (2–10%), and other streptococcal spp. (3–9%) [63].

Quinolones such as gatifloxacin, levofloxacin, and moxifloxacin have proved safe and effective in treating patients with acute bacterial rhinosinusitis. Recent studies have shown that 5-day treatment regimens of quinolones are as effective as 10-day treatment courses of other drug classes. For instance, a recent three-arm study comparing gatifloxacin 400 mg once daily for 5 days to gatifloxacin 400 mg once daily for 10 days to amoxicillin-clavulanate 875 mg twice daily for 10 days found no statistical difference in clinical efficacy between either of the three treatment groups [64]. Similarly, other studies have shown higher efficacy rates with quinolones when compared with longer treatment courses of macrolide antimicrobial agents [65].

Appropriate Doses

Food and Drug Administration–approved dosing recommendations for quinolones commonly used for the treatment of community-acquired respiratory tract infections are shown in Table 3.

REFERENCES

1. Domagk G. Ein Beitrag zur Chemotherapie der Bakteriellen Infektionen. Dtsch Med Wochenschr 1935; 61:250–253.
2. 20th Century Seer. Time. 1944; XLIII:61–68.
3. Sande MA, Mandell GL. Antimicrobial Agents. In: Goodman Cilma A, Rall TW, Nies AS, Taylor P, eds. Goodman and Gilman's: The Pharmacological Basis of Therapeutics. 8th ed. Pergamon Press, 1990:1047–1181.
4. Lesher GY, Froelich ED, Gruet MD, et al. 1,8 naphthyridine derivatives: a new class of chemotherapeutic agents. J Med Pharmacol Chem 1962; 5:1063–1068.
5. Domagala JM, Hanna LD, Heifetz CL, Hutt MP, Mitch TF, Sanchez JP, Solomon M. New structure-activity relationships of the quinolone antibacterials using the target enzyme: The development and application of a DNA gyrase assay. J Med Chem 1986; 29:394–404.
6. Domagala JM. Structure-activity and structure-side-effect relationships for quinolone antibacterials. J Antimicrob Chemother 1994; 33:685–706.
7. Brightly KE, Gootz. Chemistry and mechanism of action of the quinolone antibacterial. In: Andriole VT, ed. The Quinolones. 3d ed. Academic Press: San Diego, 37–97.
8. Philips I, King A, Shannon K. Comparative in-vitro properties of the quino-

lones. In: Andriole VT, ed. The Quinolones. 3d ed. Academic Press: San Diego, 99–137.

9. Blum MD, Graham DJ, McCloskey CA. Temafloxacin syndrome: review of 95 cases. Clin Infect Dis 1994; 18:946–950.
10. Asahina Y, Ishizaki T, Suzue S. Recent advances in structure activity relationship in new quinolones. Prog Drug Res 1992; 38:57–106.
11. Hecht DW, Wexler HM. In vitro susceptibility of anaerobes to quinolones in the United States. Clin Infect Dis 1996; 23(suppl 1):S2–S8.
12. Eagle H, Fleischman R, Levy M. Continuous vs discontinuous therapy with penicillin. N Engl J Med 1953; 238:481–486.
13. Eagle H. Effect of schedule of administration on therapeutic efficacy of penicillin: Importance of aggregate time penicillin remains at effectively bactericidal levels. Am J Med 1950; 9:280–299.
14. Eagle H, Fleischman R, Mussleman AD. Effective concentrations of penicillin in vitro and in vivo for streptococci and pneumococci and Treponema. J Bacteriol 1950; 59:625–643.
15. Shah PM, Junghanns W, Stille W. Dosis-Wirkungs-Beziehung der Bakterizidie, bei *E. coli*, *K. pneumoniae* and *Staphylococcus aureus*. Dtsch Med Wochenschr 1976; 101:325–328.
16. Kim MK, Nightingale CH. Pharmacokinetics and pharmacodynamics of the fluoroquinolones. In: Andriole VT, ed. The Quinolones. 3d ed. Academic Press: San Diego, 170–202.
17. Craig WA. Pharmacodynamics of antimicrobials: general concepts and applications, *P*1-22. In: Nightingale CH, Murakawa T, Ambrose PG, eds. Antimicrobial Pharmacodynamics in Theory and Clinical Practice. New York, N.Y.: Marcel Dekker, Inc.
18. Leggett JE, Ebert S, Fantin B, et al. Comparative dose-effect relations at several dosing intervals for beta-lactam, aminoglycoside, and quinolone antibiotics against gram-negative bacilli in murine thigh-infection and pneumonitis models. Scand J Infect Dis 1991; 74:179–184.
19. Peloquin CA, Cumbo TJ, Nix DE, et al. Evaluation of intravenous ciprofloxacin in patients with nosocomial lower respiratory tract infections. Arch Intern Med 1989; 149:2269–2273.
20. Drusano GL, Johnson DE, Rosen M, et al. Pharmacodynamics of a fluoroquinolone antimicrobial agent in a neutropenic rat model of *Pseudomonas sepsis*. Antimicrob Agents Chemother 1993; 37:483–490.
21. Forrest A, Nix DE, Ballow CH, Schentag JJ. Pharmacodynamics of intravenous ciprofloxacin in seriously ill patients. Antimicrob Agents Chemother 1993; 37:1073–1081.
22. Lacy MK, Lu W, Xu X, Nicolau DP, Quintiliani R, Nightingale CH. Pharmacodynamic comparison of levofloxacin, ciprofloxacin and ampicillin against *Streptococcus pneumoniae* in an in vitro model of infection. Antimicrob Agents Chemother 1999; 43:672–677.
23. Lister PD, Sanders CC. Pharmacodynamics of levofloxacin and ciprofloxacin against *Streptococcus pneumoniae*. J Antimicrob Chemother 1999; 43:79–86.

24. Lister PD. Pharmacodynamics of garenoxacin against *Streptococcus pneumoniae*. J Antimicrob Agents Chemother. In press.
25. Lister PD, Sanders CC. Pharmacodynamics of moxifloxacin, levofloxacin, and sparfloxacin against *Streptococcus pneumoniae* in an in vitro pharmacodynamic model. J Antimicrob Chemother 2001; 47:811–818.
26. Onyeji CO, Bui KQ, Owens RC Jr, Nicolau DP, Quintiliani R, Nightingale CH. Comparative efficacies of levofloxacin and ciprofloxacin against *Streptococcus pneumoniae* in a mouse model of experimental septicemia. Int J Antimicrob Agents 1999; 12:107–114.
27. Craig WA, Andes DR. Correlation of the magnitude of the $AUC_{24}MIC$ for 6 fluoroquinolones against *Streptococcus pneumoniae* with survival and bactericidal activity in an animal model. In: Program and Abstracts of the 40th Interscience Conference on Antimicrobial Agents and Chemotherapy, Toronto, Canada, September 17–21, 2000.
28. Preston SL, Drusano GL, Berman AL, Fowler CL, Chow AT, Dornseif B, Reichi V, Natarajan J, Wong WA, Corrado M. Pharmacodynamics of levofloxacin: a new paradigm for early clinical trials. JAMA 1997; 279:125–129.
29. Woodnut G. Pharmacodynamics to combat resistance. J Antimicrob Chemother 2000; 46:25–31.
30. Ambrose PG, Grasela DM, Grasela TH, Passarell J, Mayer HB, Pierce PF. Pharmacodynamics of fluoroquinolones against *Streptococcus pneumoniae* in patients with community-acquired respiratory tract infections. Antimicrob Agents Chemother 2001; 45:2793–2797.
31. Thomas JK, Forrest A, Bhavnani SM, et al. Pharmacodynamic evaluation of factors associated with the development of bacterial resistance in acutely ill patients during therapy. Antimicrob Agents Chemother 1998; 42:521–527.
32. Craig WA, Ebert SC. Protein binding and its significance in antibacterial therapy. Infect Dis Clin North Am 1989; 3:407–414.
33. Stahlmann R, Lode H. Safety overview: toxicity, adverse effects, and drug interactions. In: Andriole VT, ed. The Quinolones. 3d Ed. Academic Press: San Diego, 397–453.
34. Marutani K, Matsumoto M, Otabe Y, et al. Reduced phototoxicity of a fluoroquinolone antibacterial agent with methoxy group at the 8 position in mice irradiated with long wavelength (UV) light. Antimicrob Agents Chemother 1993; 37:2217–2223.
35. Akahana U, Sekiguchi M, Tsutomu U, et al. Structure-epileptogenicity relationship of quinolones with special reference to their interaction with gamma-aminobutyric acid receptor sites. Antimicrob Agents Chemother 1989; 33:1704–1708.
36. Bowie WR, Willetts V, Jewesson PJ. Adverse reactions in a dose-ranging study with a new long-acting fluoroquinolone, fleroxacin. Antimicrob Agents Chemother 1989; 33:1778–1782.
37. Bowie WR, Willetts V, Megran DW. Dose-ranging study of fleroxacin for treatment of uncomplicated Chlamydia trachomatis genital infections. Antimicrob Agents Chemother 1989; 33:1774–1777.

38. Kimura N, Miyazaki E, Matsuno O, et al. Drug-induced pneumonitis with eosinophilic inflitration due to tosufloxacin tosilate. Nihon Kokyuki Gakkai Zasshi 1998; 36:618–622.
39. Owens RC Jr. Risk assessment for antimicrobial agent-induced QTc interval prolongation and torsades de pointes. Pharmacotherapy 2001; 21:301–319.
40. Kang J, Wang L, Chen X-L, Triggle DJ, Rampe D. Interactions of a series of fluoroquinolone antibacterial drugs with the human cardiac K^+ channel HERG. Mol Pharmacol 2001; 59:122–126.
41. Ruskin JN. Antibiotic cardiotoxicity [abstr]. In: Program and abstracts of the 41st Interscience Conference on Antimicrobial Agents and Chemotherapy, Chicago, Illinois. Washington, DC: American Society for Microbiology, December 16–19, 2001:41.
42. De Ponti F, Poluzzi E, Cavalli A, Recanatini M, Montanaro N. Safety of non-antiarrhythmic drugs that prolong the QT interval or induce torsade de pointes. Drug Safety 2002; 25:263–286.
43. Bertino JS, Owens RC Jr, Carnes TD, Iannini PB. Gatifloxacin-associated corrected QT interval prolongation, torsades de pointes, and ventricular fibrillation in patients with known risk factors. Clin Infect Dis 2002; 34:861–863.
44. Shaffer D, Singer S, Korvick J, Honig P. Concomitant risk factors in reports of torsades de pointes associated with macrolide use: Review of the United States Food and Drug Administration Adverse Event Reporting System. Clin Infect Dis 2002; 35:197–200.
45. Frothingham MD. Rates of torsades de pointes associated with ciprofloxacin, ofloxacin, levofloxacin, gatifloxacin, and moxifloxacin. Pharmacotherapy 2001; 21:1468–1472.
46. Anriole VT. The quinolones; prospects. In: VT Andriole, ed. The Quinolones. 3d ed. Academic Press: San Diego, 47–495.
47. Iannini PB, von Seggern K, Wikler MA. Safety of gatifloxacin in patients with cardiovascular disease [abstr]. In: Program and abstracts of the 40th Interscience Conference on Antimicrobial Agents and Chemotherapy, Toronto, Ontario, Canada. Washington, DC: American Society for Microbiology, September 17–20, 2000.
48. Iannini P, Kubin R, Reiter C. Over 10 million patient uses: An update on the safety profile of oral moxifloxacin. In: Program and abstracts of the 42nd Interscience Conference on Antimicrobial Agents and Chemotherapy, San Diego, California. Washington, DC: American Society for Microbiology, September 27–30, 2002.
49. Gleason PP. The emerging role of atypical pathogens in community-acquired pneumonia. Pharmacotherapy 2002; 22:2S–11S.
50. Jones RN, Rubino CM, Bhavnani BM, Ambrose PG. Worldwide antimicrobial susceptibility patterns and pharmacodynamic comparisons of gatifloxacin and levofloxacin against *Streptococcus pneumoniae*: Report from the antimicrobial resistance rate epidemiology study team. Antimicrob Agents Chemother 2003; 47:292–296.

51. Owens RC, Ambrose PG. Minimum efficacy and mutation prevention exposure target attainment rates against *Streptococcus pneumoniae* for levofloxacin 500 mg and 750 mg and moxifloxacin 400 mg. In: Program and abstracts of the 40th Infectious Disease Society of America, Chicago, Illinois, October, 2002.
52. Ambrose PG, Jones RN, Gajjar DA, Van Wart S, Rubino CM, Bhavnani SM, Grasela DM. Use of Monte Carlo simulation to evaluate the antibacterial activity of garenoxacin against Gram-positive bacteria. In: Program and abstracts of the 42nd Interscience Conference on Antimicrobial Agents and Chemotherapy. San Diego, California, September 27–30, 2002.
53. Davidson R, Cavalcanti R, Bruton JL, et al. Resistance to levofloxacin and failure of treatment of pneumococcal pneumonia. N Engl J Med 2002; 346:747–750.
54. Nicolson P, Anderson P. The patients' burden: physical and psychological effects of acute exacerbations of chronic bronchitis. J Antimicrob Chemother 2000; 45:25–32.
55. Niederman MS, McCombs JS, Unger AN, Kumar A, Popovian R. Treatment of acute exacerbations of chronic bronchitis. Clin Ther 1999; 21:576–591.
56. Sethi S. Infectious etiology of acute exacerbations of chronic bronchitis. Chest 2000; 117(suppl):380S–385S.
57. Adams SG, Anzueto A. Antibiotic therapy in acute exacerbations of chronic bronchitis. Semin Respir Infect 2000; 15:234–247.
58. Andriole CL, Andriole VT. Are all quinolones created equal? Mediguide Infect Dis 2002; 21:1–5.
59. Langan CE, Zuck P, Vogel F, et al. Randomized, double blind study of short course grepafloxacin versus clarithromycin in patients with acute exacerbations of chronic bronchitis. J Antimicrob Ther 1999; 43:529–539.
60. Langan CE, Cranfield R, Breisch S, Pettit R. Randomized, double blind study of grepafloxacin versus amoxicillin in patients with acute exacerbations of chronic bronchitis. J Antimicrob Agents Chemother 1997; 40:63–72.
61. Shal PM, Maesen F, Colmann A, Vetter N, Fiss E, Wesch R. Levofloxacin versus cefuroxime axetil in the treatment of acute exacerbations of chronic bronchitis: results of a randomized double blind study. J Antimicrob Chemother 1999; 43:529–539.
62. Wilson R, Kubin R, Ballin I, et al. Five day moxifloxacin therapy compared with 7-day clarithromycin therapy for the treatment of acute exacerbations of chronic bronchitis. J Antimicrob Chemother 1999; 44:501–513.
63. Sinus and Allergy Health Partnership. Antimicrobial treatment guidelines for acute bacterial rhinosinusitis. Otolaryngol Head Neck Surg 2000; 123: S1–S38.
64. Sher LD, McAdoo MA, Bettis RB, Turner MA, Li NF, Pierce PF. A multicenter, randomized, investigator-blinded study of 5- and 10-day gatifloxacin versus 10-day amoxicillin/clavulanate in patients with acute bacterial sinusitis. Clin Ther 2002; 24:269–281.
65. Sher LD, Poole MD, Von Seggern K, Wikler MA, Nicholson SC, Pankey GA. Community-based treatment of acute uncomplicated bacterial rhinosinusitis with gatifloxacin. Otolaryngol Head Neck Surg 2002; 127:182–189.

7

Treatment of Community-Acquired Respiratory Tract Infections with Penicillins and Cephalosporins

Sandra L. Preston and George L. Drusano
Albany Medical College
Albany, New York, U.S.A.

Penicillins and cephalosporins belong to the β-lactam class of antimicrobials. Benzylpenicillin has been utilized since 1941 and cephalosporins began to be used clinically in the 1960s. Because of their spectrum of activity, the penicillins and cephalosporins have utility in treatment of community-acquired respiratory tract infections. This chapter will discuss the mechanism of action, pharmacokinetics, and pharmacodynamics of the penicillins and cephalosporins, as well as the utility of these drugs in the treatment of community-acquired respiratory tract infections. The number of β-lactams available for clinical use is extensive, so this chapter will limit discussion to the agents that are indicated and used clinically for treatment of community-acquired respiratory tract infections.

STRUCTURE ACTIVITY RELATIONSHIPS

The β-lactam agents have in common a basic structure, which includes the β-lactam ring. Penicillins have a thiazolidine ring and a side chain (Fig. 1).

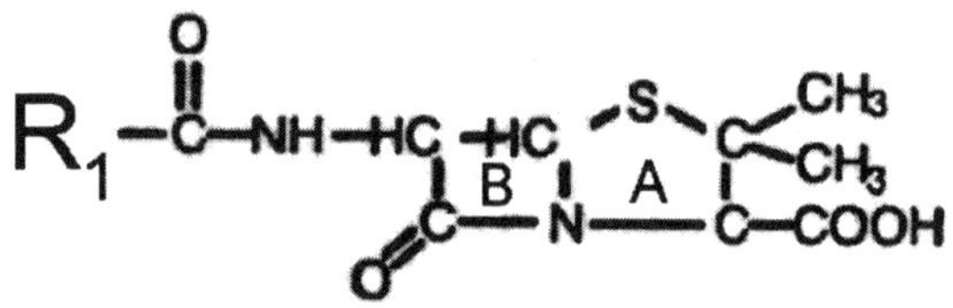

FIGURE 1 Penicillin structure. A-thiazolidine ring; B-beta-lactam ring; R_1- acyl side chain.

Manipulations of the side chain can help to sterically protect the β-lactam ring from hydrolysis by β-lactamase, thereby enhancing the activity of some penicillins against organisms such as *Staphylococcus aureus* or gram-negative rods with specific types of β-lactamase. The side chain can also protect against gastric acid degradation and lead to increased permeability of the compound, thus enhancing the oral absorption [1].

Cephalosporins are characterized by a dihydrothiazine ring, a β-lactam ring, and variations on two side chains (R-1 or C-7 and R-2 or C-3) (Fig. 2). Substitutions at the R-1 side chain can confer increased activity against β-lactamase–producing organisms by enhancing stability against some of these enzymes. The addition of a methoxy group at this position increases activity versus anaerobic bacteria, as seen with the cephamycins, cefoxitin and cefotetan. Substitutions at the R-2 side chain can extend the half-life of the drug, but the methylthiotetrazole (MTT) side chain at this position has been associated with hypoprothrombinemia and bleeding due to competitive inhibition of vitamin K–dependent clotting factors [2]. Drugs that contain this side chain at C3 are cefotetan, cefmetazole, cefomandole, and cefoperazone.

MECHANISM OF ACTION

The β-lactams are bactericidal drugs that inhibit bacterial cell wall synthesis by binding to enzymes called β-lactam (penicillin)-binding proteins (PBPs)

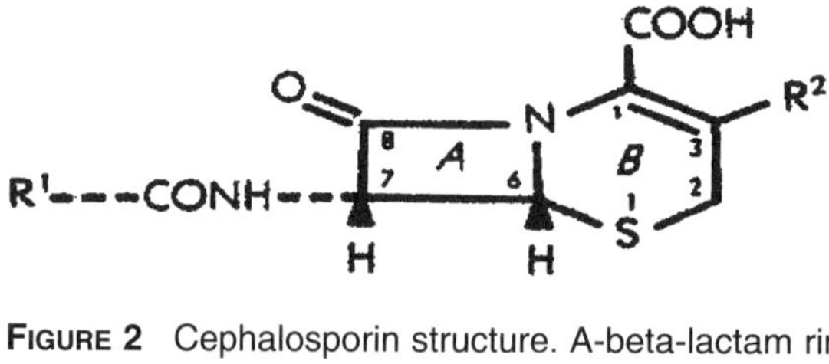

FIGURE 2 Cephalosporin structure. A-beta-lactam ring; B-dihydrothiazine ring; R_1 and R_2-positions for side chains.

located beneath the cell wall of bacteria. This binding inhibits a main component of the cell wall, peptidoglycan cross-linkage, which weakens the cell wall [3,4]. Binding to different PBPs can produce different morphologic changes. This is best seen in the effects on the morphology of gram-negative bacilli. The ability of the drug to penetrate the cell wall and, in gram-negative organisms, the outer membrane plus the ability to bind to the PBPs differs among drugs. For instance, penicillin G does not penetrate the cell wall of many gram-negative organisms; therefore, there is limited activity against these organisms. Alterations in PBPs can lead to resistance as seen in penicillin-resistant *Streptococcus pneumoniae*. Interestingly, these changes are not driven by classical mutational mechanisms. Rather, pneumococci take in the altered PBP DNA of other oral streptococci that have become β-lactam resistant to produce mosaic chromosomes. Classically, these organisms have mutations in PBP 2b and PBP 2x.

MECHANISMS OF RESISTANCE

There are three main mechanisms of resistance for the β-lactams, including (1) enzymatic degradation of the β-lactam, (2) alteration of the PBP target site, and (3) decreased permeability of the drug through the outer membrane. This latter mechanism primarily involves gram-negative organisms and will not be the focus of this discussion.

Enzymatic Degradation

Production of β-lactamase can hydrolyze the β-lactam ring and lead to loss of antimicrobial activity of the drug. Both gram-positive and gram-negative organisms can produce β-lactamases. The most relevant organisms that produce β-lactamases in community-acquired respiratory tract infection are *H. influenzae* and *M. catarrhalis*. These gram-negative bacteria secrete β-lactamases into the periplasmic space and hydrolyze the drug before it can acylate its target, the active site serine of the β-lactam binding proteins.

Alteration in Penicillin-Binding Proteins (PBP)

The primary mechanism of resistance of *Streptococcus pneumoniae* to β-lactams is an alteration in the PBP after sequential chromosomally mediated mutations in several high-molecular-weight PBPs. These mutations lead to a decreased ability of the β-lactam to bind to the PBP [5]. Since not all β-lactams bind to the same PBPs, there may be differences in susceptibility between agents of the class. The mechanism of resistance is complex and involves gene transfer events from closely related commensal *Streptococcus* species, leading to the presence of mosaic genes [6].

ANTIMICROBIAL ACTIVITY

The most common community-acquired respiratory pathogens are *Streptococcus pneumoniae, Haemophilus influenzae, Moraxella catarrhalis*, and the atypical organisms, *Mycoplasma pneumoniae, Legionella pneumophila*, and *Chlamydia pneumoniae*. The penicillins are classified into different groups according to antimicrobial spectrum characteristics and other similarities (Table 1). The natural penicillins, penicillin G and penicillin VK, have activity against *Streptococcus pneumoniae*. The aminopenicillins, ampicillin and amoxicillin, are drugs that have further manipulation of the side chain, and have enhanced activity against gram-negative organisms, specifically non–β-lactamase producing *Haemophilus influenzae*. Because β-lactamase is commonly produced by *H. influenzae* isolates, the combination of a β-lactamase inhibitor, clavulanate, with amoxicillin (Augmentin), can inhibit the β-lactamases carried and allow these organisms to be killed by clinically achievable concentrations of amoxicillin.

The penicillinase-resistant penicillins are active against *Staphylococcus aureus* and *Staphylococcus epidermidis* that produce penicillinase. The extended-spectrum penicillins include the carboxypenicillins (carbenicillin and ticarcillin), the ureidopenicillins (azlocillin and mezlocillin), and the piperazine penicillin (piperacillin). These agents have excellent coverage against gram-negative bacilli and anaerobes and are used primarily for nosocomial respiratory tract infection and other indications. The β-lactams are not active against the atypical pathogens or *Staphylococcus* unless accompanied by a β-lactamase inhibitor.

The cephalosporins are somewhat arbitrarily divided into four "generations" based on their spectrum of activity (Table 2). First-generation cephalosporins are active against gram-positive cocci, including penicillinase-

TABLE 1 Classification of Penicillins

Natural penicillins	Penicillinase-resistant	Aminopenicillins	Extended-spectrum
Penicillin G	Cloxacillin	Ampicillin	Piperacillin
Penicillin VK	Dicloxacillin	Bacampicillin	Mezlocillin
	Nafcillin	Amoxicillin	Ticarcillin
	Oxacillin	Ampicillin/sulbactam	Carbenicillin
		Amoxicillin/clavulanate	Ticarcillin/clavulanate
			Piperacillin/tazobactam

TABLE 2 Classification of Cephalosporins

First generation	Second generation	Third generation	Fourth generation
Cefadroxil	Cefaclor	Cefdinir	Cefepime
Cephalexin	Cefprozil	Cefixime	
Cefazolin	Cefuroxime	Ceftibuten	
Cephradine	Cefamandole	Cefpodoxime	
	Cefoxitin	Cefotaxime	
	Cefotetan	Ceftizoxime	
	Loracarbef	Ceftriaxone	
		Cefoperazone	
		Ceftazidime	
		Cefditoren	

producing and penicillinase non-producing *Staphylococcus aureus*, as well as *Streptococcus* sp. Second-generation cephalosporins are active against the organisms susceptible to first-generation agents plus activity against *Haemophilus influenzae*, including ampicillin-resistant strains. The agents cefoxitin and cefotetan also exhibit some useful anaerobic activity. The third-generation cephalosporins are less active against gram-positive organisms but exhibit enhanced gram-negative activity, particularly for Enterobacteriacae. Activity against *Streptococcus pneumoniae* is quite adequate, and ceftriaxone is commonly used for community-acquired respiratory tract infection. Other third-generation agents, ceftazidime and cefoperazone, have activity against *Pseudomonas aeruginosa*. The fourth-generation cephalosporin, cefepime, has expanded gram-negative coverage compared with the third-generation agents against organisms producing inducible β-lactamases, and also is active against *Pseudomonas aeruginosa*. This drug is generally not used in treatment of community-acquired respiratory tract infection; however, it does have good activity against *S. pneumoniae* and could be used empirically in the setting of severe CAP when gram-negative rods are also a possibility as the infecting organism.

The oral cephalosporins with the best antimicrobial activity against *Streptococcus pneumoniae* with MIC_{50}s of ≤ 0.1 mg/L are cefuroxime axetil, cefditoren, and cefpodoxime . Cefaclor, cephalexin, cefixime, and loracarbef have MIC_{50}s of ≤ 0.2–1 mg/L, and the least active drugs are ceftibuten and cefadroxil, with MICs of >1 mg/L [7]. Activity against *H. influenzae* varies depending on whether or not the organism produces β-lactamase. The best activity against non–β-lactamase producing strains is seen with cefixime, ceftibuten, cefditoren, and cefpodoxime. Loracarbef and cephalexin are inactive against *H. influenzae*. As with the penicillins, the activity of the cephalosporins against the atypical pathogens is poor. The antimicrobial activity of antimicrobials from clinical isolates and in vitro data versus the common respiratory pathogens are shown in Tables 3 and 4.

The ranking of these drugs solely on the basis of the MIC values can be misleading. Other factors, such as pharmacokinetic profile and protein

TABLE 3 Antimicrobial Activity for Common Respiratory Pathogens from Clinical Isolates from Surveillance Studies in North America

Drug	MIC_{50}	MIC_{90}
Streptococcus pneumoniae		
Penicillin G	0.03	1–2
Amoxicillin	0.06	1–2
Amoxicillin/clavulanate	0.25	1–2
Cefpodoxime	0.03	1–4
Cefuroxime axetil	0.06	4
Cefaclor	0.5	>64
Cefixime	0.5	>64
Ceftibuten	0.03	0.12
Cefprozil	2	8
Ceftriaxone	0.015	0.03–1
Haemophilus influenzae		
Penicillin G	0.5	>16
Amoxicillin	0.5	>8
Amoxicillin/clavulanate	0.5	1–2
Cefuroxime axetil	1	2
Cefaclor	4	16
Cefprozil	2–4	8–16
Cefixime	≤0.03	0.06
Cefpodoxime	0.06	0.12
Ceftibuten	≤0.03	0.12
Ceftriaxone	0.015	0.03
Moraxella catarrhalis		
Penicillin G	>4	16
Ampicillin	2	8
Amoxicillin/clavulanate	≤0.25	0.25
Cefuroxime axetil	1	2
Cefaclor	1	2
Cefprozil	2	8
Cefixime	0.25	0.5
Cefpodoxime	0.5	1
Ceftriaxone	0.5	1

Source: Refs. 54 through 57.

TABLE 4 In Vitro Antimicrobial Activity

Drug	MIC_{50}	MIC_{90}
Streptococcus pneumoniae[a]		
Cefuroxime	0.01	4
Cefpodoxime	0.03	4
Cefixime	0.5	32
Haemophilus influenzae[b]		
Amoxicillin/clavulanate	0.5	2
Cefuroxime	1	4
Cefixime	0.12	1
Cefpodoxime	0.06	0.125
Cefditoren	0.008	0.015
Ceftibuten	0.06	0.06
Loracarbef	2	8
Cefaclor	4	32
Moraxella catarrhalis[c]		
Amoxicillin/clavulanate	0.06	1
Cefaclor	0.5	4
Cefuroxime	0.5	2
Cefixime	0.06	0.5
Cefpodoxime	0.06	0.5
Ceftibuten	0.12	4
Cefditoren	0.03	1
Loracarbef	≤0.25	2

Includes β-lactamase positive and negative organisms.
[a] *Source*: Refs. 58 and 59
[b] *Source*: Refs. 60 through 63.
[c] *Source*: Refs. 64 through 67.

binding, will make a large difference in the relative activity of these drugs. Indeed, only free drug is microbiologically active, and the relative activity of the penicillins and cephalosporins should be graded on the fraction of the dosing interval that free drug spends above the MIC values for the target pathogens. There are differences among the β-lactams with regard to the fraction of the dosing interval necessary for coverage to achieve a specific desired endpoint (e.g., stasis or maximal cell kill). Given that true between-patient variability in pharmacokinetics exists for all drugs, the most robust way to gauge the activity of these agents for the target pathogens is to perform large Monte Carlo simulations in which the evaluative criterion is the fraction of subjects in the simulation that achieve the target free drug time above MIC.

TABLE 5 *S. pneumoniae* NCCLS Interpretive MIC Breakpoints (μg/mL)

Drug	Susceptible	Intermediate	Resistant
Penicillin	≤0.06	0.12–1	≥2.0
Amoxicillin	≤2.0	4.0	≥8.0
Amoxicillin ± clavulanate	≤2.0	4.0	≥8.0
Cefixime		No breakpoints set	
Cefpodoxime	≤0.5	1.0	≥2.0
Cefaclor	<1.0	2.0	≥4.0
Cefuroxime axetil	<1.0	2.0	≥4.0
Loracarbef	2.0	4.0	≥8.0
Ceftriaxone and cefotaxime			
non-meningeal isolates	1.0	2.0	4.0
meningeal isolates	0.5	1.0	2.0

Penicillin-Resistant *Streptococcus pneumoniae*

The current interpretive MIC breakpoints for penicillin as determined by the National Committee for Clinical Laboratory Standards (NCCLS) are ≤0.06 μg/mL (susceptible), 0.12–1.0 μg/mL (intermediate), and ≥2.0 μg/mL (resistant) [8]. Additional susceptibility breakpoints are shown in Table 5. In the United States, the prevalence of penicillin-non-susceptibility has risen from 4% in the 1980s to approximately 35% in 1997–1998 [9].

The prevalence of *Streptococcus pneumoniae* resistance to the cephalosporins is also high for cefaclor (34–78%, [10–13] and cefuroxime axetil (16–37%) [10,12–14]. Cefotaxime and ceftriaxone are more active with resistance rates of 4–11% [10,13,15]. The presence of a β-lactamase inhibitor offers no advantage in penicillin-resistant *Streptococcus pneumoniae* because the mechanism of resistance is not β-lactamase, but an altered PBP.

PHARMACOKINETICS AND PHARMACODYNAMICS

The pharmacokinetics of β-lactams vary among compounds. Amoxicillin is well absorbed with or without clavulanate. A twice-daily extended-release formulation of amoxicillin/clavulanate (Augmentin XR) has received FDA approval. The drug should be given in a dosage of 2000/125 mg twice daily (two tablets twice daily) and has the advantage of providing enhanced amoxicillin drug exposure versus resistant *Streptococcus pneumoniae*. The oral cephalosporins are commonly used in the outpatient setting for treatment of respiratory tract infection. The pharmacokinetics of the oral β-lactams commonly used for this indication is summarized in Table 6.

TABLE 6 Pharmacokinetics of Cephalosporins

Drug	Dose, mg	Cmax, mg/L	T ½, hr	Protein binding, %	Ref.
Ceftibuten	200	10.8–12.4	2.5–3.2	63	68
Cefpodoxime	200	2.5	2–3	18–33	69, 70
Cefixime	400	3.7–4.6	3–4	50–65	71, 72
Cefprozil	500	10	1–2	35–45	73, 74
Cefaclor	375	5.4	0.5–1	25	75
Cefuroxime axetil	250	4.1	1–2	33–50	76
Cefdinir	600	2.87	1.7–1.8	60–70	77
Loracarbef	400	14–15.4	1.2	25	78, 79
Cefditoren	400	4.4–4.6	1.3–2	88	80, 81
Ceftriaxone	1000	95	5.8–8.7	83–96	82, 83
Cefotaxime	1000	102	0.8–1.4	27–38	84, 85

The β-lactams exhibit relatively concentration-independent bactericidal activity, meaning that at concentrations greater than 2–4 times the MIC, no additional killing activity is seen [16]. In addition, regrowth of most organisms will occur soon after serum drug levels fall to below the level of the MIC [17], indicating that a persistent effect (PAE, PASME, etc.) is short or absent. Optimization of duration of exposure, or time that non–protein-bound serum concentrations remain above the MIC, would be the most appropriate way to maximize the likelihood of bacterial eradication and subsequently a positive outcome.

There has been a significant amount of animal model research that has examined this issue. The duration of time needed above the MIC was examined in a neutropenic mouse model infected with *Klebsiella pneumoniae* pneumonia. A bacteriostatic and bactericidal effect was seen when the time above MIC was 30–40% and 60–70%, respectively [18]. The penicillins demonstrated a slightly lower percentage of time needed above the MIC, possibly attributable to differences in rates of killing [19]. An alternative hypothesis would be that the differences among β-lactam classes (penicillins, cephalosporins, carbapenems) in the fraction of the dosing interval for which free drug concentrations need to exceed the MIC to achieve a specific endpoint (stasis, maximal cell kill, etc.) may be related to the binding to different PBPs and the manner in which they bind to the PBPs.

Streptococcus pneumoniae infection (strains that were penicillin susceptible, intermediate, and resistant) was examined in an animal model utilizing penicillins or cephalosporins. A relationship between mortality and time above MIC was developed. If the time above the MIC was 20% or less, mortality after 4 days of therapy was 80–100%. At a time above the MIC of 40–50%, the mortality was 0–20%, and at a time above the MIC of greater than 50%, the mortality was 0% [20].

A relationship between time above the MIC and bacteriological cure for patients with acute otitis media infected with *S. pneumoniae* and *H. influenzae* was developed from clinical trial data from several studies [20,21]. Time above MIC of greater than 40% was needed to achieve an 85–100% bacterial eradication rate. There did not appear to be differences in time above MIC needed between organisms.

Using a time above MIC goal of greater than 40%, common dosage regimens of several β-lactams were examined in a pediatric population to determine if sufficient drug concentrations would meet that target versus penicillin-intermediate or-resistant *Streptococcus pneumoniae* [20,21]. Amoxicillin and cefaclor were dosed 13.3 mg/kg TID and cefuroxime axetil was dosed 15 mg/kg BID. For penicillin-intermediate strains, two oral agents, cefuroxime axetil and amoxicillin, provided time above MICs for greater than 40% of the dosing interval but cefaclor did not, with a time above MIC of 0–20%. For resistant strains, only amoxicillin provided sufficient drug exposure. All parenteral β-lactams, including ampicillin, penicillin G, cefotaxime, and ceftriaxone, met the target for both intermediate and resistant organisms. In a clinical trial setting, the parenteral β-lactams performed well, even versus penicillin-resistant strains [22].

The ability of β-lactams to meet a target of serum concentrations exceeding the MIC for 40% of the dosing interval was examined using 4,489 clinical isolates of *Streptococcus pneumoniae* from a large surveillance study. For penicillin-susceptible pneumococcus, serum concentrations achieved for cefprozil, cefaclor, cefixime, cefpodoxime, and cefuroxime axetil were sufficient to meet the target. However, for penicillin-intermediate strains, only cefprozil, cefpodoxime, and cefuroxime axetil met the target. None of the drugs examined achieved sufficient concentrations for penicillin-resistant isolates [23].

The treatment guidelines for acute bacterial rhinosinusitis explicitly addressed the pharmacodynamic issue of the fraction of the time standard doses of β-lactams exceeded the MIC for 40–50% of the dosing interval for a large collection of isolates [24]. As previously demonstrated [23], many of the cephalosporins were poor in their ability to attain the target. These results are presented for the β-lactams in Table 7. Of the oral cephalosporins listed, only cefpodoxime, cefprozil, and cefuroxime attain the target at the PK/PD breakpoint for a reasonable percentage of the time (only 50–60%) for penicillin-intermediate pneumococci (n = 284). For fully penicillin-resistant

TABLE 7 Percentage of Respiratory Tract Isolates Susceptible at PK/PD Breakpoints

Drug	PK/PD Susceptibility Breakpoint (μg/mL)	Penicillin = susceptible *S. pneumoniae* (%) (n = 973)	Penicillin = intermediate *S. pneumoniae* (%) (n = 284)	Penicillin = resistant *S. pneumoniae* (%) (n = 503)	*H. influenzae* (%) (n = 1919)	*M. catarrhalis* (%) (n = 204)
High-dose amoxicillin	4	100	100	79.7	61.1	13.7
Amoxicillin/clavulanate	2	100	100	65.6	97.0	100
High-dose amoxicillin/ clavulanate	4	100	100	80.1	99.6	100
Cefaclor	0.5	47.3	7.4	0.2	2.3	5.4
Cefixime	1	95.3	28.5	0.4	99.9	100
Cefpodoxime	0.5	100	48.2	0	99.9	64.1
Cefprozil	1	99.2	57.7	0.4	18.2	6.4
Cefuroxime	1	99.8	59.9	0	79.6	37.3
Loracarbef	0.5	15.8	3.5	0	9.7	4.9

Source: Ref. 24.

pneumococci (n = 505), none of the cephalosporins attain the target, even at the 1% level. High-dose amoxicillin and amoxicillin/clavulanate, on the other hand, attain the target up to 80% of the time, even for fully penicillin-resistant isolates. For *Hemophilus influenzae* (n = 1919), only cefixime, cefuroxime, and cefpodoxime attain the target 80% of the time or more among the listed cephalosporins. It should be noted that some agents were not included in this list (ceftibutin, cefdinir, and cefditoren). Amoxicillin plus clavulanate, on the other hand, attains the target for more than 95% of the time for this pathogen.

It is clear that many oral cephalosporins are poorly active for the most important target pathogens seen in community-acquired upper and lower respiratory tract infections. If used in this setting, the agent employed should be chosen carefully, as there are major differences among these agents. Factors to consider include the severity of the illness, the possible adverse events attached to a failure of therapy, and the geographical locale, including the likelihood of encountering a strain of *Streptococcus pneumoniae* that is intermediate in its penicillin sensitivity or is fully penicillin resistant.

It should also be noted that this analysis likely overestimates the activity of all the β-lactams, as total drug concentrations were employed in the analysis. Only free drug is microbiologically active [25]. Ceftibuten, cefixime, cefdinir and cefditoren all have protein binding exceeding 50% (Table 6), indicating that correcting for free drug will, in essence, decrease the pharmacodynamic MIC breakpoint by one further dilution.

Finally, overuse of these agents (poorly active cephalosporins) may have an adverse ecological impact, in terms of amplifying the number of strains of *Streptococcus pneumoniae* that are penicillin-resistant. It has been demonstrated that utilization patterns of both macrolides and β-lactams affected the number of resistant isolates of pneumococcus found in their different areas of surveillance [26]. In this analysis, while aminopenicillin use adversely affected the number of resistant isolates, cephalosporins had a stronger association with this outcome. Again, this finding provides more importance to the idea that the overuse of all antibiotics should be avoided and that when necessary, drugs that are likely to attain the target of optimal antibacterial effect should be employed.

ADVERSE EFFECTS

Oral penicillin and cephalosporins are generally well tolerated, with the most common side effects being gastrointestinal intolerance, including nausea, vomiting, and diarrhea. The incidence of diarrhea with amoxicillin/clavulanate is approximately 12–15%. *Clostridium difficile* colitis has been reported to occur with both penicillin and cephalosporin use.

A maculopapular rash can occur in 5–10% of patients receiving amoxicillin and is generally self-limited. β-Lactam use may also be associated with an increase in liver transaminases. Other toxicities associated with cephalosporins that may occur include eosinophilia, thrombocytopenia, leukopenia, and a positive Coombs test. Cefpodoxime administration is associated with a metallic taste.

Penicillin hypersensitivity can occur in 1–10% of patients [27], and can range from a rash to anaphylaxis. Though potentially fatal, the incidence of anaphylaxis is low at about 0.004–0.015% of patients [28]. Sensitivity can result secondary to antibodies to the breakdown products of penicillin, including the major determinant (benzylpenicilloyl) and the minor determinants. These determinants can serve as an antigen to elicit an immune response [29]. The most immediate reaction is a type I or anaphylactic reaction involving IgE antibodies, which cause degranulation of mast cells and subsequent physiological reactions leading to urticaria, bronchoconstriction, and laryngeal edema [30].

Other types of hypersensitivity reactions to penicillins may occur, including a type II cytotoxic reaction resulting in a hemolytic anemia, a type III reaction resulting from antigen-antibody complexes depositing in major organs and leading to a serum sickness–like syndrome, and a type IV delayed hypersensitivity reaction of contact dermatitis or acute interstitial nephritis. Types II and III reactions usually occur after prolonged periods of penicillin use on the order of several weeks [31].

Allergic reactions may occur with cephalosporin use in a similar fashion to penicillins. The rate of cross-reactivity in patients with a penicillin allergy varies, but is usually reported to be 2–10% [32] but may be lower [33]. This may be due to the fact that the cephalosporanic acid nucleus is unstable once the β-lactam bond is lysed, resulting in the absence of minor degradation products for these agents. In patients with a history of an anaphylactic reaction to penicillin, cephalosporin use should be avoided.

Cefaclor has been associated with a serum sickness–like reaction with an incidence of 0.5%. Manifestations include a maculopapular rash or erythema multiforme, pruritis, and arthritis, arthralgia, irritability, and fever [34,35]. This syndrome is most common in patients under the age of 6 years, and management consists of drug discontinuation, antihistamines, and corticosteroids for symptomatic relief.

CLINICAL UTILITY IN TREATMENT OF COMMUNITY-ACQUIRED RESPIRATORY TRACT INFECTION

The choices for treatment of community-acquired respiratory tract infection can include several different antimicrobial classes, including macrolides, fluoroquinolones, and β-lactams. This section will focus on the utility of β-lactams for this indication.

Because *Hemophilus influenzae* is a common pathogen in community-acquired respiratory tract infections and often carries a β-lactamase, amoxicillin and penicillin VK are not commonly used for treatment of community-acquired respiratory tract infection. Instead, other β-lactam choices include amoxicillin/clavulanate and the second- and third-generation cephalosporins, cefuroxime axetil, cefpodoxime, cefaclor, loracarbef, cefixime, and ceftibuten. Common dosages for these and other agents are listed in Table 8.

Pharyngitis/Tonsillitis

The oral cephalosporins are effective in treating this infection; however there are no data on the efficacy of these agents in subsequent prevention of rheumatic fever. Penicillin V or benzathine penicillin G are still considered the drugs of choice for treatment of group A Streptococcus infection because of their prevention of primary rheumatic fever and cost considerations [36]. In patients allergic to penicillin, erythromycin is an alternative agent. A first-generation cephalosporin, such as cephalexin or cefadroxil, may be considered in patients without a history of anaphylaxis to penicillin.

Penicillin VK is dosed at 250 mg b.i.d. or t.i.d. in children. Adolescents and adults receive a dose of either 250 mg t.i.d. or q.i.d., or 500 mg b.i.d. Once-

TABLE 8 Adult Dosage of β-lactams in Treatment of Community Acquired Respiratory Tract Infections

Generic name (Brand)	Common dosage
Cefpodoxime (Vantin)	200 mg PO q.12hr × 10–14 days
Pharyngitis and tonsillitis	100 mg PO q.12hr × 5–10 days
Cefprozil (Cefzil)	250–500 mg PO q.12hr × 10 days
Cefixime (Suprax)	400 mg PO q.24hr or 200 mg PO q.12hr for 10–14 days
Cefdinir (Omnicef)	600 mg PO q.d. or 300 mg PO q.12hr for 10–14 days
Cefaclor (Ceclor)	
Acute exacerbation of chronic bronchitis	500 mg PO q.12hr × 7d
Pharyngitis/tonsillitis	375 mg PO q.12hr × 10 days
Ceftibuten (Cedax)	400 mg PO q.d. × 10 days
Cefuroxime axetil (Ceftin)	250–500 mg q.12hr × 7–10 days
Loracarbef (Lorabid)	200–400 mg PO q.12hr × 7–10 days
Cefditoren (Spectracef)	400 mg PO b.i.d. × 10 days
Ceftriaxone (Rocephin)	1–2 g I.M./I.V. q.24hr × 10–14 days

daily penicillin VK is not effective [37]. Several agents are FDA approved for once-a-day administration for streptococcal pharyngitis, including the oral cephalosporins cefadroxil, cefixime, and cefdinir and a macrolide, azithromycin.

The duration of therapy for penicillin VK is 10 days to achieve maximal rates of pharyngeal pathogen eradication. While shorter-course therapy of 5 days or less has demonstrated efficacy and has been approved by the FDA for cefdinir, cefpodoxime, and azithromycin, it is not recommended at this time because of concerns over study design and the broad spectrum of the agents and increased cost over penicillin VK [38].

Acute Exacerbation of Chronic Bronchitis

Acute exacerbation of chronic bronchitis (AECB) is a condition associated with chronic obstructive pulmonary disease (COPD) and is most commonly caused by *H. influenzae, S. pneumoniae*, and *M. catarrhalis*. Treatment with antibiotics has been shown to lengthen the exacerbation-free period [39]. Treatment is often empiric as it is not always possible to get an appropriate sample for microbiological testing due to the outpatient nature of cases of this infection. Coverage of the most common organisms causing this infection is therefore necessary.

First-line agents such as amoxicillin, doxycycline, and trimethoprim/sulfamethoxazole were used extensively in the past to treat these infections, but increasing prevalence of resistance [40], such as β-lactamase production affecting the activity of β-lactams, has limited the use of these agents, particularly in patients with comorbidities. A β-lactam/β-lactamase inhibitor combination or a cephalosporin such as cefuroxime are some alternative second-line agents that can be used to treat this infection, particularly in more complicated cases and in patients with more symptoms where β-lactam resistance is possible [41,42]. In general, these agents are more expensive that amoxicillin, but some data have suggested that they may be more cost-effective [43].

Acute Maxillary Sinusitis

Acute sinusitis is a common infection, with about 20 million cases per year in the United States [44]. Despite the fact that symptoms of acute sinusitis can improve without antibiotic therapy, antibiotics have been shown to increase the speed of symptom resolution [45] and decrease the incidence of clinical failures by as much as 50% [46]. Also, antibiotic therapy may be cost-effective [46]. It is important to note, however, that acute sinusitis is similar to acute otitis media in that high clinical success rates seen in clinical trials of antibiotics may not translate to bacteriological efficacy. This phenomenon is termed the "Pollyanna phenomenon," meaning that symptoms may resolve despite inadequate antimicrobial therapy and that these drugs may appear more effective clinically than they really are as measured by antimicrobial activity [47]. This may explain why clinical success may be discordant with predicated success based on pharmacodynamics.

The causative pathogens include *H. influenzae, S. pneumoniae*, and less frequently, *M. catarrhalis*. The β-lactams are commonly used to treat this infection. First-line therapy includes the inexpensive agents amoxicillin and trimethoprim/sulfamethoxazole. If there is suspicion of penicillin-resistant pneumococcus, the dose of amoxicillin should be increased to a maximum of 3 g/day to attempt to overcome this resistance.

Use of second-line agents such as the second- and third- generation cephalosporins (cefprozil, cefuroxime axetil, cefpodoxime) and amoxicillin/clavulanate should be considered as a first choice in therapy in patients who have received prior antibiotic therapy in the past 4–6 weeks [44], if first-line therapy failed, if the patient is younger than 2 years, if there is a smoker in the family or a child in a day-care facility, or if resistance is common in the community [48]. The utility of cefaclor and loracarbef is limited due to decreasing activity versus resistant *H. influenzae* and only fair activity against *Streptococcus pneumoniae*, particularly resistant organisms.

Community-Acquired Pneumonia

The organisms that most commonly cause community-acquired pneumonia (CAP) include *Streptococcus pneumoniae*, *H. influenzae*, *M. catarrhalis*, and the atypicals, *Mycoplasma pneumoniae, Chlamydia pneumoniae*, and *Legionella pneumophila*. The β-lactams are inactive against the atypical pathogens; therefore, empiric regimens that include a β-lactam must also be combined with a macrolide or doxycycline to provide adequate coverage for these potential pathogens.

The role of β-lactams for empiric therapy for CAP in the era of resistant *Streptococcus pneumoniae* has been supported in various levels by the Centers for Disease Control and Prevention (CDC) guidelines [49], as well as guidelines from the American Thoracic Society (ATS) [50] and Infectious Diseases Society of America (IDSA) [51]. The CDC guidelines for empiric CAP therapy include a recommendation for certain β-lactams for initial empiric therapy if the penicillin MIC is 2 mg/L or lower. The agents recommended for oral therapy include cefuroxime, cefpodoxime, high-dose amoxicillin (1g PO q8h), or amoxicillin/clavulanate 875 mg twice daily. For intravenous therapy, cefotaxime, ceftriaxone, or ampicillin/sulbactam can be used. These guidelines also illustrate the potential role of the antipneumococcal fluoroquinolones, particularly if the penicillin MIC is 4 mg/L or higher.

In developing their guidelines for empiric therapy for CAP, the ATS stratified outpatients according to presence or absence of cardiopulmonary disease or other modifying factors, such as age older than 65, immunosuppressive illness, or other comorbidities. They did not recommend a β-lactam for outpatients with no modifying factors or a history of cardiopulmonary disease. If the patient does have cardiopulmonary disease or other modifying factors, a β-lactam such as oral cefpodoxime, cefuroxime, high-dose amoxicillin, amoxicillin/clavulanate, or parenteral ceftriaxone followed by oral cefpodoxime is recommended in conjunction with a macrolide (or doxycycline) as a treatment alternative.

According to the ATS guidelines, for inpatients who are not in the intensive care unit with cardiopulmonary disease and/or modifying factors, an intravenous β-lactam such as cefotaxime, ceftriaxone, ampicillin/sulbactam, or high-dose ampicillin plus a macrolide (or doxycycline) is recommended. In hospitalized patients without cardiopulmonary disease or modifying factors, a β-lactam is recommended only in case of a macrolide allergy/intolerance. In ICU-admitted patients, an intravenous β-lactam such as ceftriaxone may be given with an intravenous macrolide.

If patients are at risk for *Pseudomonas aeruginosa* infection, choices include cefepime, imipenem, meropenem, or piperacillin/tazobactam. If resistant *Streptococcus pneumoniae* is suspected, certain β-lactams should not be used secondary to possible decreased efficacy. These agents include first-generation cephalosporins, cefaclor, and loracarbef [50].

The IDSA guidelines do not recommend a β-lactam for empiric CAP therapy for outpatients. If the patient needs hospitalization, either in a general medical ward or the ICU, a β-lactam (cefotaxime, ceftriaxone, or a β-lactam/β-lactamase inhibitor) plus a macrolide is one of two preferred choices (the other being a fluoroquinolone with anti-pneumococcal activity) [51].

For treatment of pneumonia due to penicillin-susceptible *Streptococcus pneumoniae* (MIC $\leq$ 1.0 μg/mL, amoxicillin, the oral cephalosporins (such as cefpodoxime, cefprozil, or cefuroxime), or parenteral agents such as ceftriaxone are effective [51,52]. In settings with a *Streptococcus pneumoniae* MIC of 2 μg/mL or greater, treatment can be guided on the basis of susceptibility testing; appropriate agents may include high-dose ampicillin, cefotaxime, ceftriaxone, and Augmentin XR.

H. influenzae and *M. catarrhalis* pneumonia may be treated with the β-lactams in the form of a second- or third-generation cephalosporin or a β-lactam/β-lactamase inhibitor. β-Lactam/β-lactamase inhibitor combinations are also useful for treatment of an anaerobic pneumonia [51].

Treatment outcomes associated with initial β-lactam–containing regimens for empiric treatment of pneumonia were examined in a 12,945 patient retrospective review of elderly Medicare inpatients [53]. Approximately three quarters of the population were community-dwelling, with the remainder admitted to a long-term-care facility. Of the regimens used initially, the ones associated independently with a decreased 30-day mortality included (1) a second-generation cephalosporin plus a macrolide, (2) a non-pseudomonal third-generation cephalosporin plus a macrolide, and (3) a fluoroquinolone. The regimens associated with an increase in 30-day mortality include a β-lactam/β-lactamase inhibitor plus a macrolide and an aminoglycoside plus another agent. In the 75% of patients who were community-dwelling, only initial therapy with a non-pseudomonal third-generation cephalosporin plus a macrolide was associated with decreased mortality; however, this may have been due to a smaller sample size. It is unclear why the β-lactam/β-lactamase inhibitor plus a macrolide regimen did not perform well. Possible reasons include suboptimal activity against penicillin-resistant *Streptococcus pneumoniae*, use of this regimen in patients suspected of having aspiration pneumonia, infection with an unrecognized pathogen for which the regimen was not effective, or that it was a chance finding because the study was a retrospective analysis.

SUMMARY

The penicillins and cephalosporins are commonly used for treatment of community-acquired respiratory tract infections and continue to have a role in the era of drug-resistant *Streptococcus pneumoniae*. They remain popular because of their well-defined safety profile and their activity against common respiratory pathogens. The efficacy of a specific β-lactam against specific respiratory pathogens (including drug-resistant *Streptococcus pneumoniae*) varies based on intrinsic antimicrobial activity against the infecting organism and the pharmacokinetics and pharmacodynamics of the drug.

REFERENCES

1. Price KE, Gourevitch A, Cheney LC. Biological properties of semisynthetic penicillins: structure-activity relationships. Antimicrob Agents Chemother 1966; 13:670–708.
2. Marshall WF, Blair JE. The cephalosporins. Mayo Clin Proc 1999; 74:187–195.
3. Tomasz A. The mechanism of the irreversible antimicrobial effects of penicillin: how the beta-lactam antibiotics kill and lyse bacteria. Annu Rev Microbiol 1979; 33:113–117.
4. Yocum RR, Waxman DW, Strominger JL. The mechanism of action of penicillin. J Biol Chem 1980; 255:3977–3986.
5. Markiewicz Z, Tomasz A. Variation in penicillin-binding protein patterns of penicillin-resistant clinical isolates of pneumococci. J Clin Microbiol 1989; 27: 405–410.
6. Hakenbeck R, Grebe T, Zahner D, Stock JB. β-lactam resistance in Strep-

tococcus pneumoniae: penicillin-binding proteins and non-penicillin binding proteins. Mol Microbiol 1999; 33:673–678.
7. Bacquero F, Loza E. Antibiotic resistance of micro-organisms involved in ear, nose, and throat infections. Pediatr Infect Dis J 1994; 13:S9–S14.
8. National Committee for Clinical Laboratory Standards (NCCLS). Methods for dilution antimicrobial susceptibility tests for bacteria that grow aerobically; approved standard. 6th ed. NCCLS document M7-A5. Wayne, PA: NCCLS, 2001.
9. Appelbaum PC. Resistance among *Streptococcus pneumoniae*: implications for drug selection. Clin Infect Dis 2002; 34:1613–1620.
10. Doern GV, Pfaller MA, Kugler K, Freeman J, Jones RN. Prevalence of antimicrobial resistance among respiratory tract isolates of Streptococcus pneumoniae in North America: 1997 results from the SENTRY Antimicrobial Surveillance Program. Clin Infect Dis 1998; 27:764–770.
11. Centers for Disease Control and Prevention. Geographic variation in penicillin resistance in Streptococcus pneumoniae: selected sites, United States, 1997. MMWR Morb Mortal Wkly Rep 1999; 48:656–661.
12. Doern GV, Ehilmann KP, Huynh HK, Rhomberg PR, Coffman SL, Brueggemann AB. Antimicrobial resistance among clinical isolates of Streptococcus pneumoniae in the United States during 1990–2000, including a comparison of resistance rates since 1994–1995. Antimicrob Agents Chemother 2001; 45:1721.
13. Pfaller MA, Jones RN, Doern GV, Sader HA, Kugler KC, Beach ML. Survey of blood stream infections attributable to gram-positive cocci: frequency of occurrence and antimicrobial susceptibility of isolates collected in 1997 in the United States, Canada, and Latin America from the SENTRY Antimicrobial Surveillance Program. Diagn Microbiol Infect Dis 1999; 33:283–297.
14. Jacobs MR, Bajaksouzian S, Zilles A, Lin G, Pankuch GA, Appelbaum PC. Susceptibilities of *Streptococcus pneumoniae* and *Haemophilus influenzae* to 10 oral antimicrobial agents based on pharmacodynamic parameters: 1997 US surveillance study. Antimicrob Agents Chemother 1999; 43:1901–1908.
15. Sahm DF, Thornsberry C, Mayfield DC, Jones ME, Karlowsky JA. In vitro activities of broad-spectrum cephalosporins against nonmeningeal isolates of Streptococcus pneumoniae: MIC interpretation using NCCLS M100-S12 recommendations. J Clin Microbiol 2002; 40:669–674.
16. Craig WA, Ebert SC. Killing and regrowth of bacteria in vitro: a review. Scand J Infect Dis Suppl 1991; 74:63–70.
17. Craig WA. Pharmacokinetic/ pharmacodynamic parameters: rationale for antibacterial dosing of mice and men. Clin Infect Dis 1998; 26:1–12.
18. Craig WA. Interrelationship between pharmacokinetics and pharmacodynamics in determining dosage regimens for broad-spectrum cephalosporins. Diagn Microbiol Infect Dis 1995; 22:89–96.
19. Craig WA, Ebert S, Watanabe Y. Differences in time above MIC required for efficacy of beta-lactams in animal infection models (abstract 86). In: Abstracts of the 33rd Interscience Conference on Antimicrobial Agents and Chemotherapy (San Francisco). Washington, D.C: American Society for Microbiology, 1993.
20. Craig WA. Antimicrobial resistance issues of the future. Diagn Microbiol Infect Dis 1996; 25:213–217.

21. Craig WA, Andes D. Pharmacokinetics and pharmacodynamics of antibiotics in otitis media. Pediatr Infect Dis J 1996; 15:255–259.
22. Pallares R, Linares J, Vadillo M, Cabellos C, Manresa F, Viladrich PF, Martin R, Gudiol F. Resistance to penicillin and cephalosporin and mortality from severe pneumococcal pneumonia in Barcelona, Spain. N Engl J Med 1995; 333: 474–480.
23. Mason EO, Malberth LB, Kershaw NL, Prosser BLT, Zoe A, Ambrose PG. Streptococcus pneumoniae in the United States: in-vitro susceptibility and pharmacodynamic analysis. J Antimicrob Chemother 2000; 45:623–631.
24. Sinus and Allergy Health Partnership. Antimicrobial treatment guidelines for acute bacterial rhinosinusitis. Otolaryng Head Neck Surg 2000; 123:S1–S32.
25. Merrikin DJ, Briant J, Rolinson GN. Effect of protein binding on antibiotic activity in vivo. J Antimicrob Chemother 1983; 11:233–238.
26. Garcia-Rey C, Aguilar L, Baquero F, Casal J, Sal-Re R. Importance of local variations in antibiotic consumption and geographical differences of erythromycin and penicillin resistance in *Streptococcus pneumoniae*. J Clin Microbiol 2002; 40:159–164.
27. Deswarte RD. Drug allergy—problems and strategies. J Allergy Clin Immunol 1984; 74:209–221.
28. Idsoe O, Guthe T, Wilcox RR, Weck AL. Nature and extent of penicillin side reactions with particular reference to fatalities from anaphylactic shock. Bull WHO 1968; 38:159–188.
29. Levine BB. Immunologic mechanisms of penicillin allergy. A haptenic model system for the study of diseases in man. N Engl J Med 1966; 275:1115–1125.
30. O'Leary MR, Smith MS. Penicillin anaphylaxis. Am J Emerg Med 1986; 4:241–247.
31. Sher TH. Penicillin hypersensitivity—a review. Pediatr Clin North Am 1983; 30:161–176.
32. Petz LD. Immunologic cross-reactivity between penicillins and cephalosporins: a review. J Infect Dis 1978; 137(suppl):74–79.
33. Anne S, Reisman RE. Risk of administering cephalosporin antibiotics to patients with histories of penicillin allergy. Ann Allergy Asthma Immunol 1995; 74:167–170.
34. Hebert AA, Sigman ES, Levy ML. Serum sickness-like reactions from cefaclor in children. J Am Acad Dermatol 1991; 25:805–808.
35. Reynolds R. Cefaclor and serum sickness-like reaction. JAMA 1996; 276:950–951.
36. Bisno AL, Gerber MA, Gwaltney JM Jr, Kaplan EL, Schwartz RH. Practice guidelines for the diagnosis and management of group A streptococcal pharyngitis. Clin Infect Dis 2002; 35:113–125.
37. Gerber MA, Randolph MF, Demeo K, Feder HM Jr, Kaplan EL. Failure of once-daily penicillin V therapy for streptococcal pharyngitis. Am J Dis Child 1989; 143:153–155.
38. Gerber MA, Tanz RR. New approaches to the treatment of group A streptococcal pharyngitis. Curr Opin Pediatr 2001; 13:51–55.

39. Adams SG, Melo J, Luther M, Anzueto A. Antibiotics are associated with lower relapse rates in outpatients with acute exacerbations of COPD. Chest 2000; 117:1345–1352.
40. Jorgensen J, Doern G, Maher L, Howell AW, Redding JS. Antimicrobial resistance among respiratory isolates of *Haemophilus influenzae, Moraxella catarrhalis*, and *Streptococcus pneumoniae* in the United States. Antimicrob Agents Chemother 1990; 34:2075–2080.
41. Balter M. Recommendations on the management of chronic bronchitis: a practical guide for Canadian physicians. Can Med Assoc J 1994; 151(Suppl):1–23.
42. Akalin HE. The place of antibiotic therapy in the management of chronic acute exacerbations of chronic bronchitis. Int J Antimicrob Agents 2001; 18:S49–S55.
43. Destache CJ, Dewan N, O'Donohue WJ, et al. Clinical and economic considerations in the treatment of acute exacerbations of chronic bronchitis. J Antimicrob Chemother 1999; 43(Suppl A):107–113.
44. Fendrick AM, Saint S, Brook I, Jacobs MR, Pelton S, Sethi S. Diagnosis and treatment of upper respiratory tract infections in the primary care setting. Clin Ther 2001; 23:1683–1706.
45. Gwaltney JM Jr. State-of-the-art: acute community-acquired sinusitis. Clin Infect Dis 1996; 23:1209–1223.
46. Benninger MS, Sedory Holzer SE, Lau J. Diagnosis and treatment of uncomplicated acute bacterial rhinosinusitis: Summary of the Agency for Health Care Policy and Research evidence-based report. Otolaryngol Head Neck Surg 2000; 122:1–7.
47. Marchant CD, Carlin SA, Johnson CE, Shurin PA. Measuring the comparative efficacy of antibacterial agents for acute otitis media: the "Polyanna phenomenon." J Pediatr 1992; 120:72–77.
48. Brook I, Gooch WM, Jenkins SG, Pichichero ME, Reiner SA, Sher L, Yamauchi T. Medical management of acute bacterial sinusitis. Recommendations of a clinical advisory committee on pediatric and adult sinusitis. Ann Otol Rhinol Laryngol 2000; 109:2–20.
49. Whitney CG, Farley MM, Hadler J, Harrison LH, Lexau C, Reingold A, Lefkowitz L, Cieslak PR, Cetron M, Zell ER, Jorgenson JH, Schuchat A. Increasing prevalence of multidrug-resistant *Streptococcus pneumoniae* in the United States. N Engl J Med 2000; 343:1917–1924.
50. Guidelines for the Management of Adults with Community-Acquired Pneumonia. Am J Respir Crit Care Med 2001; 163:1730–1754.
51. Bartlett JG, Dowell SF, Mandell LA, File TM Jr, Musher DM, Fine MJ. Practice guidelines for the management of community-acquired pneumonia in adults. Clin Infect Dis 2000; 31:347–382.
52. Kaplan SL, Mason EO Jr. Management of infections due to antibiotic-resistant *Streptococcus pneumoniae*. Clin Microbiol Rev 1998; 11:628.
53. Gleason PP, Meehan TP, Fine JM, Galusha DH, Fine MF. Associations between initial antimicrobial therapy and medical outcomes for hospitalized elderly patients with pneumonia. Arch Intern Med 1999; 159:2562–2572.
54. Thornsberry C, Sahm DF, Kelly LJ, Critchley IA, Jones ME, Evagelista AT,

Karlowsky JA. Regional trends in antimicrobial resistance among clinical isolates of *Streptococcus pneumoniae, Haemophilus influenzae*, and *Moraxella catarrhalis* in the United States: results from the TRUST surveillance program, 1999–2000. Clin Infect Dis 2002; 34(suppl 1):S4–S16.

55. Mathai D, Lewis MT, Kugler KC, Pfaller MA, Jones RN, and the SENTRY Participants Group (North America). Diagn Microb Infect Dis 2001; 39:105–116.
56. Jacobs MR, Bajaksouzian S, Zilles A, Lin G, Pankuch GA, Appelbaum PC. Susceptibilities of *Streptococcus pneumoniae* and *Haemophilus influenzae* to 10 oral antimicrobial agents based on pharmacodynamic parameters: 1997 US surveillance study. Antimicrob Agents Chemother 1999; 43:1901–1908.
57. Hoban DJ, Doern GV, Fluit C, Roussel-Delvallez M, Jones RN. Worldwide prevalence of antimicrobial resistance in *Streptococcus pneumoniae*, *Haemophilus influenzae*, and *Moraxella catarrhalis* in the SENTRY antimicrobial surveillance program, 1997–1999. Clin Infect Dis 2001; 32(suppl 2).
58. Janknegt R, van der Meer JWM. Antimicrobial practice-sequential therapy with intravenous and oral cephalosporins. J Antimicrob Chemother 1994; 33: 169–177.
59. Cunha BA. Third-generation cephalosporins: a review. Clin ther 1992; 14:616–647.
60. Debbia EA, Schito GC, Pesce A. Antibacterial activity of ceftibuten, a new third generation cephalosporin. J Chemother 1991; 3:209–225.
61. Klepser ME, Marangos MN, Patel KB, Nicolau DP, Quintiliani R, Nightingale CH. Clinical pharmacokinetics of newer cephalosporins. Clin Pharmacokinet 1995; 28:361–384.
62. Felmingham D, Robbins MJ, Ghosh G, Bhogal H, Mehta MD, Leakey A, Clark S, Dencer CA, Ridgway GL, Gruneberg RN. An in vitro characterization of cefditoren, a new oral cephalosporin. Drug Exp Clin Res 1994; 20:127–147.
63. Williams JD, Powell M, Fah YS, Seymour A, Yuan M. In vitro susceptibility of *Haemophilus influenzae* to cefaclor, cefixime, cefetamet, and loracarbef. Eur J Clin Microb Infect Dis 1992; 11:748–751.
64. Doern GV, Vautour R, Parker D, Tubert T, Torres B. In vitro activity of loracarbef (LY 163892), a new oral carbacephem antibacterial agent, against respiratory isolates of *H. influenzae* and *M. catarrhalis*. Antimicrob Agents Chemother 1991; 35:1504–1507.
65. Jones RN. Ceftibuten: a review of antimicrobial activity, spectrum and other microbiologic features. Pediatr Infect Dis J. 1993; 12:S37–S44.
66. Sarubbi FA, Verghese A, Caggiano C, Holtsclaw-Berk S, Berk SL. In vitro activity of cefpodoxime proxetil (U-76,252, CS 807) against clinical isolates of *Branhamella catarrhalis*. Antimicrob Agents Chemother 1989; 33:113–114.
67. Dabernat H, Avril JL, Boussougant Y. In-vitro activity of cefpodoxime against pathogens responsible for community-acquired respiratory tract infections. J Antimicrob Chemother 1990 Dec; 26(suppl E):1–6.
68. Radwanski E, Teal M, Affrime M, Cayen M, Lin CC. Multiple dose phar-

macokinetics of ceftibuten in healthy adults and geriatric volunteers. Am J Ther 1994; 1:42–48.
69. Borin MT, Hughes GS, Spillers CR, Patel RK. Pharmacokinetics of cefpodoxime in plasma and skin blister fluid following oral dosing of cefpodoxime proxetil. Antimicrob Agents Chemother 1990; 34:1094–1099.
70. O'Neill P, Nye K, Douce G, Andrews J, Wise R. Pharmacokinetics and inflammatory fluid penetration of cefpodoxime proxetil in volunteers. Antimicrob Agents Chemother 1990; 34:232–234.
71. Faulkner RD, Yacobi A, Barone JS, Kaplan SA, Silber BM. Pharmacokinetic profile of cefixime in man. Pediatr Infect Dis J 1987; 6:963–970.
72. Brittain DC, Scully BE, Hirose T, Neu HC. The pharmacokinetic and bactericidal characteristics of oral cefixime. Clin Pharmacol Ther 1985; 38:590–594.
73. Barbhaiya RH, Shukla UA, Gleason CR, Shyu WC, Wilber RB, Martin RR, Pittman KA. Phase I study of multiple-dose cefprozil and comparison with cefaclor. Antimicrob Agents Chemother 1990; 34:1198–1203.
74. Barbhaiya RH, Shukla UA, Gleason CR, Shyu WC, Wilber RB, Pittman KA. Comparison of cefprozil and cefaclor pharmacokinetics and tissue penetration. Antimicrob Agents Chemother 1990; 34:1204–1209.
75. Glynne A, Goulbourn RA, Ryden R. A human pharmacology study of cefaclor. J Antimicrob Chemother 1978; 4:343–348.
76. Nix DE, Symonds WT, Hyatt JM, Wilton JH, Teal MA, Reidenberg P, Affrime MB. Comparative pharmacokinetics of oral ceftibuten, cefixime, cefaclor, and cefuroxime axetil in healthy volunteers. Pharmacotherapy 1997; 17(1):121–125.
77. Appelbaum PC: Cefdinir. A review of its antibacterial and therapeutic potential in community-acquired infections. Clin Drug Invest 1996; 9(suppl):54–64.
78. Nahata MC, Koranyi KI. Pharmacokinetics of loracarbef in pediatric patients. Eur J Metabol Pharmaco 1992; 17:201–204.
79. Therasse DG, Farlow DS, Davidson RL, Quadracci LJ, Hatcher BL, Cerimele BJ, DeSante KA. Effects of renal dysfunction on the pharmacokinetics of loracarbef. Clin Pharmacol Ther 1993; 54:311–316.
80. Li JT, Hou F, Lu H, Li TY, Li H. Phase I clinical trial of cefditoren pivoxil (ME 1207): pharmacokinetics in healthy volunteers. Drugs Exp Clin Res 1997; 23(5–6):145–150.
81. Felmingham D, Robbins MJ, Ghosh G, Bhogal H, Mehta MD, Leakey A, Clark S, Dencer CA, Ridgway GL, Gruneberg RN. An in vitro characterization of cefditoren, a new oral cephalosporin. Drugs Exp Clin Res 1994; 20(4):127–147.
82. Pickup ME, Bird HA, Lowe JR, Lees L, Wright W. A pharmacokinetic and tolerance study of Ro 13-9904, a new cephalosporin antibiotic. Br J Clin Pharmacol 1981; 12:111–115.
83. Product Information: Rocephin(R), ceftriaxone. Roche Laboratories, Nutley, NJ, 2000.
84. Product Information: Claforan(R), cefotaxime. Hoechst-Roussel Pharmaceuticals, Kansas City, MO, 2000.
85. Patel KB, Nicolau DP, Nightingale CH, et al. Pharmacokinetics of cefotaxime in healthy volunteers and patients. Diagn Microbiol Infect Dis 1995; 22:49–55.

8

Treatment of Community-Acquired Respiratory Tract Infections with Other Antibiotics

William A. Craig and David R. Andes
University of Wisconsin
Madison, Wisconsin, U.S.A.

Besides the β-lactams, macrolides, and fluoroquinolones, a variety of drugs have been used to treat community-acquired pulmonary infections: the tetracyclines (primarily doxycycline), clindamycin, trimethoprim-sulfamethoxazole, vancomycin, and linezolid. The appearance of strains of *Streptococcus pneumoniae* resistant to some of these drugs has limited their current use in upper respiratory tract infections, acute exacerbations of chronic bronchitis, and community-acquired pneumonia [1]. Others such as vancomycin have been used primarily in hospitalized patients with severe pneumococcal pneumonia. The optimal dosing of these drugs for respiratory infections is dependent on the drug's pharmacokinetics and pharmacodynamics (PK/PD) against the infecting pathogens. For upper respiratory tract infections such as sinusitis and otitis media, concentrations in serum are often predictive of efficacy [2]. However, for pulmonary infections, there is increasing evidence that the concentrations in lung secretions, such as epithelial lining fluid (ELF), are very important for determining the outcome of treatment. This chapter will review the current available data on the activity of these drugs against respiratory pathogens and their distribution in respiratory tissues.

TETRACYCLINES

The tetracyclines have been used for respiratory tract infections for many years. Doxycycline is the primary tetracycline derivative used for community-acquired pneumonia. It is recommended by the American and Canadian Thoracic Societies, the Infectious Diseases Society of America (IDSA), and the Canadian Infectious Disease Society as an alternative to macrolides for mild to moderate disease in patients treated as outpatients [3–5]. It has also been shown to be effective in hospitalized patients with community-acquired pneumonia [6]. However, the increasing appearance of tetracycline-resistant *S. pneumoniae* has called into question the empiric use of doxycyline in community-acquired pneumonia. The incidence of tetracycline resistance in North America with pneumococci has varied between 12% and 17% in the large surveillance studies [7–9]. However, higher rates of resistance have been reported in Asia, Europe, Latin America, and some locations in the United States [8–10]. However, doxycycline is more potent than tetracycline, and lower resistance rates have been observed when doxycycline susceptibility is determined. For example, Shea and Cunha [11] observed 20% resistance to tetracycline but only 5% resistance to doxycycline in a survey of drug susceptibility for 256 strains of *S. pneumoniae*. Doxycyline has maintained good activity against *Haemophilus influenzae* and *Moraxella catarrhalis*. MICs are usually less than 2 μg/mL for both organisms. The drug also has excellent activity against the common atypical pathogens.

The pharmacodynamics of doxycycline against strains of *S. pneumoniae* with varying MICs has recently been evaluated in the neutropenic murine thigh-infection model [12,13]. The drug does not exhibit concentration-dependent killing, but it does produce prolonged postantibiotic effects (PAEs). The 24-hr AUC/MIC ratio is the important PK/PD parameter determining efficacy of doxycyline [12]. More limited studies have demonstrated similar findings with minocycline [14]. The magnitude of the 24-hr AUC/MIC required for a bacteriostatic effect varies from 12 to 55 with a mean of 25 when free drug is used for calculation of the AUC [13]. This magnitude or target is very similar to the 24-hr AUC/MIC of free drug required for efficacy of various macrolides [15]. The presence of neutrophils in the mouse model enhances the activity of doxycycline approximately two- to three-fold [16]. If one translates the data from the mouse model to the pharmacokinetics of doxycyline in humans, dosing regimens of 100 mg twice daily would provide therapeutic free drug concentrations in plasma for organisms with MICs up to 2 μg/mL. However, there are few if any clinical data with tetracycline-resistant strains of *S. pneumoniae* to determine if organisms with MICs above 2 μg/mL have a high failure rate in patients with community-acquired pneumonia.

The concentrations of doxycycline in respiratory secretions are generally reported to be lower than in either serum or plasma. For example, sputum, middle ear fluid, and sinus fluid concentrations of doxycycline are usually 17–57% of serum values [17–19]. Although ELF levels of doxycyline have not been reported, bronchial secretions of minocycline are 3 to 5 times higher than in serum [18]. One would expect the concentrations of doxycycline in bronchial secretions to be of similar magnitude. High concentrations in respiratory secretions might increase the efficacy of empiric doxycycline therapy even when some resistant strains are present. High penetration of macrolides into respiratory secretions has been used as an explanation for the small number of clinical failures despite high levels of resistance in microbiology surveys [20]. Moderately large clinical trials with doxycycline have shown equivalent efficacy to macrolides and fluoroquinolones [21–23]. However, the drug's efficacy against tetracycline-resistant strains in not known.

CLINDAMYCIN

Clindamycin has been used more for the therapy of aspiration pneumonia and lung abscesses than for treatment of community-acquired pneumonia. It has also occasionally been used for pneumococcal otitis media. Clindamycin is active against many pneumococci, but its activity against *H. influenzae*, *M. catarrhalis*, and atypical pathogens is less than that of the tetracyclines and macrolides [9]. In Europe, most macrolide-resistant pneumococci are also resistant to clindamycin [8,9]. This is because macrolide resistance in Europe is due primarily to the presence of *Erm* genes and the methylation of the 23s ribosome. In North America, 70–80% of macrolide-resistant *S. pneumoniae* are susceptible to clindamycin. Drug efflux due to the presence of *Mef* genes is the primary mechanism of macrolide resistance in North America, and clindamycin is not a substrate for the efflux pump.

The penetration of clindamycin into bronchial secretions is only about 60% of drug concentrations in serum [17,19]. The amount or AUC of clindamycin distributing into pleural fluid is also similar to values observed in serum [19,24]. However, the peak levels in pleural fluid are lower than in serum, whereas the trough levels are higher in pleural fluid than in serum. One would also expect the concentrations of clindamycin in middle ear fluid to be similar to that in serum. Initial studies on the pharmacodynamics of clindamycin in the neutropenic murine thigh-infection model suggested that the important PK/PD parameter was time above MIC [25]. On the other hand, recent studies with multiple isolates of *S. pneumoniae* suggest that the 24-hr AUC/MIC is the major determinant of in vivo efficacy [26]. The magnitude of the 24-hr AUC/MIC using free drug required for a bacteriostatic effect ranged from 16 to 30. The presence of neutrophils reduced the target requirement at least four-fold [16]. Based on human drug concentrations and protein binding of 78%, a dose of 300 mg 3 times a day would provide a 24-hr AUC/MIC that would exceed the target value generated in animal models for organisms with MICs of 0.5 μg/mL or less. Thus, this dose should be very effective for susceptible *S. pneumoniae* for which the MICs are usually 0.25 μg/mL or less [9]. Trials of clindamycin in pneumococcal pneumonia have validated the high efficacy of the drug for this infection [27].

TRIMETHOPRIM-SULFAMETHOXAZOLE

Trimethoprim-sulfamethoxazole has been one of the major drugs for treatment of exacerbations of chronic bronchitis. In the pediatric age group, it has also been a commonly used drug for treatment of otitis media and community-acquired pneumonia. However, resistance rates to trimethoprim-sulfamethoxazole of *S. pneumoniae* have been significantly increasing over the past decade. In the large surveillance studies, trimethoprim-sulfamethoxazole resistance in North America for *S. pneumoniae* has ranged from 20% to 38% [8,9]. Resistance has been higher in Asia and Latin America [8]. Trimethoprim-sulfamethoxazole resistance has also been observed for *H. influenzae* at a frequency of 14–18% in most areas, but 31% in Latin America [9].

Trimethoprim penetrates better into respiratory secretions than sulfamethoxazole. Concentrations in sputum, middle ear fluid, and sinus fluid are about 119–173% of serum for trimethoprim and only 20–27% of serum for sulfamethoxazole [18,19]. Trimethoprim concentrations in bronchial secretions are 4 to 10 times those in serum [28]. Sulfamethoxazole exhibits concentrations in bronchial secretions that are 60–100% of those in serum. Very little is known about the pharmacodynamics of trimethoprim-sulfamethoxazole. The drug exhibits concentration-independent or time-dependent killing and produces moderate to prolonged postantibiotic effects [29]. Thus, one would predict that 24-hr AUC/MIC would be the important PK/PD parameter determining efficacy. However, there are no animal or human studies specifically designed to characterize the pharmacodynamics of this drug combination. Nevertheless, eradication rates in otitis media and sinusitis due to *S. pneumoniae* and *H. influenzae* using a double-tap methodology were very high (88–100%) for susceptible strains and very low (27–50%) for resistant strains [30,31].

Clinical trials in developing countries with trimethoprim-sulfamethoxazole for community-acquired pneumonia in children have demonstrated the drug's equivalent efficacy to penicillin, ampicillin, and chloramphenicol

[32,33]. In one clinical trial in Pakistan, trimethoprim-sulfamethoxazole was less effective than amoxicillin in severe pneumonia [34]. However, there was no correlation of outcome with the presence or absence of trimethoprim-sulfamethoxazole resistance in *S. pneumoniae*. It is possible that the high respiratory tract concentrations of trimethoprim maintained some efficacy even in the presence of resistant strains.

VANCOMYCIN

Vancomycin is used primarily in severe community-acquired pneumonia, often with other agents. The drug is added to ensure effective therapy even against multiple drug-resistant *S. pneumoniae*. Such strains are still 100% susceptible to vancomycin at concentrations of 0.5 μg/mL or less. Vancomycin is not active against *H. influenzae*, *M. catarrhalis*, and atypical pathogens.

Vancomycin is a very water-soluble drug and penetrates poorly into respiratory secretions. Mean epithelial lining fluid concentrations have ranged from 10% to 18% of serum concentrations [35,36]. Penetration was higher in patients with lung inflammation (25%) than in patients without inflammation (14%) [36]. Thus, one needs vancomycin serum concentrations of 15–20 μg/mL to ensure ELF levels of 2 μg/mL.

A variety of pharmacodynamic studies have been performed with vancomycin. In a murine peritoneal infection with *S. pneumoniae*, the peak level and AUC were both important for efficacy [37]. Studies in the murine thigh-infection model found that the AUC was the major determinant of in vivo efficacy [25]. The magnitude of the peak/MIC and the 24-hr AUC/MIC required for efficacy were 5.7 and 6.4 for free drug, respectively [37]. However, Moise et al. [38] found in patients with ventilator-acquired pneumonia due to *S. aureus* that the 24-hr AUC/MIC required for clinical and bacteriologic cure was 345 and 850, respectively. These higher 24-hr AUC/MIC targets in the pneumonia model are likely due to both the protein binding of vancomycin and its poor penetration into respiratory secretions. Because the MICs for vancomycin against *S. pneumoniae* are about four-fold lower than for *S. aureus*, current dosages of 1 g twice daily should provide adequate concentrations in ELF for most strains. On the other hand, *S. aureus* infections will likely require higher concentrations to ensure that concentrations above the MIC are maintained in ELF. Continuous infusion of vancomycin has been recommended to maintain constantly adequate concentrations of vancomycin in ELF for most strains of *S. aureus*.

LINEZOLID

Linezolid is the first oxazolidinone approved for treatment of community-acquired pneumonia [39,40]. The drug is active against *S. pneumoniae*, *H.*

influenazae, *M. catarrhalis*, and atypical pathogens. Linezolid is also active against penicillin-, macrolide, and quinolone-resistant strains of *S. pneumoniae*. The drug has excellent bioavailability and is available for both oral and intravenous administration. However, the cost of the drug precludes its routine use in community-acquired pneumonia.

Linezolid differs from vancomycin in that the drug has enhanced penetration into respiratory secretions. Epithelial lining fluid concentrations are about three-fold higher than simultaneous concentrations in serum [41]. The pharmacodynamics of linezolid against *S. pneumoniae* and *S. aureus* has been studied in the murine thigh-infection model [42]. The 24-hr AUC/MIC is the PK/PD parameter determining efficacy of the drug. The magnitude or target required for efficacy ranged from 22 to 97 for multiple strains of both organisms. A dose of linezolid at 600 mg b.i.d. would provide a 24-hr AUC/MIC value in serum of 120 for organisms with MICs of 1 μg/mL. Because ELF concentrations are significantly higher, linezolid should be very effective for treatment of *S. pneumoniae* and *S. aureus* pulmonary infections.

Clinical trials of linezolid have demonstrated superior activity to ceftriaxone in pneumococcal pneumonia with bacteremia and superior activity to vancomycin for MRSA in ventilator-acquired pneumonia [40,43]. The drug has also been effective in eradicating penicillin-resistant pneumococci from the middle ears of gerbils and chinchilla [44,45]. However, linezolid was not effective in eradication of *H. influenzae* [45].

REFERENCES

1. File TM. Appropriate use of antimicrobials for drug-resistant pneumonia: focus on the significance of beta-lactam resistant *Streptococcus pneumoniae*. Clin Infect Dis 2002; 34(suppl 1):17–26.
2. Craig WA, Andes D. Pharmacokinetics and pharmacodynamics of antibiotics in otitis media. Pediatr Infect Dis J 1996; 115:255–259.
3. Bartlett JG, Dowell SF, Mandell LA, File TM Jr, Musher DM, Fine MJ. Practice guidelines for the management of community acquired pneumonia in adults. Infectious Diseases Society of America. Clin Infect Dis 2000; 31:347–382.
4. Mandell LA, Marrie TJ, Grossman RF, Chow AW, Hyland RH. Summary of Canadian guidelines for the initial management of community acquired pneumonia: an evidence based update by the Canadian Infectious Disease Society and the Canadian Thoracic Society. Can Respir J 2000; 7:371–382.
5. Niederman MS, Mandell LA, Anzueto A, Bass JB, Broughton WA, Campbell GD, Dean N, File T, Fine MJ, Gross PA, Martinez F, Marrie TJ, Plouffe JF, Ramirez J, Sarosi GA, Torres A, Wilson R, Yu VL. Guidelines for the management of adults with community acquired pneumonia. Diagnosis, assessment of severity, antimicrobial therapy, and prevention. Am J Respir Crit Care Med 2001; 163:1730–1754.

6. Ailani RK, Agastya G, Ailani RK, Mukunda BN, Shekar R. Doxycycline is a cost effective therapy for hospitalized patients with community acquired pneumonia. Arch Intern Med 1999; 159:266–270.
7. Doern GV, Heilmann KP, Huynh HK, Rhomberg PR, Coffman SL, Brueggemann AB. Antimicrobial resistance among clinical isolates of *Streptococcus pneumoniae* in the United States during the 1999–2000, including a comparison of resistance rates since 1994–1995. Antimicrob Agents Chemother 2001; 45:1721–1729.
8. Felmingham D, Reinert RR, Hirakata Y, Rodloff A. Increasing prevalence of antimicrobial resistance among isolates of *Streptococcus pneumoniae* from the PROTEKT surveillance study, and comparative in vitro activity of the ketolide, telithromycin. J Antimicrob Chemother 2002; 50(suppl 1):25–37.
9. Hoban DJ, Doern GV, Fluit AC, Roussel-Delvallez M, Jones RN. Worldwide prevalence of antimicrobial resistance in *Streptococcus pneumoniae*, *Haemophilus influenzae*, and *Moraxella catarrhalis* in the SENTRY antimicrobial surveillance program, 1997–1999. Clin Infect Dis 2001; 32(suppl 2):81–93.
10. Lederman ER, Gleeson TD, Driscoll T, Wallace MR. Doxycycline sensitivity of *S. pneumoniae* isolates. Clin Infect Dis 2003; 36:1091.
11. Shea KW, Cunha BA. Doxycycline activity against *Streptococcus pneumoniae*. Chest 1995; 108:1775–1776.
12. Christianson J, Andes D, Craig WA. Characterization of the pharmacodynamics of doxycycline against *Streptococcus pneumoniae* in a murine thigh-infection model. 41th Interscience Conference on Antimicrobial Agents and Chemotherapy, American Society for Microbiology, 2001.
13. Christianson J, Andes D, Craig WA. Magnitude of the 24-hr AUC/MIC required for efficacy of doxycycline against *Streptococcus pneumoniae* in a murine thigh infection model. 39th Annual Meeting of the Infectious Diseases Society of America, IDSA, 2001.
14. van Ogtrop ML, Andes D, Stamstad TJ, Conklin B, Weiss WJ, Craig WA, Vesga O. In-vivo pharmacodynamic activity of two glycylcyclines (GAR-936 and WAY 152,288) against various gram-positive and gram-negative bacteria. Antimicrob Agents Chemother 2000; 44:943–949.
15. Craig W, Kiem S, Andes D. Free drug 24-hr AUC/MIC is the PK/PD target that correlates with in vivo efficacy of macrolides, azalides, ketolides and clindamycin. 42nd Interscience Conference on Antimicrobial Agents and Chemotherapy, American Society for Microbiology, 2002.
16. Christianson J, Andes D, Craig WA. Impact of neutrophils on pharmacodynamic activity of clindamycin and doxycycline against *Streptococcus pneumoniae*. 42nd Interscience Conference on Antimicrobial Agents and Chemotherapy, American Society for Microbiology, 2002.
17. Cunha BA. Antibiotic pharmacokinetic considerations in pulmonary infections. Semin Respir Infect 1991; 6:168–182.
18. Gerding DN, Hughes CE, Bamberger DM, Foxworth J, Larson TA. Extravascular antimicrobial distribution and the respective blood concentrations in humans. In: Lorian VL, ed. Antibiotics in Laboratory Medicine: Williams & Wilkins, 1996:835–599.

19. Hitt JA, Gerding DN. Sputum antimicrobial levels and clinical outcome in bronchitis. Semin Respir Infect 1991; 6:122–128.
20. Rodvold KA, Gotfried MH, Danziger LH, Servi RJ. Intrapulmonary steady-state concentrations of clarithromycin and azithromycin in healthy adult volunteers. Antimicrob Agents Chemother 1997; 41:1399–1402.
21. Biermann C, Loken A, Riise R. Comparison of spiramycin and doxycycline in the treatment of lower respiratory infections in general practice. J Antimicrob Chemother 1988; 22(suppl B):155–158.
22. Harazim H, Wimmer J, Mittermayer HP. An open randomized comparison of ofloxacin and doxycycline in lower respiratory tract infections. Drugs 1987; 34(suppl 1):71–73.
23. Norby SR, the Nordic Atypical Pneumonia Study Group. Atypical pneumonia in the Nordic countries: aetiology and clinical results of a trial comparing fleroxacin and doxycycline. J Antimicrob Chemother 1997; 39:499–508.
24. Teixeira LR, Sasse SA, Villarino MA, Nguyen T, Mulligan ME, Light RW. Antibiotic levels in empyemic pleural fluid. Chest 2000; 117:1734–1739.
25. Craig WA. Pharmacokinetic/pharmacodynamic parameters: rationale for antibacterial dosing of mice and men. Clin Infect Dis 1998; 26:1–12.
26. Christianson J, Andes D, Craig WA. Characterization of the pharmacodynamics of clindamycin against *Streptococcus pneumoniae* in a murine thigh-infection model. 41th Interscience Conference on Antimicrobial Agents and Chemotherapy, American Society for Microbiology, 2001.
27. Schreiner A. Use of clindamycin in lower respiratory tract infections. Scand J Infect Dis 1984; 43:56–61.
28. Dubar V, Lopez I, Gosset P, Aerts C, Voisin C, Wallaert B. The penetration of co-trimoxazole into alveolar macrophages and its effect on inflammatory and immunoregulatory functions. J Antimicrob Chemother 1990; 26:791–802.
29. Gudmundsson S, Craig WA. Postantibiotic effect. In: Lorian VL, ed. Antibiotics in Laboratory Medicine: Williams & Wilkins, 835–899.
30. Harmory BH, Sande MA, Sydnor A, Seale DL, Gwaltney JM. Etiology and antimicrobial therapy of acute maxillary sinusitis. J Infect Dis 1979; 139:197–202.
31. Leiberman A, Leibovitz E, Piglansky L, Raiz S, Press J, Yagupsky P, Dagan R. Bacteriologic and clinical efficacy of trimethoprim-sulfamethoxazole for treatment of acute otitis media. Pediatr Infect Dis J 2001; 20:260–264.
32. Campbell H, Byass P, Forgie IM, O'Neill KP, Lloyd-Evans N, Greenwood BM. Trial of co-trimoxazole versus procaine penicillin with ampicillin in treatment of community acquired pneumonia in young Gambian children. Lancet 1988; 8621:1182–1184.
33. Mulholland EK, Falade AG, Corrah PT, Omosigho C, N'Jai P, Giadom B, Adegbola RA, Tschappeler H, Todd J, Greenwood BM. A randomized trial of chloramphenicol vs. trimethoprim-sulfamethoxazole for the treatment of malnourished children with community acquired pneumonia. Pediatr Infect Dis J 1995; 14:959–965.
34. Straus WL, Qazi SA, Kundi Z, Nomani NK, Schwartz B. Antimicrobial re-

sistance and clinical effectiveness of co-trimoxazole versus amoxycillin for pneumonia among children in Pakistan: randomized controlled trial. Pakistan Co-trimoxazole Study Group. Lancet 1998; 352:270–274.

35. Georges H, Leroy O, Alfandari S, Guery B, Roussel-Delvallez M, Dhennain C, Beaucaire G. Pulmonary disposition of vancomycin in critically ill patients. Eur J Clin Microbiol Infect Dis 1997; 16:385–388.
36. Lamer C, de Beco V, Soler P, Calvat S, Fagon JY, Dombret MC, Farinotti R, Chastre J, Gilbert C. Analysis of vancomycin entry into pulmonary lining fluid by bronchoalveolar lavage in critically ill patients. Antimicrob Agents Chemother 1993; 37:281–286.
37. Knudsen JD, Fuursted K, Raber S, Espersen F, Frimodt-Moller N. Pharmacodynamics of glycopeptides in the mouse peritonitis model of *Streptococcus pneumoniae* or *Staphylococcus aureus* infection. Antimicrob Agents Chemother 2000; 44:1247–1254.
38. Moise PA, Forrest A, Bhavnani SM, Birmingham MC, Schentag JJ. Area under the inhibitory curve and a pneumonia scoring systemic for predicting outcomes of vancomycin therapy for respiratory infections by *Staphylococcus aureus*. Am J Health Syst Pharm 2000; 57(suppl 2):4–9.
39. Kaplan SL, Patterson L, Edwards KM, Azimi PH, Bradley JS, Blumer JL, Tan TQ, Lobeck FG, Anderson DC. Linezolid Pediatric Pneumonia Study Group. Linezolid for the treatment of community acquired pneumonia in hospitalized children. Pediatr Infect Dis J 2001; 20:488–494.
40. San Pedro GS, Cammarata SK, Oliphant TH, Todisco T, the Linezolid Community Acquired Pneumonia Study Group. Linezolid versus ceftriaxone/cefpodoxime in patients hospitalized for the treatment of *Streptococcus pneumoniae* pneumonia. Scand J Infect Dis 2002; 34:720–728.
41. Conte JE, Golden JA, Kipps J, Zurlinden E. Intrapulmonary pharmacokinetics of linezolid. Antimicrob Agents Chemother 2002; 46:1475–1480.
42. Andes D, Peng J, Craig WA. In-vivo characterization of the pharmacodynamics of a new oxazolidinone (linezolid). Antimicrob Agents Chemother 2002; 46:3484–3489.
43. Wunderink R, Cammarata SK, Croos-Darbera RV, Kollef M. Linezolid vs vancomycin: predictors of outcome in methicillin-resistant *Staphylococcus aureus* nosocomial pneumonia. 40th Infectious Diseases Society of America, 2002.
44. Humphrey WR, Shattuck MH, Zielinski RJ, Kuo MS, Biermacher JJ, Smith DP, Jensen JL, Schaadt RD, Zurenko GE, Richards IM. Pharmacokinetics and efficacy of linezolid in a gerbil model of *Streptococcus pneumoniae* induced acute otitis media. Antimicrob Agents Chemother 2003; 47:1355–1363.
45. Pelton SI, Figueira M, Albut R, Stalker D. Efficacy of linezolid in experimental otitis media. Antimicrob Agents Chemother 2000; 44:654–657.

9

Acute Community-Acquired Rhinosinusitis

James A. Hadley
University of Rochester Medical Center
Rochester, New York, U.S.A.

INTRODUCTION

Acute and chronic rhinosinusitis represent some of the most prevalent disorders encountered by physicians in ambulatory care environments and are among the most common diagnoses for which antibiotics are prescribed [1,2]. The high prevalence of this disease accounts for a large contribution of health-care resource consumption and costs, and yet the incidence of this disorder seems to be increasing [3,4]. Because the etiology and pathophysiology remain obscure, rhinosinusitis poses a considerable challenge for physicians in the overall management of the problem.

Sinus disease remains one of the most common reasons for antimicrobial prescriptions in the United States. Data from the National Ambulatory Medical Care Survey [5] show that sinusitis is the fifth most common diagnosis for which antibiotics are prescribed. Health-care expenditures attributable to a primary diagnosis of acute or chronic rhinosinusitis were estimated to be $3.39 billion in 1996.

Treatment has traditionally been based on empiric data aimed at the most common pathogens (i.e., *Streptococcus pneumoniae*, *Haemophilus influenzae*, and *Moraxella catarrhalis*), and prescriptions for broad-spectrum antimicrobials have generally been utilized [6]. Due to prior overuse of these agents, the development of resistant bacteria has become a problem. *Streptococcus pneumoniae* remains the most important pathogen, and it has steadily acquired resistance to a majority of the currently available antibacterial agents.

Although the majority of these infections are mild and are community acquired during the respiratory season, they often lead to significant morbidity and loss of productivity in school or work environments. The disruption of the patient's quality of life from the symptoms leads these patients to seek early medical management. In addition, this health-care problem has been increasing in incidence and consequently poses a major economic burden.

Rhinosinusitis is a complex disease and the management of the disorder is controversial. Even though the majority of these infections begin as viral upper respiratory diseases, patients demand antimicrobial therapy for fear of developing the more serious complications of this disorder. Antibiotic therapy is most often administered empirically without factual knowledge of the type of pathogen potentially causing the infection. Injudicious usage and indiscriminate prescription of antibiotics has fostered the rapid development of antibiotic-resistant organisms over the past two decades. Appropriate medical management of this common problem requires a systemic approach to the diagnosis, reasonable and swift management, and the considerations of adjunctive medical therapy.

Definition of rhinosinusitis: Acute community-acquired rhinosinusitis is most often preceded by a common viral upper respiratory tract infection. Common cold symptoms are characterized by sneezing, rhinorrhea, nasal congestion, facial pressure, postnasal drip, cough, sore throat, fever, and myalgia. Bacterial superinfection may occur at any time during the course of this viral infection. The term sinusitis is used to describe any inflammatory response involving the sinus cavities with resultant clinical symptoms. In 1996, the American Academy of Otolaryngology–Head and Neck Surgery (AAO-HNS) Task Force for Rhinosinusitis developed working definitions of this disorder in order for health-care providers to communicate appropriately regarding this disease [7].

The term rhinosinusitis was found to be more appropriate than sinusitis alone because the mucous membranes of the nasal passages and paranasal sinuses are contiguous and are histologically identical, and infection or inflammation of the sinus cavities is commonly preceded by rhinitis [7]. Infection of the sinus cavities alone is rare. Rhinosinusitis, then, can be clinically defined as an inflammatory response involving the mucous membranes of the nasal cavity and paranasal sinuses, the fluids within these cavities, and the underlying bone.

Acute community-acquired bacterial rhinosinusitis (ABRS) is an inflammatory event that is the result of bacterial infection within the sinus cavities and commonly follows an acute upper respiratory viral episode. Recent guidelines for the medical management of this disorder have been established by the Sinus and Allergy Health Partnership [1]. Because of the high rates of respiratory infections and bacterial resistance, this group established bacterial efficacy rates and used mathematic modeling to develop a rational algorithm for the treatment of this very common disorder.

Chronic rhinosinusitis (CRS) remains poorly defined. Although many articles describe therapeutic measures for CRS, there are no established characteristics of the symptoms of this entity [8]. In fact, the Federal Drug Administration does not consider this diagnosis when planning medication trials. CRS has been characterized as an inflammation and infection of the sinus cavities, which is defined by the length of time of the patient's symptoms (longer than 3 months). Still, the pathophysiology and pathology of CRS remain somewhat indeterminate.

EPIDEMIOLOGY

According to national governmental statistics, 32 million persons were told they had sinusitis in 1997 [4], and 16.3% of the United States population over the age of 18 had sinusitis. These rates were highest among women and people living in the South. The number of physician visits annually reached 11.7 million for this diagnosis in the year 2000. Hospital outpatient visits totaled 1.2 million in the same year [9].

The development of acute community-acquired rhinosinusitis is related to a series of environmental and host factors [7]. These are listed in Table 1. Not all patients present with a similar cause, and a variety of factors may coexist in any given patient. There are many risk factors, and these may be associated with viral infections, distorted nasal and sinus anatomy, and allergic and nonallergic rhinitis.

In essence, there are multiple and various causes of rhinosinusitis, and many different factors may be present, which makes it difficult to determine the precise cause in any given patient. Host factors, genetic predisposition, cystic fibrosis, allergic/immune conditions, anatomic abnormalities, endocrine and metabolic disorders, environmental causes, infectious/viral agents, chemicals, medications, and surgery or trauma are all included in the etiology.

ETIOLOGY

In the United States, adults will experience an average of two to three, and children will experience six to eight, viral respiratory illnesses annually [9].

TABLE 1 Multifactorial Causes of Rhinosinusitis

Environmental factors
Infectious/viral agents
Trauma
Noxious chemicals (occupational exposure)
Iatrogenic
Medications
Surgery
Host Factors
Genetic/congential conditions
Cystic fibrosis
Immotile cilia syndrome
Allergic/immune conditions
Anatomic abnormalities
Systemic diseases
Endocrine
Metabolic
Neuromechanisms
Neoplasm

Source: Ref. 7.

Viral rhinosinusitis for the most part is self-limiting, and symptoms normally improve within 5–7 days. Secondary bacterial infection may occur at any time throughout the course of a viral infection and may complicate approximately 2% of cases of viral rhinosinusitis.

Community-acquired acute rhinosinusitis, then, is the development of a bacterial infection that follows inflammation of a viral episode, the sinus cavities being colonized with bacterial pathogens common to the community.

Studies involving direct cultures of the maxillary antrum during both acute and chronic infections demonstrate the typical bacterial responsible for the infections. Maxillary sinus aspirations performed under controlled circumstances demonstrate contamination by *Streptococcus pneumonia*, *Haemophilus influenzae*, and other bacteria, including *Moraxella catarrhalis*, as the prevalent pathogens in acute bacterial rhinosinusitis. These pathogens have been investigated by many authors [10] (see Table 2). The bacteria responsible for chronic rhinosinusitis are somewhat different; although *Streptococcus pneumonia* remains a pathogen, other bacteria include anaerobic pathogens and *Staphylococcus* species [11–13].

TABLE 2 Common Pathogens in Acute Maxillary Rhinosinusitis

Bacterial species/positive cultures in 383 pretreatment sinus aspirates	
Strep pneumococcus	41%
H. influenzae	35%
Anaerobes	7%
Strep. species	7%
Moraxella catarrhalis	3.5%
Staph. aureus	3.0%
Others	3.5%

Source: Ref. 11.

PATHOGENESIS

The development of acute community-acquired rhinosinusitis involves damage to the integrity of the mucosa and/or ostial obstruction, which then predisposes the paranasal sinuses to infection from bacteria.

Normal Anatomy and Physiology

In order to understand the physiology of infection, it is helpful to review the normal physiology and anatomy of the paranasal sinuses.

The paranasal sinuses represent paired, air-filled cavities in the mid-face that are lined with respiratory mucosa. With the exception of the sphenoid sinus, the paranasal sinuses arise as evaginations from the nasal cavity, developing mostly after birth. The various ostia of the sinuses drain into the nasal cavity and potentially can become obstructed. The maxillary sinus is the largest, and its ostia drains into the lateral nasal wall under the middle nasal turbinate. The ethmoid sinuses are the most complex; they represent a group of small sinus cavities that may vary greatly in number and are believed to represent the origin of the majority of paranasal sinus diseases. The anterior ethmoid sinuses drain into the middle meatus, under the middle turbinate. The posterior ethmoid sinuses usually drain into the spheno-ethmoid recess posteriorly. The frontal sinuses vary greatly in size and are usually only secondarily involved in acute respiratory tract infections. The sinuses drain into the anterior nasal-fronto-ethmoid recess. (See Figs. 1 and 2.)

The mucosa of the nasal cavity and the paranasal sinuses represents a continuum of the mucosa of the respiratory tract. This mucosa is a ciliated, pseudostratified, columnar epithelium, and it also contains mucosal glands

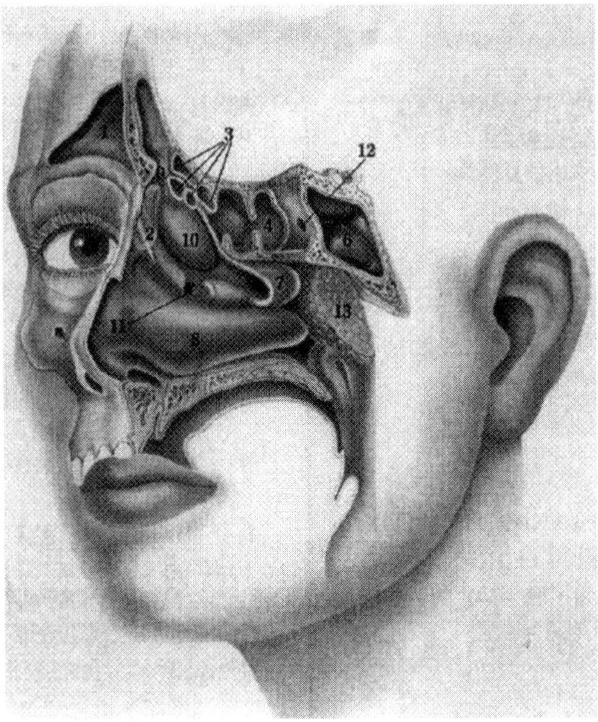

FIGURE 1 Front view of paranasal sinuses demonstrating narrow pathways and relationship of drainage from maxillary sinus into nasal cavity.

and goblet cells. The goblet cells and mucosal glands produce the mucus and serous layers of the mucous blanket that lines this epithelium. The cilia move the mucus gradually to the natural ostia of the paranasal sinus cavities and then into the nasopharynx.

Nasal mucus has numerous functions and represents the means of humidification, warming of air, and filtration of inspired air, the important roles of the nasal cavities. Nasal mucus also is involved in the immune defense of the upper respiratory tract: not only does it contain inflammatory cells, it also provides inflammatory chemical mediators that upregulate and modify the immune response.

The function of the cilia is to gradually sweep the nasal mucus toward the natural sinus ostia. Normal ciliary function results in clearance of the sinus cavities within a short period of time. Normal transport time from the front of the nose to the posterior nasopharynx is approximately 20 min. Cilia stasis may occur or during the acute inflammatory reaction, or may be in-

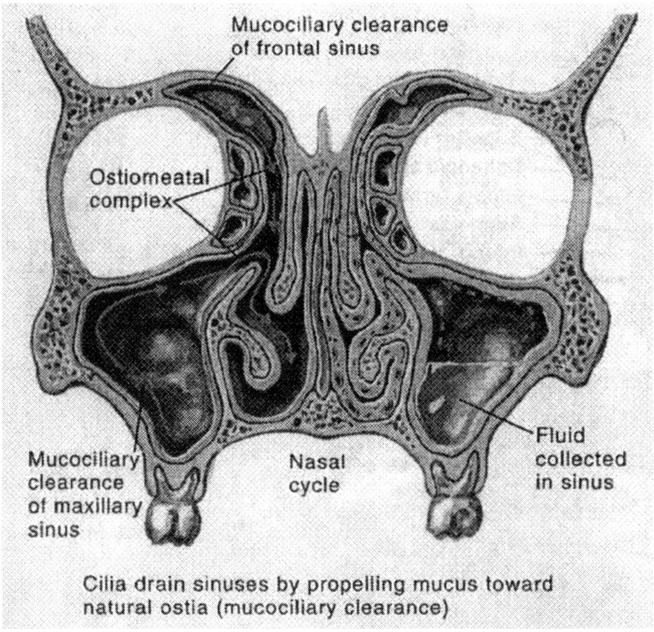

FIGURE 2 Cut view of paranasal sinuses showing normal mucociliary clearance on one side and obstruction secondary to inflammatory blockage on the other side of the paranasal sinuses. It is clear that the narrow drainage pathways lead to a potential for obstruction and stasis of secretions. (Courtesy CIBA-Geigy collection.)

duced by other toxic agents. With a decrease in ciliary function, the normal nasal mucus stagnates and forms a nidus for secondary infection.

Mucous stasis and obstruction of the ostia may allow decreased oxygenation within the paranasal sinus cavities. The lowered oxygen tension favors the development of bacterial secondary infection. Gas exchange within the obstructed sinus cavities is inhibited, and this may favor the growth of bacteria in an anaerobic environment.

With obstruction of the sinus ostia, there is a transient decrease in the pressure within the large sinus cavities. Transudation results from the lowered pressure and may lead to significant edema, bleeding, and sinus pain. The initial decrease in partial pressure within the sinus cavity may be followed by an increase in pressure from the development of the secondary infection causing pressure on the sinus cavity walls. These pressure differentials may explain the facial discomfort experienced by persons who are descending from altitudes or deep sea diving [14].

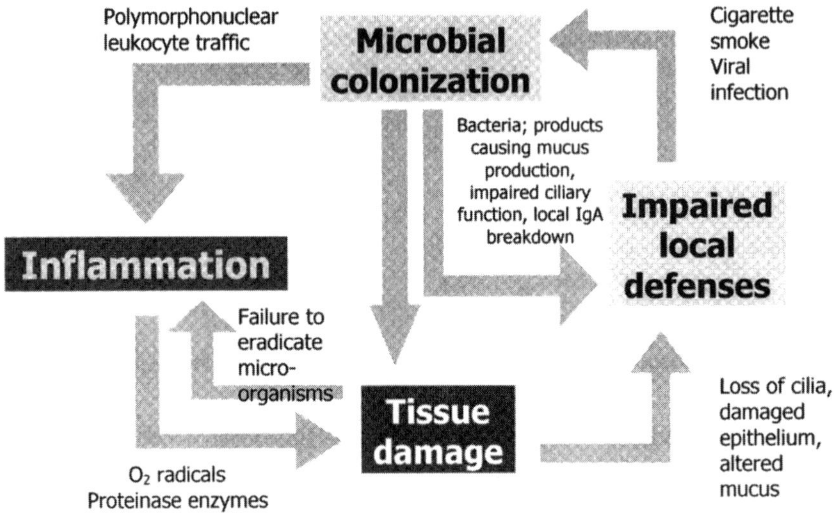

FIGURE 3 Vicious cycle of respiratory infections. (From Ref. 16)

Pathophysiologically, the inflammation from an inciting event causes swelling with the narrow drainage pathways of the sinuses. A partial or total obstruction of the ostia induces stagnation and stasis of the normal mucus, which then serves as a medium for the growth of resident pathogenic bacteria. Inflammatory mediators are liberated and lead to the development of patient symptoms. A vicious cycle may then develop as a result of continued mediator release. (See Fig. 3 [16].)

Antimicrobial therapy is usually indicated to resolve the inflammatory cascade and break this vicious circle. Once appropriate antibiotics and other anti-inflammatory measures are instituted, there is usually complete healing and resolution of symptoms.

CLINICAL MANIFESTATIONS

In clinical practice, the diagnosis of acute community-acquired rhinosinusitis is based on patient symptoms and potential findings on physical examination [15]. Too often, however, the clinical findings are difficult to determine on every presentation, and differentiation from viral rhinosinusitis and bacterial rhinosinusitis is challenging without culture data.

The signs and symptoms, as defined by the Task Force on Rhinosinusitis, include facial pain/pressure, facial congestion/fullness, nasal obstruction, nasal/postnasal discharge, hyposmia/anosmia, fever, halitosis, fatigue, dental pain, cough and otalgia [16].

Acute community-acquired rhinosinusitis typically manifests itself as an upper respiratory tract infection that persists beyond 5–7 days, and the patient has persistent symptoms lasting longer than ten days. A patient's symptoms of nasal congestion and postnasal discharge that last only a few days are more characteristic of a viral disorder, such as a rhinovirus or an adenovirus.

A common misconception is that the presence of discolored nasal secretions predictably indicates a bacterial infection. Patients with viral infections and chronic rhinitis alone may also have discolored nasal discharge, and the diagnostic specificity of discolored nasal discharge was reported to be only 52% [17].

A broad definition of the clinical symptoms incorporates the following (see Table 3):

Percussion of the sinuses in addition to the presence of other factors may also assist the clinician in predicting the presence of an acute infection. Increased maxillary facial pain and pressure while the patient bends the head forward may be another positive sign.

The diagnosis of acute community-acquired rhinosinusitis in children is more difficult. Children experience up to six or more episodes of viral upper respiratory tract infections per year, and these may take longer to resolve. The incidence of viral infections is greater among children attending day-care or school [1]. The symptoms are similar to the adult major and minor factors, but children demonstrate persistent rhinorrhea of a mucopurulent nature and can develop an associated nocturnal cough. Symptoms of rhinosinusitis in

TABLE 3 Clinical Symptoms of Acute Community-Acquired Rhinosinusitis

Major symptoms	Minor symptoms
Facial congestion/fullness	Headache
Nasal discharge/purulence/discolored nasal discharge	Halitosis
Facial pain/pressure[a]	Dental Pain
Nasal obstruction/blockage	Ear pain/fullness/pressure
Hyposmia/anosmia	Fever
Fever (acute rhinosinusitis only)[b]	Fatigue
	Cough (in children)

[a] Facial pain/pressure alone does not constitute a suggestive history of acute rhinosinusitis in the absence of another major sign or symptom.
[b] Fever in acute rhinosinusitis alone does not constitute a suggestive history of acute rhinosinusitis in the absence of another major sign or symptom.
Source: Ref. 7.

children usually consist of a "cold" lasting more than 10 days, sometimes associated with low-grade fever; thick, yellow-green nasal discharge; headache, irritability, or fatigue [18,19]. Foul-smelling nasal discharge and halitosis are common findings with poor resolution despite at-home remedies.

Early recognition and appropriate management are extremely important in prevention of the more serious complications of rhinosinusitis. Sinus infection may potentially spread to the orbit and meninges either by direct extension or by venous thrombophlebitis. Direct and immediate referral to an otolaryngologist in warranted in immunocompromised patients with serious sinus symptoms or impending signs of orbital cellulitis.

Diagnostic Modalities

Physical examination of the patient usually provides little information to assist the clinician in the diagnosis. The clinical diagnosis of acute community-acquired rhinosinusitis is also clouded by the lack of uniformity among physicians in regard to classification of the disease. There are many professionals involved in the diagnosis and management of this disease, including primary care physicians, otolaryngologists, pediatricians, and other specialists.

A number of diagnostic techniques, however, can assist the clinician in determination of the presence of community-acquired rhinosinusitis.

Anterior Rhinoscopy

An evaluation of the anterior nasal chamber, the nasal turbinates, and perchance the middle meatus with either a nasal speculum (see Fig. 4) or an oto-

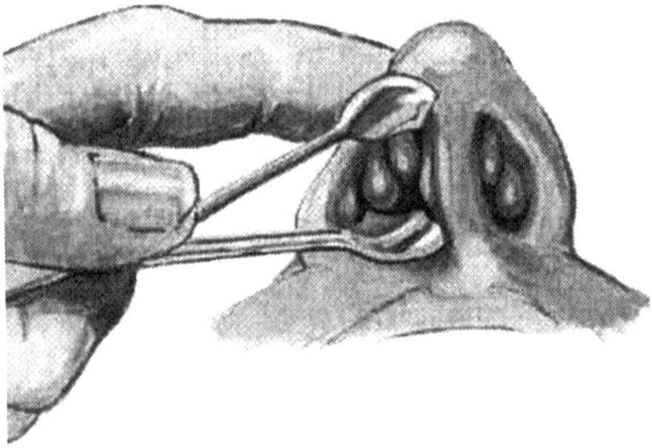

FIGURE 4 View of anterior rhinoscopy with nasal speculum demonstrating relationship of inferior and middle turbinates. (Courtesy R. Netter Collection.)

scope may document turbinate swelling, mucopurulent nasal secretions, and purulence stemming from the sinus drainage pathways. A thorough examination of this area is helpful in determining the presence or absence of clinical disease [15].

Diagnostic nasal endoscopy is the method favored by otolaryngologists in the diagnosis of disorders of the nose and sino-nasal tract and is the primary evaluation strategy for patients with recurrent or chronic symptoms. Nasal endoscopy employs the use of rigid or flexible nasal endoscopes to examine the entire nasal cavity and may allow microbiologic culture [13]. Systemic nasal endoscopy can demonstrate the normal sinus drainage pathways or show aberrant anatomy and active mucopurulent secretions (see Fig. 5). Direct culture of purulent secretions from the area of the middle meatus has been demonstrated to correlate with cultures obtained directly from the maxillary sinuses [20,21].

Transillumination

This technique is no longer utilized widely: it is subject to operator variability and does not differentiate bacterial from viral infection.

Ultrasound

Not widely used, and subject to false-negative results, ultrasonography uses acoustic imaging to detect reflection of sound waves off two media with

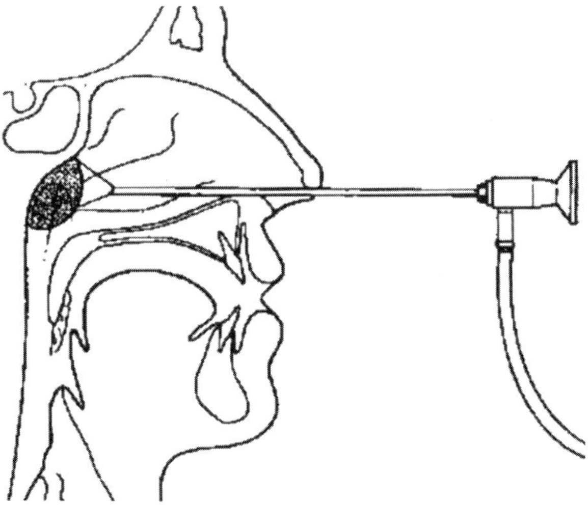

FIGURE 5 View of a nasal endoscope which can visualize the entire nasal cavity.

differing acoustic characteristics. This technique may be used to help follow the course of the disease, especially in frontal or maxillary sinus disease.

Radiography

Plain x-ray evaluation of the sinuses was once the diagnostic procedure of choice but has been recently shown to provide an inaccurate assessment of the extent of sinus inflammation [22]. Air-fluid levels and opacification may enhance the diagnosis of acute rhinosinusitis in the patient with acute symptoms. As an adjunct to diagnosis, plain x-rays are helpful but should not be utilized as the sole criteria for selecting methods of treatment (see Fig. 6).

Computed Tomography (CT)

Considered the gold standard for imaging of paranasal sinuses, CT scans are particularly useful for displaying the extent of the inflammation, which may be missed by nasal endoscopy. This technique is extremely sensitive, but lacks specificity because many viral infections may also produce CT abnormalities [22]. However, recommendations are made to consider CT scans in patients who fail to respond to adequate medical management after appropriate medical therapy. In addition, they are recommended in face of any impending complication of infection of the sinuses (see Fig. 7).

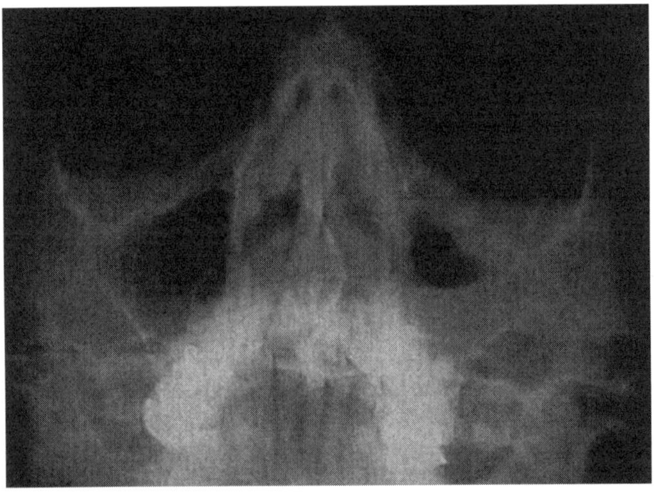

FIGURE 6 Radiograph of Water's view of paranasal sinuses and air-fluid level on left.

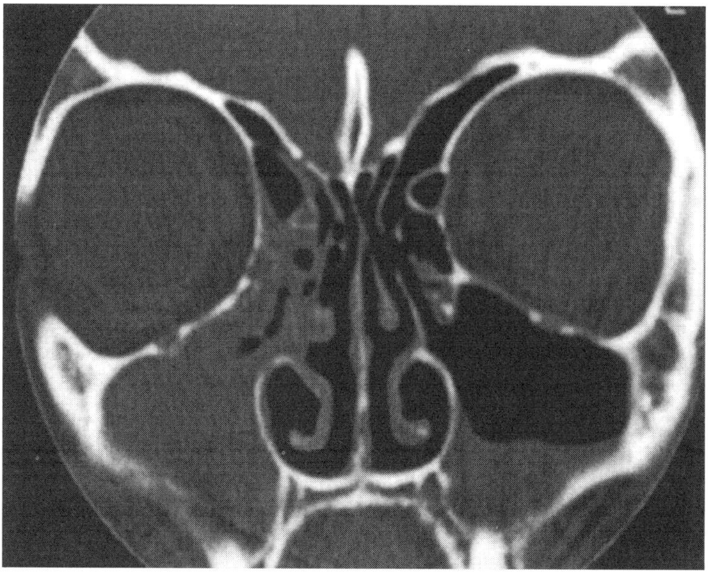

FIGURE 7 CT scan of anterior nasal sinuses which demonstrates opacification of maxillary and partial ethmoid sinuses on the right and air-fluid level on the left.

The use of CT scans in community-acquired rhinosinusitis should be limited.

MRI Scan

The imaging provided by magnetic resonance demonstrates excellent visualization of the soft tissue, but little information regarding the cortical bone. MRI scans are useful for evaluation of regional and intracranial complications of infection prior to surgical and medical management.

Culture Techniques

The routine use of nasal cultures in identifying the cause of bacterial rhinosinusitis has not proved useful, due to lack of reliability. The paranasal sinuses are relatively inaccessible and thus microbiological specimens are difficult to obtain. The maxillary sinus (antral) tap has been the recommended approach, and samples are sent for culture for both aerobic and anaerobic pathogens (see Fig. 8). Nasal endoscopic cultures, however, have been shown to correlate well with findings on maxillary sinus tap [20,23] (see Fig. 9).

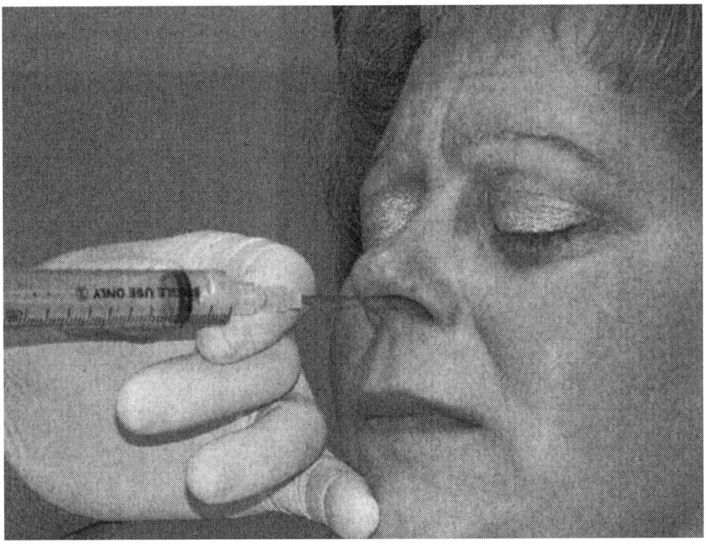

FIGURE 8 Transmaxillary aspiration through the nasal cavity at the level of inferior meatus. This is the "gold-standard" of maxillary sinus culture study.

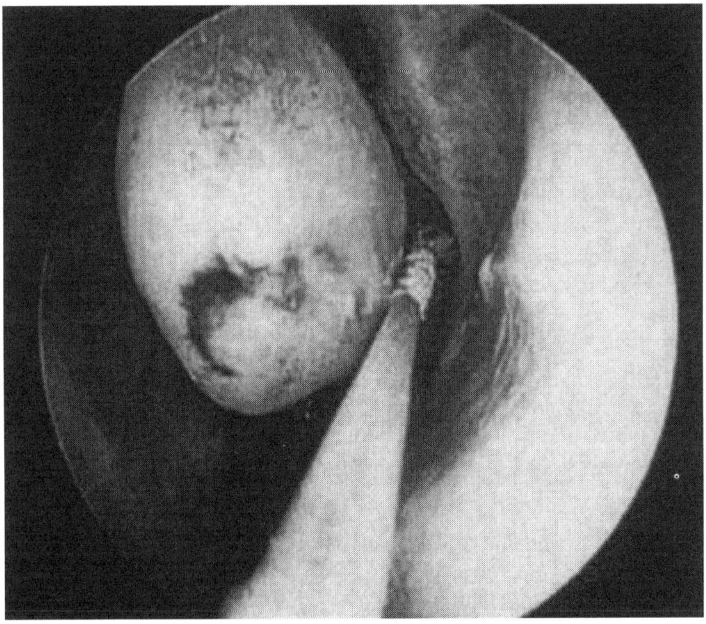

FIGURE 9 Nasal endoscopic view of swab taking a culture through the nose at the level of the maxillary sinus drainage pathway.

Temporal Aspects of Rhinosinusitis

The typical progression of acute community acquired rhinosinusitis may proceed along one of four scenarios: complete resolution without aftereffects, development of adverse sequelae, transition to symptomatic chronic rhinosinusitis, or development of silent chronic rhinosinusitis.

In order to facilitate the diagnosis and treatment of acute community acquired rhinosinusitis, definitions based on the temporal nature of the disease were developed and subsequently adopted by the Agency for Healthcare Research and Quality [16,24] (see Table 4).

Acute Adult Rhinosinusitis

This is the most common presentation and is usually characterized by the worsening of symptoms after 5–7 days and then persistence of major or minor factors for at least 10 days. The symptoms resolve completely after 4 weeks. Common denominators of the positive history include facial pain, pressure, and purulent nasal discharge that persist after a common viral episode.

Subacute Adult Rhinosinusitis

The continuum of symptoms, or the progression of symptoms after 4 weeks and lasting up to 12 weeks, defines this form of rhinosinusitis. Patients may not have been managed appropriately during the acute stage, or the symptoms may have been not severe enough to warrant antimicrobial therapy. This stage usually resolves completely after effective medical management.

Recurrent Acute Adult Rhinosinusitis

The symptoms are the same as those of adult rhinosinusitis, but the patient may experience up to four episodes in a year. The symptoms usually completely resolve between episodes. Antimicrobial therapy is not generally required during the interim.

TABLE 4 Temporal Aspects of Rhinosinusitis

Acute Lasts up to 4 weeks, with total resolution of symptoms
Nasal discharge/purulence/discolored postnasal drainage
Subacute Lasts longer than 4 weeks but less than 12 weeks
Recurrent Acute 4 or more episodes per year, with resolution in between attacks
Chronic 12 weeks or more of signs/symptoms

Source: Ref. 7.

Chronic Adult Rhinosinusitis

Chronic rhinosinusitis occurs when symptoms last 12 or more weeks. Patients may experience acute exacerbations with sudden worsening of the baseline symptoms, or the development of new symptoms during this stage.

COMPLICATIONS

Untreated acute community-acquired rhinosinusitis may potentially lead to severe, and perhaps fatal, complications. Rhinosinusitis may spread to important neighboring structures, including the eye, with development of periorbital cellulititis, subperiosteal abscess, orbital cellulititis, or orbital abscess and blindness (see Fig. 10). Severe intracranial complications may occur such as meningitis and brain abscess, primarily from ethmoid and frontal sinus infection. Patients with impending complications require immediate

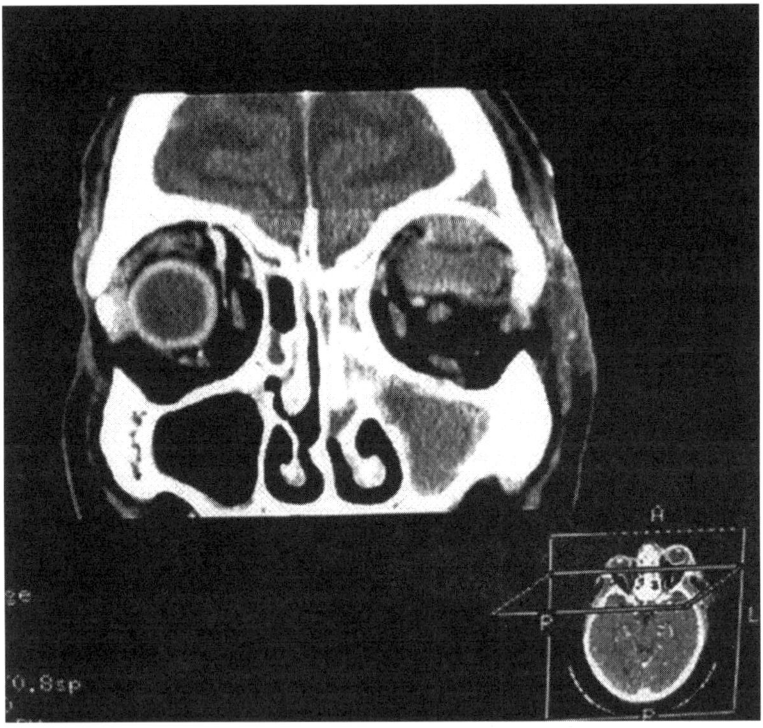

FIGURE 10 CT scan of patient with acute rhinosinusitis on the left which has progressed to involve the orbit and formation of an abscess of the orbit.

treatment and referral to appropriate specialists. Aggressive itravenous antibiotics and hospitalization are required.

Clinical signs of complications include symptoms of sepsis—chills, high fever, severe headache, excessive eyelid swelling, chemosis or proptosis of the eye, or restriction of ocular movement. Affected patients require urgent consultation with an otolaryngologist for appropriate management of their impending complications and potential immediate surgical drainage of the infection.

MANAGEMENT

The main strategy of management of acute community-acquired rhinosinusitis resolves around relief of symptoms and eradication of the underlying cause of the infection. The goals are to reduce the inflammation and tissue swelling, promote sinus drainage and maintain the ostia of the normal sinus drainage pathways. Treatment regimens should interrupt the pathologic vicious circle that can lead to recurrent infection, complications, or development of chronic rhinosinusitis.

Antimicrobial Management

Acute community-acquired rhinosinusitis is managed with antimicrobials directed against the common pathogens involved in the infection. The organisms have changed little over the past 50 or more years. *Streptococcus pneumoniae* and *Haemophilus influenzae* are the predominant pathogens and make up more than 70% of all bacterial species isolated [10,25]. *Moraxella catarrhalis* is another causative pathogen, but its clinical impact remains limited because infection with this pathogen tends to resolve spontaneously.

Bacterial resistance has become a major problem in the treatment of these infections over the past decade. The reader is referred to the other chapters in this book regarding this problem. Suffice it to say that the empiric choice of an antimicrobial is no longer recommended. The clinician needs to recognize the potential for resistant bacteria and choose an appropriate antibiotic that will be effective in killing the responsible pathogen (see Table 5).

The Sinus and Allergy Health Partnership recently developed guidelines as an educational tool for clinicians who are involved in treating patients with acute bacterial rhinosinusitis [1] (see Table 6). The objective was to provide a systematic approach for the diagnosis and management of this disorder.

Antimicrobial selection is now based on consideration of a bacterial efficacy model. The Poole therapeutic model [26] was introduced as a mathematical method for determination of the efficacy of a chosen antimicrobial. Based on patient distribution, pathogen distribution, spontaneous resolution

TABLE 5 Antimicrobials for Rhinosinusitis

Antimicrobial	
Fluoroquinolones (95%)	↑ More effective, More antibiotic use
HD Amoxicillin/clavulanate (94%)	
Amoxicillin/clavulanate (91%)	
HD Amoxicillin (88%)	
Cefpodoxime proxetil (85%)	
Cefdinir (85%)	
Cefixime (83%)	
Cefuroxime axetil (82%)	
TMP/SMX (78%)	
Macrolides (72%)	
Placebo (60%)	↓ Less effective, Less antibiotic use

rate, and the resolution based on current susceptibility data for each organism at pharmacokinetic/pharmacodynamic breakpoints, we can calculate an estimated efficacy for any given antimicrobial therapy. Considerations utilized in the development of the treatment guidelines included patient age, severity of disease, prior use of antibiotics, and the relative rank order of predicted efficacy.

Antimicrobial therapy thus can be placed into a relative rank order of predicted efficacy in adult patients with community-acquired acute bacterial rhinosinusitis. Antimicrobials showing a greater than 90% efficacy include amoxicillin/clavulanate, and the fluoroquinolones. Those showing 80–90% efficacy include high-dose amoxicillin, cefdinir, cefuroxime axetil, and cefpodoxime proxetil. Antibiotics showing 70–80% resolution include clindamycin (based on gram-positive coverage only), cefprozil, azithromycin, clarithromycin, and erythromycin. Based on the fact that the predicted spontaneous resolution rate in untreated adults with acute bacterial rhinosinusitis is 46.6%, recommendations to use other antimicrobials are not justified based on this efficacy data.

Amoxicillin remains effective for penicillin-intermediate and -resistant *Streptococcus pneumoniae* but is less effective against β-lactamase producing organisms. Addition of clavulanic acid with amoxicillin provides coverage against all three important pathogens in acute bacterial rhinosinusitis. Second-generation cephalosporins have adequate activity against penicillin-intermediate *Streptococcus pneumoniae*, *Haemophilus influenza*, and *Moraxella catarrhalis* but have limited activity against penicillin-resistant *Streptococcus pneumoniae*. Trimethoprim/sulfamethoxazole and the macrolides have limited indications in the treatment of acute bacterial rhinosinusitis. Increasing resistance to *Streptococcus pneumoniae* has limited their use for upper respiratory tract infections. Clindamycin remains effective against

TABLE 6 Suggested Antimicrobials for Adult Rhinosinusitis

Severity	Prior antibiotics	Initial therapy	Predicted efficacy (% of patients)	Switch options
Mild	No	Amoxicillin/clavulanate*	93.3	Fluoroquinolone; reevaluate patient
↓	↓	Amoxicillin*	88.8	Amox/clav, fluoroquinolone, cefpodoxime, cefixime
		Cefpodoxime/cefdinir	86.7	Amoxicillin, clindamycin, fluoroquinolone
		Cefuroxime	84.4	Amox/clav, fluoroquinolone, combination
		β-Lactam allergic: TMP/SMX, Doxycycline, Macrolide		Fluoroquinolone, combination
Mild OR	Yes OR	Amoxicillin/clavulanate	93.3	Fluoroquinolone; reevaluate patient
		Amoxicillin	88.8	Amox/clav, fluoroquinolone, cefpodoxime, cefixime
Moderate	No			
↓	↓	Cefpodoxime/cefdinir	86.7	Amoxicillin, clindamycin, fluoroquinolone
		Cefuroxime	84.4	Amox/clav, fluoroquinolone, combination
		β-Lactam allergic: Fluoroquinolone		Reevaluate patient
Moderate	Yes	Fluoroquinolone	95.1	Reevaluate patient
↓	↓	Amoxicillin/clavulanate	94.4	Fluoroquinolone, reevaluate patient
		Combination		Fluoroquinolone, reevaluate patient

gram-positive pathogens and certain anaerobes, but it is ineffective against the majority of gram-negative pathogens.

Ancillary Management

Ancillary therapy should enhance the drainage of the infected sinus cavities and help relieve facial pain, pressure, nasal congestion, postnasal discharge, and the other systemic symptoms.

Nonpharmacologic therapy is indicated for patients with acute community acquired rhinosinusitis as an adjunct to antibiotic management. The adjunctive use of topical nasal saline has been shown to have significant impact in reduction of the tenacity and thickness of the nasal and sinus secretions. In addition, household remedies such as the use of steam-tents may also give patients some relief. Hypertonic saline has been shown to increase mucociliary clearance and ciliary frequency, as well as mucociliary transit times of saccharin [27,28]. The use of hypertonic saline in children was associated with statistically significant improvement in symptoms compared with nasal saline alone.

Adjunctive pharmacologic therapy may include the use of topical nasal decongestants. To avoid rebound rhinitis, it is recommended that the patient use these topical decongestants for less than 5 to 7 days. Antihistamine therapy is not usually recommended, although patients who have a significant history of inhalant upper respiratory allergies may potentially use these medications in a preventive fashion. Mucolytic therapy with the use of guaifenesin has also been shown to give some benefit. Patients may actually feel some relief with a guaifenesin/pseudoephedrine combination product.

Although intranasal steroids are currently not indicated in cases of acute bacterial rhinosinusitis, their theoretic value lies in their ability to decrease inflammation. Topical nasal corticosteroid therapy has been both discouraged and recommended for adjunctive therapy. An investigation of children diagnosed with acute bacterial rhinosinusitis reported improvement in a group that used intranasal budesonide compared with a group receiving oral pseudoephedrine [29]. Topical intranasal steroids have a marked anti-inflammatory action that decreases vascular permeability and inhibits the release of chemical mediators, especially histamine, leukotrienes, and others. They reduce the cellular influx to the inflammatory sites and modify both the early-phase and the late-phase response in inflammatory rhinitis. Topical nasal steroids are advocated for patients with hyperplastic polypoid rhinosinusitis [30]; these drugs reduce polyp inflammation but unfortunately they do not reduce the expression of pro-inflammatory cytokines. Combination therapy with systemic steroids and topical intranasal steroids has a dramatic increase in effect, but unfortunately it does not change the need for consideration of surgical intervention [31].

Oral systemic corticosteroids are extremely effective in reducing the inflammation secondary to rhinosinusitis. They dramatically reduce the edema from increased capillary permeability and reduce the cellular influx. These medications are generally not recommended in cases of acute bacterial rhinosinusitis. The potential risk of development of a more fulminant infection suggests that their use be reserved for more chronic disease states.

Leukotriene receptor antagonists have also been recently advocated for consideration of therapy in patients with rhinosinusitis. These medications are perhaps better suited to patients with the more chronic forms of inflammation rather than patients who have an acute bacterial infection.

Role of Surgery

Surgical intervention for acute bacterial sinus infections generally is reserved for patients with recurrent acute or chronic rhinosinusitis who have not responded to appropriate medical therapy, or in cases where there is a potential for the development of an acute complication. There are more than 150,000 sinus surgeries performed per year in the United States. However, surgery is not recommended for the typical case of acute community-acquired rhinosinusitis.

Most surgical procedures are performed on patients with complications of the disorder or other forms of rhinosinusitis, including extensive nasal polyposis, or chronic rhinosinusitis with persistence of abnormal findings on CT scans.

Endoscopic sinus surgery theoretically aims to restore the natural drainage patterns of the paranasal sinuses, open the blocked ostiomeatal complex, and allow for drainage of the anterior ethmoid cells. This "functional" surgical technique is used to restore the mucociliary clearance and ventilation through the ostia. Computer-assisted sinus surgery now also allows for precise identification of areas within the sinuses and may be useful for

TABLE 7 Absolute Indications for Surgery in Adult Rhinosinusitis

Bilateral extensive and massive obstructive nasal polyposis with complications
Complications of adult rhinosinusitis
Subperiosteal or orbital abscess
Meningitis
Brain abscess
Chronic adult rhinosinusitis with mucocele or mucopyocele formation
Invasive or allergic fungal adult rhinosinusitis
Diagnosis of tumor of nasal cavity and paranasal sinuses
Cerebrospinal fluid rhinorrhea

potential extended applications. Surgical success is defined as the resolution or the improvement of preoperative symptoms with absence of recurrence for 6 or more months.

The absolute indications for surgery for rhinosinusitis are listed in Table 7. Still, there are no real indications for any surgical intervention in uncomplicated cases of acute community-acquired rhinosinusitis [32,33].

The antral sinus tap is the standard of diagnosis of acute maxillary rhinosinusitis, and the adjunctive use of saline irrigation can be of significant benefit to reestablish the clearance of sinus secretions from the obstructed sinus cavity.

PREVENTION

Although it may not be possible to prevent all episodes of acute community-acquired rhinosinusitis, it may be possible to reduce the severity and number of attacks of rhinosinusitis and to prevent the acute form from progressing to a more chronic stage.

The following recommendations can be utilized [34]:

Adequate hydration to ensure fluidity of nasal secretions
Topical intranasal saline mist to moisten nasal mucosa
Humidification of room air, especially in the winter months
Avoidance of chemical irritants such as cigarette smoke or other environmental pollutants
Use of a topical decongestant for a few days at the onset of symptoms
Oral decongestant therapy to shrink swollen nasal mucosa
Avoidance of air travel, or use of topical nasal decongestants to prevent sinus blockage from airplane cabin pressure changes
Increased frequency of hand washing to prevent unknown sources of infection and to reduce contamination from respiratory infections
Investigation of relationship of upper respiratory allergy in persons with suspicion that seasonal or perennial allergens may precipitate infections.
Immunization of patients for viral pathogens with vaccines.

CONCLUSIONS

Acute community-acquired rhinosinusitis plays a major role in overall general health concerns. The frequency of these common upper respiratory tract infections have led to the overprescription of antibiotics to assist in the reduction of patient symptoms despite the fact that the majority of these cases begin as common viral illnesses. The diagnosis of acute bacterial rhinosinusitis should not be made until the symptoms of a viral upper respiratory tract infection last for at least 10 days, or the symptoms worsen after 5 to 7 days. The most common pathogens in this disorder include *Streptococcus pneumoniae*, *Haemophilus influenza*, and *Moraxella catarrhalis*.

The prevalence of antimicrobial resistance, particularly penicillin-resistant *S. pneumoniae* and β-lactamase–producing organisms, constitutes a major concern in the treatment of these upper respiratory tract infections. Appropriate evaluation of the antimicrobials based on antibiotic susceptibility and efficacy offers the clinician an appropriate choice rather than strict empiric therapy in antimicrobial management of these patients. The guidelines developed by the Sinus and Allergy Health Partnership provided significant recommendations for the treatment of ABRS.

REFERENCES

1. Sinus & Allergy Health Partnership. Antimicrobial treatment guidelines for acute bacterial rhinosinusitis. Sinus and Allergy Health Partnership. Otolaryngol Head Neck Surg 2000; 123(1 pt 2):5–31.
2. Gwaltney JM Jr, Jones JG, et al. Medical management of sinusitis: educational goals and management guidelines. The International Conference on Sinus Disease. Ann Otol Rhinol Laryngol Suppl 1995; 167:22–30.
3. Benninger MS, Sedory Holzer SE, et al. Diagnosis and treatment of uncomplicated acute bacterial rhinosinusitis: summary of the Agency for Health Care Policy and Research evidence-based report. Otolaryngol Head Neck Surg 2000; 122(1):1–7.
4. Ray NF, Baraniuk JN, Thamer M, et al. Healthcare expenditures for sinusitis in 1996: contributions of asthma, rhinitis, and other airway disorders. J Allergy Clin Immunol 1996; 103:408–414.
5. McCaig LF, Besser RE, et al. Trends in antimicrobial prescribing rates for children and adolescents. JAMA 2002; 287(23):3096–3102.
6. Poole MD. A focus on acute sinusitis in adults: changes in disease management. Am J Med 1999; 106(5A):38S–47S; discussion 48S–52S.
7. Lanza D, Kennedy D. Adult rhinosinusitis defined. Otolaryngol Head Neck Surg 1997; 117(suppl):S1–S7.
8. Bhattacharyya N. The role of infection in chronic rhinosinusitis. Curr Allergy Asthma Rep 2002; 2(6):500–506.
9. Faststats cdc.gov/nchs/fastats.
10. Gwaltney JM Jr, Acute community-acquired sinusitis. Clin Infect Dis 1996; 23(6):1209–1223; quiz 1224–1225.
11. Gwaltney JM Jr, Scheld WM, et al. The microbial etiology and antimicrobial therapy of adults with acute community-acquired sinusitis: a fifteen-year experience at the University of Virginia and review of other selected studies. J Allergy Clin Immunol 1992; 90(3 pt 2):457–461; discussion 462.

12. Brook I, Thompson DH, et al. Microbiology and management of chronic maxillary sinusitis. Arch Otolaryngol Head Neck Surg 1994; 120(12):1317–1320.
13. Hartog B, Degener JE, et al. Microbiology of chronic maxillary sinusitis in adults: isolated aerobic and anaerobic bacteria and their susceptibility to twenty antibiotics. Acta Otolaryngol 1995; 115(5):672–677.
14. Brook I, Frazier EH, et al. Microbiology of chronic maxillary sinusitis: comparison between specimens obtained by sinus endoscopy and by surgical drainage. J Med Microbiol 1997; 46(5):430–432.
15. Aust R, Falck B, et al. Studies of the gas exchange and pressure in the maxillary sinuses in normal and infected humans. Rhinology 1979; 17(4):245–251.
16. Cappelletty D. Microbiology of bacterial respiratory infections. Pediatr Infect Dis J 1998; 17(8 suppl):S55–S61.
17. Hadley JA, Schaefer SD. Clinical evaluation of rhinosinusitis: History and physical examination. Otolaryngol Head Neck Surg 1997; 117(3 pt 2):8–11.
18. Report of the Rhinosinusitis Task Force Committee Meeting. Alexandria, Virginia, August 17, 1996. Otolaryngol Head Neck Surg 1997; 117(3 pt 2):S1–S68.
19. Williams JW Jr, Simel DL, Roberts L, Smasa GP. Clinical evaluation for sinusitis: Making the diagnosis by history and physical examination. Ann Intern Med 1992; 117:705–710.
20. Dowell SF, Schwartz B, et al. Appropriate use of antibiotics for URIs in children: Part I. Otitis media and acute sinusitis. The Pediatric URI Consensus Team. Am Fam Physician 1998; 58(5):1113–1118 (1123).
21. Dowell SF, Schwartz B, et al. Appropriate use of antibiotics for URIs in children: part II. Cough, pharyngitis and the common cold. The Pediatric URI Consensus Team. Am Fam Physician 1998; 58(6):1335–1342 (1345).
22. Gold SM, Tami AT. Role of middle meatus aspiration culture in the diagnosis of chronic sinusitis. Laryngoscope 1997; 107(12 pt 1):1586–1589.
23. Talbot GH, Kennedy DW, et al. Rigid nasal endoscopy versus sinus puncture and aspiration for microbiologic documentation of acute bacterial maxillary sinusitis. Clin Infect Dis 2001; 33(10):1668–1675.
24. Zinreich SJ. Rhinosinusitis: radiologic diagnosis. Otolaryngol Head Neck Surg 1997; 117(3 pt 2):S27–S34.
25. Vogan JC, Bolger WE, et al. Endoscopically guided sinonasal cultures: a direct comparison with maxillary sinus aspirate cultures. Otolaryngol Head Neck Surg 2000; 122(3):370–373.
26. AHCPR. Diagnosis and treatment of acute bacterial rhinosinusitis. Rockville, Md: Agency for Healthcare Policy and Research, 1999.
27. Lusk SL. Agency for Health Care Policy and Research guidelines on rhinosinusitis and depression. Aaohn J 1999; 47(12):586–588.
28. Brook I, Yocum P, et al. Bacteriology and beta-lactamase activity in acute and chronic maxillary sinusitis. Arch Otolaryngol Head Neck Surg 1996; 122(4): 418–422; discussion 423.
29. Poole MD, Jacobs MR, et al. Antimicrobial guidelines for the treatment of acute bacterial rhinosinusitis in immunocompetent children. Int J Pediatr Otorhinolaryngol 2002; 63(1):1–13.

30. Talbot AR, Herr TM, et al. Mucociliary clearance and buffered hypertonic saline solution. Laryngoscope 1997; 107(4):500–503.
31. Jones NS. Current concepts in the management of paediatric rhinosinusitis. J Laryngol Otol 1999; 113(1):1–9.
32. Yilmaz G, Varan B, et al. Intranasal budesonide spray as an adjunct to oral antibiotic therapy for acute sinusitis in children. Eur Arch Otorhinolaryngol 2000; 257(5):256–259.
33. Hamilos DL, Thawley SE, Kramper MA, Kamil A, Hamid QA. Effect of intranasal fluticasone on cellular infiltration, endothelial adhesion molecule expression and proinflammatory cytokine mRNA in nasal polyp disease. J All Clin Immunol 1999; 103:79–87.
34. Damm M, Jungehulsing M, et al. Effects of systemic steroid treatment in chronic polypoid rhinosinusitis evaluated with magnetic resonance imaging. Otolaryngol Head Neck Surg 1999; 120(4):517–523.

10

Otitis Media

Scott F. Dowell
U.S. Centers for Disease Control and Prevention
and Thai Ministry of Public Health
Nonthaburi, Thailand

Of all community-acquired respiratory tract infections, otitis media remains the leading indication for antimicrobial therapy among children in the United States. The rate of prescribing declined remarkably during the 1990s, probably a result of broad-based efforts to improve the specificity of the diagnosis and to limit antimicrobial therapy to those patients who are likely to benefit from it. The recent past has also seen substantial changes in the antimicrobial susceptibility patterns of the leading agents—pneumococcus in particular—and in the perception of the importance of viral agents. Clinicians caring for patients with otitis media now need to carefully consider such options as deferring antimicrobial treatment for many patients, prescribing a shortened course for some, and recommending topical therapy with newer agents for others. Many patients meeting diagnostic criteria for acute otitis media should still be treated with an appropriate course of an antimicrobial agent with efficacy against the major pathogens, although efforts are under way to promote watchful waiting for certain patients.

DIAGNOSIS

It may appear self-evident that an accurate diagnosis informs and directs appropriate therapy, but it should be appreciated that the accurate diagnosis of acute otitis media remains one of the most technically demanding skills required of the office-based clinician [1]. The presence of a perforated tympanic membrane or tympanostomy tubes, with drainage from the middle ear, or of otitis externa, should be confirmed through careful examination, as some of the treatment options differ if these conditions are present. The appearance and mobility of the tympanic membrane is used to identify the presence of a middle ear effusion. In the presence of middle ear effusion, the critical issue is differentiating acute otitis media (AOM), which may warrant antimicrobial treatment, from otitis media with effusion (OME), which does not [2].

Acute otitis media is diagnosed when the patient has a documented middle ear effusion, accompanied by signs or symptoms of acute inflammation [2–4]. Establishing the presence of middle ear effusion is one of the most technically demanding aspects of the ear examination, and requires the consistent use of a properly fitted and maintained pneumatic otoscope, with an attached bulb, a bright light, and an appropriate sized ear speculum [1,3]. Even with the proper equipment, determining if an effusion is present is a challenge. In a comparative study of pediatric residents and otolaryngologists, there was only slight agreement between tympanometry and residents on the presence of effusion (kappa statistic 0.20), and the agreement between tympanometry and otolaryngologists was not much better (kappa 0.32) [5]. The correlation between the two groups on the overall diagnosis of otitis media was fair (kappa 0.30).

In the presence of a middle ear effusion, signs and symptoms of acute inflammation supporting the diagnosis of AOM include fever, a bulging red or yellow tympanic membrane, or ear pain [2,6,7]. If a middle ear effusion is present but acute inflammation is not, the diagnosis is otitis media with effusion (OME), and antimicrobial therapy is not indicated [2]. Antimicrobial therapy for OME has marginal short-term benefit in terms of resolution of the effusion, but there is not evidence that children treated with antibiotics are better off than those treated with placebo when assessed one or more months after the effusion is noted [8,9].

PATHOGENS

Therapy should be directed on the basis of a thorough understanding of the likely pathogens and their predicted susceptibility patterns, as culture-directed therapy is rarely possible or even indicated. The most likely bacterial pathogens to cause AOM have changed very little in tympanocentesis studies conducted over the past several decades, which have consistently identified *Streptococcus pneumoniae* in about 35% of cases, *Haemophilus influenzae* in about 30%, and *Moraxella catarrhalis* in about 10% (Table 1) [10–13]. Documentation of the role of respiratory viruses, long presumed to be important co-pathogens, has come with the more recent widespread use of nucleic acid amplification techniques (Table 1). The role of antimicrobial resistance, which had become a concern with the emergence of β-lactamase producing strains of *M. catarrhalis* and *H. influenzae* in the 1970s, was recognized as increasingly important and resulted in changes in practice with the emergence of multiply resistant strains of *S. pneumoniae* in the 1990s.

Of the major pathogens, the pneumococcus is not only the most commonly identified, it is also the one most commonly associated with treatment failures, and the least likely to resolve spontaneously if no therapy or inadequate therapy is given. In patients randomized to the placebo or no-treatment arm of otitis media treatment trials, approximately 80% of patients infected with *M. catarrhalis* and 50% of those infected with *H. influenzae* have sterile middle ear fluid on reevaluation 3–10 days later, whereas only 20% of similarly untreated patients infected with pneumococci have the infection

TABLE 1 Pathogens Implicated in Acute Otitis Media

Pathogen	Approximate % of patients
Bacteria	
Streptococcus pneumoniae	25–65
Haemophilus influenzae	20–40
Moraxella catarrhalis	5–15
Group A streptococci	1–6
Other bacteria	1–8
Viruses	
Respiratory syncytial virus	6–18
Influenza virus	3–10
Rhinoviruses	2–24
Parainfluenzae viruses	2–8
Other viruses	3–8

Other bacteria include *Chlamydophila pneumoniae*, *Staphylococcus aureus*, atypical mycobacteria, and others. Other viruses include respiratory adenoviruses, coronaviruses, rhinoviruses, enteroviruses, and others. Numbers do not add to 100% because more than one agent may be identified in a single patient.
Source: Refs. 13, 23, 28, 34, 35, and 102.

resolve without therapy [14,15]. Thus, the pneumococcus is the pathogen of primary concern when selecting an antimicrobial agent, and the presence and antimicrobial susceptibilities of the other pathogens are additional secondary considerations.

In the United States, approximately 30% of all invasive pneumococcal isolates are nonsusceptible to penicillin, and most of these nonsusceptible strains also have reduced susceptibility to many of the agents commonly used for the treatment of AOM (Table 2). The mechanism of resistance is important. Pneumococcal resistance to penicillins and cephalosporins is mediated by changes in penicillin-binding proteins, and it can be overcome by moderate increases in the dosage or the use of more active agents [16,17]. Other types of resistance, such as the methylation of ribosomal subunits that results in high-level macrolide resistance, or the double mutations in DNA topoisomerase that results in fluoroquinolone resistance, tend to confer absolute resistance to the drug or class of drugs involved [16,18,19].

Haemophilus influenzae has maintained a steady second position to pneumococcus as an important pathogen in acute otitis media, and antimicrobial agents used to treat AOM should be selected with this pathogen in mind. The dramatic decreases in invasive *H. influenzae* type b disease that

TABLE 2 Antimicrobial Susceptibility of *Streptococcus pneumoniae* to Agents Commonly Used to Treat Acute Otitis Media

	Streptococcus pneumoniae susceptibility according to penicillin-susceptibility category		
Agent	Susceptible (75%)	Intermediate (10%)	Resistant (16%)
Amoxicillin	+++	+++	+
Cefprozil	+++	++	–
Cefpodoxime	+++	++	–
Cefuroxime	+++	+	–
Cefaclor	+++	–	–
Cefixime	+++	–	–
Ceftibuten	+++	–	–
Ceftriaxone (injection)	+++	+++	++
Macrolides[a]	+++	+	–
Trimethoprim-sulfamethoxazole	++	–	–

Note. Estimated percentage of pneumococci covered by agent is as follows: +++, at least 90%; ++, >75%; +, >50%; – <50%.

[a] "Macrolides" refers to erythromycin, clarithromycin, and azithromycin.

Source: Refs. 13, 17, 59, 103, and 104.

followed widespread use of the conjugate vaccine did little to decrease *Haemophilus* in otitis media, because most middle ear fluid isolates are nontypeable. During the 1970s and 1980s, the proportion of *H. influenzae* that produce β-lactamase increased to approximately one-third of all strains, but this proportion did not change appreciably during the 1990s [20,21].

Moraxella catarrhalis is consistently identified in a minority of middle ear fluid specimens from patients with AOM. The proportion of strains producing β-lactamase is now greater than 90% in most studies [20,22]. In spite of this, treatment with agents to which *M. catarrhalis* is not susceptible (such as amoxicillin) rarely results in treatment failures from persisting *M. catarrhalis* [12,23,24]. Presumably this is because of the high rate of spontaneous resolution of AOM associated with *M. catarrhalis* [14].

Other bacteria are occasionally isolated from middle ear fluid of patients with AOM, including group A streptococci, *Staphylococcus aureus*, and gram-negative rods. Recently, *Chlamydophila pneumoniae* has been detected in approximately 10% of middle ear aspirates by polymerase chain reaction [25] or by culture [26]. If these findings are confirmed in other studies, it may be necessary to consider efficacy against *C. pneumoniae* in future antimicrobial treatment guidelines.

The fact that respiratory viruses can be detected in middle ear fluid and play a role in the pathogenesis of acute otitis media has been appreciated for several decades [27–29], but the more recent finding that influenza vaccines may substantially reduce the incidence of acute otitis media has led to renewed interest in the role of viruses and the opportunities for prevention [30–33]. Children often present with AOM during or after an upper respiratory infection, and it is easy to demonstrate the presence of respiratory viruses in the nasopharynx and occasionally the middle ear fluid of such children [34,35]. The most commonly identified viruses are respiratory syncytial virus, influenza virus, human rhinoviruses, and parainfluenza viruses [34,35], but enteroviruses, adenoviruses, coronaviruses, herpex simplex virus, cytomegalovirus, human herpesvirus-6, and others have occasionally been identified as well [35–37]. Experimental studies with human volunteers and observational studies on children with colds have documented that viral infection of the middle ear cavity can lead to negative pressure and eustachian tube dysfunction, presumed to be an initiating event in facilitating entry of bacterial pathogens from the nasopharynx to the middle ear space [38,39]. Often, both viruses and bacterial pathogens are detected in the middle ear fluid at the same time, and there is evidence to suggest that such co-infection is associated with an increased risk of treatment failure [28,40]. It is not clear that viruses alone are an important cause of AOM.

Whether viruses act as cofactors, initiating and exacerbating bacterial AOM, or whether they act alone, it seems clear that controlling viral infections is likely to substantially reduce the incidence of AOM. Early findings that immunization of children with injected subunit influenza vaccines was associated with reductions in AOM of 30% to 36% [30,31] have been confirmed and extended by studies of the newer, live attenuated intranasal influenza vaccines [32,33]. Vaccines against other respiratory viruses are in various stages of testing, and it seems likely that vaccines against respiratory syncytial virus in particular, but perhaps also those against the parainfluenza viruses or others, will contribute substantially to the control of AOM in the future.

TREATMENT

First-Line Antimicrobial Therapy

There is no doubt that antimicrobial therapy benefits patients with documented AOM. It also is true that most episodes of AOM will resolve with or without therapy. Traditional estimates of the benefit of treatment are modest—on the order of 15% (80% of AOM episodes treated with placebo will resolve by 14 days, compared with 95% treated with an appropriate agent) [41,42]. Some now argue that even these modest estimates of efficacy are too high, that the true benefit is even smaller, and that this small benefit does not outweigh the potential adverse effects of unnecessary treatment, such as carriage or invasive disease caused by resistant organisms [43–45]. However, the newer estimates of efficacy are still in the same range as traditional estimates (i.e., 13% [45] and 12% [44]), and there is clear evidence in these trials of measurable clinical benefit in terms of shortened duration of fever and reduced pain.

In nonsevere cases in a randomized trial, more than 90% of episodes were significantly improved by 48 hr, whether treated with amoxicillin or placebo. Initial treatment failure (persistent fever of ≥38°C or severe pain after 48 hr) occurred in 3.9% of amoxicillin-treated patients and 7.7% of those treated with placebo ($P = 0.009$) [46]. Finally, there is now some evidence that the rates of mastoiditis may be higher in the Netherlands and other countries where antimicrobial therapy is not routinely prescribed [47].

In view of the documented benefit from antimicrobial treatment for a minority of patients, in terms of accelerated eradication of the pathogen, shortening of the duration of ear pain and fever, and potentially in terms of reduction in the likelihood of mastoiditis or other complications, it seems reasonable to prescribe an antimicrobial agent to certain patients appropriately diagnosed with AOM, and the question becomes, "which children?" and "which antibiotic?"

The reduction in pneumococcal disease observed with the use of the new conjugate pneumococcal vaccine may also influence the risk/benefit considerations involved in weighing the decision to treat children with AOM. Reductions in AOM on the order of 6–8% have been seen in the controlled trials of the vaccine [48]. Although the magnitude of reduction is small, there is also evidence that widespread use of the vaccine may result in reductions in multiply resistant pneumococci and in serotype replacement by nonvaccine serotypes.

Young children with documented AOM should be treated. The American Academy of Pediatrics is considering adopting watchful waiting as an option for certain low-risk older children. These might include those who are 2 years of age or older, are otherwise healthy, have no history of recurrent AOM, no craniofacial abnormalities, no evidence of immune compromise, and have only mild to moderate symptoms.

The primary consideration in selecting an antimicrobial agent is efficacy against the major pathogens. Secondary considerations are cost, palatability, convenience of dosing schedules, and effects on antimicrobial resistance. Efficacy is best measured by microbiological outcomes in studies that include tympanocentesis to identify the organism and repeat tympanocentesis for patients who have treatment failures documented on days 3 through 5. Such studies have now established that early eradication of pathogens from middle ear fluid is associated with improved clinical outcome [49]. On the other hand, comparison of efficacy using less precisely defined measures of outcome often lead to the false conclusion that the two agents being compared have equivalent efficacy, an observation aptly dubbed the "Pollyanna phenomenon" after the blind optimism of the heroine of the novel by that name [50].

Antimicrobial efficacy correlates with clinical efficacy. Patients infected with penicillin-nonsusceptible pneumococci were more likely to have documented bacteriological failure of treatment with cefuroxime, and even more likely to fail treatment with cefaclor, a cephalosporin with relatively low activity against nonsusceptible pneumococci [17]. In this study and others like it, bacteriologic failure was consistently correlated with clinical failure [17,49,51].

Amoxicillin remains the first-line agent for treating uncomplicated acute otitis media, despite the many changes in antimicrobial susceptibility of the leading bacterial pathogens. Of the available oral agents, amoxicillin has among the highest antibacterial efficacy for *S. pneumoniae*, the major pathogen of concern, especially when given at the high dosages currently recommended (80–90 mg/kg/day) [52–55]. Amoxicillin also has good antimicrobial and clinical efficacy against two-thirds of *H. influenzae* and occasional *M. catarrhalis*, but this latter pathogen is very likely to resolve on its own even without treatment. Amoxicillin is also inexpensive and well tolerated, and it enjoys a strong safety record as the leading agent for otitis media treatment over more than 3 decades of use [55].

Second-line Agents

Second-line agents should be considered for patients who return with persisting symptoms during amoxicillin treatment, for those with documented penicillin allergy, and for those known to be at increased risk for infection with resistant strains.

Treatment outcome should be assessed in children who are not improved by day 3, not at the traditional 10-day ear recheck. Patients who return with persistent and unimproved signs and symptoms at day 3 are likely to have microbiological treatment failure, and should have antimicrobial treatment optimized at that time [41]. A 10-day recheck is likely to be too late to influence the duration of pain or fever with a change in therapy, because these symptoms resolve in most patients within the first week, even among patients treated with placebo. Furthermore, more than 70% of patients will have a persistent effusion at 10–14 days, despite successful treatment of the AOM episode and eradication of the pathogen [56,57].

One might anticipate that patients who return after failing therapy with amoxicillin would be more likely to be infected with β-lactamase–producing strains of *H. influenzae* or *M. catarrhalis*, because those strains would not be eradicated by amoxicillin, whereas the drug is highly active against pneumococci. However, even in cases where amoxicillin treatment has failed, pneumococci remain predominant pathogens, with β-lactamase–producing strains of *H. influenzae* or *M. catarrhalis* present to a lesser extent [23]. Presumably this is related to the increased likelihood of spontaneous resolution of *H. influenzae* or *M. catarrhalis* compared with pneumococci, but it has implications for the selection of agents for children with treatment failure. Such agents must be active against pneumococci, including penicillin-nonsusceptible strains, as well as having β-lactamase stability.

In 1999 the Centers for Disease Control and Prevention (CDC) recommended three agents with appropriate antimicrobial coverage and documented clinical efficacy for patients who fail amoxicillin therapy: amoxicillin-clavulanate, cefuroxime axetil, and intramuscular ceftriaxone (Table 3) [41]. Each of these agents has good activity against intermediate-penicillin-susceptible pneumococci and is stable against β-lactamase–producing strains of *H. influenzae* and *M. catarrhalis*. However, amoxicillin-clavulanate is expensive, cefuroxime axetil has a bitter taste, and cefriaxone requires an injection.

In the years since these recommendations were made, additional information on these and other agents and on the likely pathogens in cases of treatment failure has become available, and has reinforced the importance of treating with agents effective against nonsusceptible pneumococci and β-lactamase–producing *H. influenzae* [23,48,58]. Recent anecdotal reports of treatment failure with cefuroxime and surveillance information about its

TABLE 3 Treatment Recommendations for Acute Otitis Media

Antibiotics in prior month	Day 0	Treatment failure[a] on day 3	Treatment failure[a] on days 10–28
No	Amoxicillin[b]	Amoxicillin/clavulanate[b]; cefuroxime axetil; I.M. ceftriaxone[c]	Amoxicillin/clavulanate[b]; cefuroxime axetil; I.M. ceftriaxone[c]
Yes	Amoxicillin[b]; amoxicillin/clavulanate[b]; cefuroxime axetil	I.M. ceftriaxone[c]; clindamycin[d]; or tympanocentesis-guided therapy	Amoxicillin/clavulanate; cefuroxime axetil; I.M. ceftriaxone[c], or tympanocentesis-guided therapy

Note. Strong evidence for efficacy of these agents was available in 1999. Other drugs that may also be effective are discussed in the text.

[a] Treatment failure is defined as a lack of clinical improvement in signs and symptoms such as ear pain, fever, and tympanic membrane findings of redness, bulging, or otorrhea. Persisting middle ear effusion is expected in up to 70% of appropriately treated patients at 10–28 days and should not be considered as evidence of treatment failure.

[b] Amoxicillin and amoxicillin/clavulanate should generally be given at 80 to 90 mg/kg/day. The clavulanate component should be given at 6.4 mg/kg/day (requires newer formulations or combination with amoxicillin).

[c] Intramuscular ceftriaxone in one to three daily injections of 50 mg/kg.

[d] Clindamycin is not effective against *Haemophilus influenzae* or *Moraxella catarrhalis.*

Source: Ref. 55.

possibly decreased efficacy against penicillin nonsusceptible pneumococci have led some authorities to question its inclusion as a second-line agent [59–61]. Ceftriaxone can be given as either 1-day injection or a 3-day course, and some evidence now exists that the single dose is comparable clinically to 10 days of amoxicillin-clavulanate [62]. However, in direct comparison using bacteriological efficacy as an outcome measure, the 3-day course is superior [51]. High-dose amoxicillin-clavulanate does appear to be bacteriologically and clinically efficacious against penicillin-nonsusceptible pneumococci and *H. influenzae* [53], although it has a substantial effect on subsequent nasopharyngeal colonization with resistant organisms [63].

In addition to the three agents listed above, newer information indicates that other agents may meet these criteria. Cefdinir, for example, is active against β-lactamase–producing strains of *H. influenzae* or *M. catarrhalis* and has the advantage of palatability and convenient dosing, although some evidence indicates the efficacy against intermediate susceptible pneumococci may not be as good as amoxicillin-clavulanate or ceftriaxone [64–66]. Cefprozil and cefpodoxime have reasonable in vitro activity against intermediate pneumococci [41]. A recent comparison of cefprozil with amoxicillin clavulanate reported similar clinical efficacy, although the more sensitive microbiological efficacy outcome was not assessed [67].

Second-line agents may also be considered for patients who present with an increased likelihood of infection with resistant pathogens. Such patients include those who present with AOM within one month of completing a course of an antibiotic, those with well-documented previous treatment failures, and those on long-term antimicrobial prophylaxis.

For patients with a history of a serious allergic reaction to penicillin, other classes of agent must be considered. In this context, the macrolides and related agents (azithromycin, clarithromycin, and erythromycin) would be appropriate alternatives. For those children who have a history of rash or other nonspecific symptoms following treatment with amoxicillin, it may be more appropriate to select one of the cephalosporins with better efficacy against nonsusceptible pneumococci, as cross-reactivity between the penicillins and cephalosporins is approximately 15% [68]. In cases where there is tympanic membrane perforation or a tympanostomy tube in place, topical treatment with fluoroquinolone or other otic drops may also be an appropriate approach [69].

Less Useful Agents

Some agents that may have been useful in the past may no longer be appropriate for treatment of AOM. Trimethoprim-sulfamethoxazole was considered a first-line agent for many years [70,71], but increasing resistance and recent evidence of bacteriologic and clinical failure make this agent a poor choice for most areas where resistant pneumococci are a concern. In U.S. and international pneumococcal surveillance studies, resistance to trimethoprim-sulfamethoxazole ranges from 30% to more than 60% [13,59,72]. A study using repeat tympanocentesis documented bacteriological failure in 73% of those infected with a trimethoprim-sulfamethoxazole–resistant pneumococcus, and these bacteriological failures correlated directly with clinical failure [72].

Erythromycin and related agents have similarly been useful drugs for AOM treatment in the past, but the utility of these agents is also threatened by increasing antimicrobial resistance. Macrolide resistance among pneumococci has increased rapidly in recent years, doubling from 10% to 20% in association with a 320% increase in prescribing to young children in one U.S. national study [73]. Much of the resistance observed is due to the less concerning efflux mechanism, rather than the higher-level resistance associated with ribosomal methylation, but the degree of resistance associated with efflux has also increased, with increasing minimal inhibitory concentrations (MICs) even among those isolates with efflux mediated resistance [59,73]. Repeat tympanocentesis studies have documented a strong correlation between high azithromycin MICs among pneumococci and bacteriological and clinical treatment failure for AOM [54,74] and worrisome failures to eradicate *H. influenzae* as well [54]. In regions where macrolide resistance is less of a concern and in patients with penicillin allergy, the macrolide agents are likely to remain attractive options, especially because of the convenient dosing and palatability of the newer agents.

Several of the oral cephalosporins approved for treatment of AOM are also suboptimal choices in the era of increasing pneumococcal resistance because of their poor activity against nonsusceptible pneumococci. These agents include cefaclor, cefixime, loracarbef, and ceftibuten (Table 2) [17,41,74].

Adjunctive treatment of AOM with antihistamines and decongestants has often been prescribed despite mixed evidence for efficacy. Most carefully conducted controlled trials have found no benefit, some have documented worrisome side effects. A recent systematic review found no evidence for efficacy of either antihistamines or decongestants, and marginal benefits only in some less rigorous trials of combination therapy [75]. In view of the documented and significant increase in side effects [75], these agents should have little or no future role in AOM treatment.

OTHER TREATMENT OPTIONS

Deferring Antibiotic Therapy

Some authorities now argue that deferring antimicrobial therapy for children with AOM is the preferred option [43], and that parents and physicians are willing to forgo antibiotic treatment of AOM because of concerns about antimicrobial resistance [76]. As discussed above, the evidence that 12% to 15% of children will benefit with decreased duration of pain and fever, prompt eradication of the pathogen, and possibly lower risk of complications argues that antimicrobial treatment of AOM remains appropriate for many children. Older children with mild AOM and no history of recurrent AOM, craniofacial abnormalities, or immune compromise may be managed with watchful waiting for 2–3 days as long as follow-up is assured. As well, children with OME should be clearly differentiated, and deferral of antimicrobial therapy for this condition is the appropriate option [2,58].

Several controlled community trials have demonstrated that antimicrobial use for respiratory tract infections can be reduced by 10% to 30% in a single year with education directed at physicians and patients [77–80]. These decreases are encouraging and come in addition to the substantial annual declines of 8% to 10% in prescribing seen in the control groups in all of these trials. The declines in prescribing in the control groups reflect a wider trend in the United States and elsewhere to use antimicrobial agents more judiciously, as advocated by many [81–84]. These efforts have paid dividends in terms of reduced prescribing. For otitis media, prescribing on a population basis throughout the United States decreased by a remarkable 47% between 1990 and 2000 [85].

Short-Course Therapy

One way of reducing excessive antimicrobial use is to shorten the prescribed course from the traditional 10 days, and this approach has the added benefit of simplifying treatment for parents and potentially increasing compliance. A number of randomized trials have compared outcomes with shortened courses and reported favorable comparison to traditional regimens [86–91]. Recommendations from the CDC and American Academy of Pediatrics in 1998 endorsed shortened courses for children 2 years or older with mild and uncomplicated AOM [2] and a meta-analysis published in that year lent support to the recommendations [92].

Since that time, concerns about antimicrobial resistance and resulting treatment failures have increased. Additional information from large trials has reenforced earlier findings that full 10-day courses of treatment are measurably superior to shorter courses, although the differences are most pronounced in the younger children and those more prone to treatment failure [93–95]. On the other hand, the proposed benefit of shortened courses of therapy on reduced carriage of resistant strains has been substantiated [96]. Treatment of selected children with 5- to 7-day courses of antimicrobial agents remains an appropriate option, but children younger than 2 years of age, those with perforated tympanic membranes, craniofacial abnormalities or other underlying conditions predisposing to otitis media, and those with chronic or recurrent otitis media should not be considered candidates for shortened courses of therapy. These considerations apply to shortened courses of therapy with traditional 10-day oral β-lactam regimens, not to the previously discussed 3-day regimen of intramuscular ceftriaxone or 5-day courses of azithromycin, both of which have prolonged half-lives and may therefore provide antimicrobial effects well beyond the last administered dose.

Topical Therapy

For patients with otitis externa, topical therapy with otic drops containing aminoglycosides or other antimicrobial agents, often in combination with corticosteroids and mechanical removal of fluid and cerumen, has been the traditional treatment of choice. With the availability of newer fluoroquinolone topical preparations, attention has turned to a broadened set of indications for topical therapy with these agents, including patients with chronic suppurative otitis media, AOM with tympanic membrane perforation, and AOM with tympanostomy tubes in place, in addition to those with otitis externa [69,97].

Controlled trials comparing topical fluoroquinolone treatment with traditional therapy are limited, but it appears that topical therapy with ciprofloxacin or ofloxacin offers comparable or slightly improved bacteriological efficacy to traditional topical preparations for otitis externa or chronic suppurative otitis media [98–100]. In addition, topical ofloxacin appears to offer comparable cure rates and a broadened spectrum of coverage compared to oral amoxicillin-clavulanate for patients with AOM who have tympanostomy tubes in place [69,101]. More direct comparisons of topical with oral therapy are warranted before topical therapy can be recommended as a preferred option. In the meantime, clinicians caring for patients with tympanostomy tubes and/or drainage in the ear canal in the era of increasing antimicrobial resistance may welcome the additional treatment option provided by the newer topical agents.

CONCLUSIONS

National campaigns to reduce unnecessary antibiotic use have been highly successful; nevertheless, otitis media remains a leading indication for antimicrobial use. Efforts to further reduce unnecessary antimicrobial use continue, including the anticipated promotion of watchful waiting for low-risk children with acute otitis media. Observation with analgesia and careful follow-up is an option for selected older children. All antimicrobial agents are not equally efficacious. If tympanocentesis is used to document bacteriological eradication, some agents can be shown to be clearly superior, and others ineffective. High-dose amoxicillin remains the first-line drug of choice, and several other β-lactam agents are reasonable second-line options. Deferral of antimicrobial therapy for patients without clear evidence of AOM, short-course therapy for low-risk patients, and topical treatment for those with nonintact tympanic membranes are viable options that should be considered.

REFERENCES

1. Block S. Accurately diagnosing acute otitis media: "dispose of the disposables." Pediatr Infect Dis J 1998; 17:1179–1180.
2. Dowell SF, Marcy SM, Phillips WR, Gerber MA, Schwartz B. Otitis media—principles of judicious use of antimicrobial agents. Pediatrics 1998; 101:165–171.
3. Faden H, Duffy L, Boeve M. Otitis media: back to basics. Pediatr Infect Dis J 1998; 17:1105–1112; quiz 1112–3.
4. Isaacson G. The natural history of a treated episode of acute otitis media. Pediatrics 1996; 98:968–971.
5. Steinbach WJ, Sectish TC, Benjamin DK Jr, Chang KW, Messner AH. Pediatric residents' clinical diagnostic accuracy of otitis media. Pediatrics 2002; 109:993–998.
6. Schwartz RH, Rodriguez WJ, Brook I, Grundfast KM. The febrile response in acute otitis media. JAMA 1981; 245:2057–2058.
7. McCormick DP, Lim-Melia E, Saeed K, Baldwin CD, Chonmaitree T. Otitis media: can clinical findings predict bacterial or viral etiology? Pediatr Infect Dis J 2000; 19:256–258.
8. Williams RL, Chalmers TC, Stange KC, Chalmers FT, Bowlin SJ. Use of antibiotics in preventing recurrent acute otitis media and in treating otitis media with effusion. A meta-analytic attempt to resolve the brouhaha. JAMA 1993; 270:1344–1351.
9. Rosenfeld RM, Post JC. Meta-analysis of antibiotics for the treatment of otitis media with effusion. Otolaryngol Head Neck Surg 1992; 106:378–386.
10. Mortimer E, Watterson R. A bacteriologic investigation of otitis media in infancy. Pediatrics 1956; 17:359–366.
11. Jacobs MR. Increasing importance of antibiotic-resistant *Streptococcus pneumoniae* in acute otitis media. Pediatr Infect Dis J 1996; 15:940–943.
12. Harrison CJ, Marks MI, Welch DF. Microbiology of recently treated acute otitis media compared with previously untreated acute otitis media. Pediatr Infect Dis J 1985; 4:641–646.
13. Jacobs MR, Dagan R, Appelbaum PC, Burch DJ. Prevalence of antimicrobial-resistant pathogens in middle ear fluid: multinational study of 917 children with acute otitis media. Antimicrob Agents Chemother 1998; 42: 589–595.

14. Klein JO. The "in vivo sensitivity test" for acute otitis media revisited. The Pediatr Infect Dis J 1998; 17:774–775.
15. Howie VM, Dillard R, Lawrence B. In vivo sensitivity test in otitis media: efficacy of antibiotics. Pediatrics 1985; 75:8–13.
16. Schrag SJ, Beall B, Dowell SF. Limiting the spread of resistant pneumococci: biological and epidemiologic evidence for the effectiveness of alternative interventions. Clin Microbiol Rev 2000; 13:588–601.
17. Dagan R, Abramson O, Leibovitz E, et al. Impaired bacteriologic response to oral cephalosporins in acute otitis media caused by pneumococci with intermediate resistance to penicillin. Pediatr Infect Dis J 1996; 15:980–985.
18. Bedos JP, Rieux V, Bauchet J, Muffat-Joly M, Carbon C, Azoulay-Dupuis E. Efficacy of trovafloxacin against penicillin-susceptible and multiresistant strains of Streptococcus pneumoniae in a mouse pneumonia model. Antimicrob Agents Chemother 1998; 42:862–867.
19. Berry V, Thorburn CE, Knott SJ, Woodnutt G. Bacteriological efficacies of three macrolides compared with those of amoxicillin-clavulanate against Streptococcus pneumoniae and Haemophilus influenzae. Antimicrob Agents Chemother 1998; 42:3193–3199.
20. Hoban DJ, Doern GV, Fluit AC, Roussel-Delvallez M, Jones RN. Worldwide prevalence of antimicrobial resistance in Streptococus pneumoniae, Haemophilus influenzae, and Moraxella catarrhalis in the SENTRY Antimicrobial Surveillance Program, 1997–1999. Clin Infect Dis 2001; 32:S81–S93.
21. Barnett ED, Klein JO. The problem of resistant bacteria for the management of acute otitis media. Pediatr Clin North Am 1995; 42:509–517.
22. Berk SL, Kalbfleisch JH. Antibiotic susceptibility patterns of community-acquired respiratory isolates of Moraxella catarrhalis in western Europe and in the USA. The Alexander Project Collaborative Group. J Antimicrobiol Chemother 1996; 38(suppl A):85–96.
23. Block SL, Hedrick JA, Tyler RD, Smith RA, Harrison CJ. Microbiology of acute otitis media recently treated with aminopenicillins. Pediatr Infect Dis J 2001; 20:1017–1021.
24. Gehanno P, N'Guyen L, Derriennic M, Pichon F, Goehrs JM, Berche P. Pathogens isolated during treatment failures in otitis. Pediatr Infect Dis 1998; 17:885–890.
25. Storgaard M, Ostergaard L, Jensen JS, et al. Chlamydia pneumoniae in children with otitis media. Clin Infect Dis 1997; 25:1090–1093.
26. Block SL, Hammerschlag MR, Hedrick J, et al. Chlamydia pneumoniae in acute otitis media. Pediatr Infect Dis J 1997; 16:858–862.
27. Klein BS, Dollete FR, Yolken RH. The role of respiratory syncytial virus and other viral pathogens in acute otitis media. J Pediatr 1982; 101:16–20.
28. Chonmaitree T, Owen MJ, Patel JA, Hedgpeth D, Horlick D, Howie VM. Effect of viral respiratory tract infection on outcome of acute otitis media. J Pediatr 1992; 120:856–862.
29. Ruuskanen O, Heikkinen T. Viral-bacterial interaction in acute otitis media. Pediatr Infect Dis J 1994; 13:1047–1049.

30. Heikkinen T, Ruuskanen O, Waris M, Ziegler T, Arola M, Halonen P. Influenza vaccination in the prevention of acute otitis media in children. Am J Dis Child 1991; 145:445–448.
31. Clements DA, Langdon L, Bland C, Walter E. Influenza A vaccine decreases the incidence of otitis media in 6- to 30-month-old children in day care. Arch Pediatr Adolesc Med 1995; 149:1113–1117.
32. Belshe RB, Gruber WC. Safety, efficacy and effectiveness of cold-adapted, live, attenuated, trivalent, intranasal influenza vaccine in adults and children. Philos Trans R Soc Lond B Biol Sci 2001; 356:1947–1951.
33. Marchisio P, Cavagna R, Maspes B, et al. Efficacy of intranasal virosomal influenza vaccine in the prevention of recurrent acute otitis media in children. Clin Infect Dis 2002; 35:168–174.
34. Pitkaranta A, Virolainen A, Jero J, Arruda E, Hayden FG. Detection of rhinovirus, respiratory syncytial virus, and coronavirus infections in acute otitis media by reverse transcriptase polymerase chain reaction. Pediatrics 1998; 102:291–295.
35. Heikkinen T, Thint M, Chonmaitree T. Prevalence of various respiratory viruses in the middle ear during acute otitis media. N Engl J Med 1999; 340: 260–264.
36. Barone SR, Kaplan MH, Krilov LR. Human herpesvirus-6 infection in children with first febrile seizures. J Pediatr 1995; 127:95–97.
37. Chonmaitree T, Owen MJ, Patel JA, Hedgpeth D, Horlick D, Howie VM. Presence of cytomegalovirus and herpes simplex virus in middle ear fluids from children with acute otitis media. Clin Infect Dis 1992; 15:650–653.
38. Buchman CA, Doyle WJ, Skoner D, Fireman P, Gwaltney JM. Otologic manifestations of experimental rhinovirus infection. Laryngoscope 1994; 104: 1295–1299.
39. Winther B, Hayden FG, Arruda E, Dutkowski R, Ward P, Hendley JO. Viral respiratory infection in schoolchildren: effects on middle ear pressure. Pediatrics 2002; 109:826–832.
40. Sung BS, Chonmaitree T, Broemeling LD, et al. Association of rhinovirus infection with poor bacteriologic outcome of bacterial-viral otitis media. Clin Infect Dis 1993; 17:38–42.
41. Dowell SF, Butler JC, Giebink GS. Acute otitis media: management and surveillance in an era of pneumococcal resistance. Drug-Resistant Streptococcus Pneumoniae Therapeutic Working Group. Nurse Pract 1999; 24:1–9; quiz 15-6.
42. Rosenfeld RM, Vertrees JE, Carr J, et al. Clinical efficacy of antimicrobial drugs for acute otitis media: metaanalysis of 5400 children from thirty-three randomized trials. J Pediatr 1994; 124:355–367.
43. Culpepper L, Froom J. Routine antimicrobial treatment of acute otitis media: is it necessary? JAMA 1997; 278:1643–1645.
44. Takata GS, Chan LS, Shekelle P, Morton SC, Mason W, Marcy SM. Evidence assessment of management of acute otitis media: I. The role of antibiotics in treatment of uncomplicated acute otitis media. Pediatrics 2001; 108:239–247.

45. Damoiseaux RA, van Balen FA, Hoes AW, Verheij TJ, de Melker RA. Primary care based randomised, double blind trial of amoxicillin versus placebo for acute otitis media in children aged under 2 years. BMJ 2000; 320:350–354.
46. Kaleida PH, Casselbrant ML, Rockette HE, et al. Amoxicillin or myringotomy or both for acute otitis media: results of a randomized clinical trial. Pediatrics 1991; 87:466–474.
47. Van Zuijlen DA, Schilder AG, Van Balen FA, Hoes AW. National differences in incidence of acute mastoiditis: relationship to prescribing patterns of antibiotics for acute otitis media? Pediatr Infect Dis J 2001; 20:140–144.
48. Klein JO. Management of otitis media: 2000 and beyond. Pediatr Infect Dis J 2000; 19:383–387.
49. Dagan R, Leibovitz E, Greenberg D, Yagupsky P, Fliss DM, Leiberman A. Early eradication of pathogens from middle ear fluid during antibiotic treatment of acute otitis media is associated with improved clinical outcome. Pediatri Infect Dis J 1998; 17:776–782.
50. Marchant CD, Carlin SA, Johnson CE, Shurin PA. Measuring the comparative efficacy of antibacterial agents for acute otitis media: the "Pollyanna phenomenon." J Pediatr 1992; 120:72–77.
51. Leibovitz E, Piglansky L, Raiz S, Press J, Leiberman A, Dagan R. Bacteriologic and clinical efficacy of one day vs. three day intramuscular ceftriaxone for treatment of nonresponsive acute otitis media in children. Pediatr Infect Dis J 2000; 19:1040–1045.
52. Pelton SI. Acute otitis media in an era of increasing antimicrobial resistance and universal administration of pneumococcal conjugate vaccine. Pediatr Infect Dis J 2002; 21:599–604; discussion 613-4.
53. Dagan R, Hoberman A, Johnson C, et al. Bacteriologic and clinical efficacy of high dose amoxicillin/clavulanate in children with acute otitis media. Pediatr Infect Dis J 2001; 20:829–837.
54. Dagan R, Johnson CE, McLinn S, et al. Bacteriologic and clinical efficacy of amoxicillin/clavulanate vs. azithromycin in acute otitis media. Pediatr Infect Dis J 2000; 19:95–104.
55. Dowell SF, Butler JC, Giebink GS, et al. Acute otitis media: management and surveillance in an era of pneumococcal resistance—a report from the Drug-resistant Streptococcus pneumoniae Therapeutic Working Group. Pediatr Infect Dis J 1999; 18:1–9.
56. Klein JO. Otitis media. Clin Infect Dis 1994; 19:823–833.
57. Teele DW, Klein JO, Rosner BA. Epidemiology of otitis media in children. Annals of Otology, Rhinology, & Laryngology - Supplement 1980; 89:5–6.
58. Klein JO. Review of consensus reports on management of acute otitis media. Pediatr Infect Dis J 1999; 18:1152–1155.
59. Whitney CG, Farley MM, Hadler J, et al. Increasing prevalence of multidrug-resistant Streptococcus pneumoniae in the United States. N Engl J Med 2000; 343:1917–1924.
60. Dowell SF, Smith T, Leversedge K, Snitzer J. Failure of treatment of

pneumonia associated with highly resistant pneumococci in a child. Clin Infect Dis 1999; 29: 462–463.

61. Hoberman A, Marchant CD, Kaplan SL, Feldman S. Treatment of acute otitis media consensus recommendations. Clin Pediatr (Phila) 2002; 41:373–390.
62. Cohen R, Navel M, Grunberg J, et al. One dose ceftriaxone vs. ten days of amoxicillin/clavulanate therapy for acute otitis media: clinical efficacy and change in nasopharyngeal flora. Pediatr Infect Dis J 1999; 18:403–409.
63. Ghaffar F, Muniz LS, Katz K, et al. Effects of large dosages of amoxicillin/clavulanate or azithromycin on nasopharyngeal carriage of Streptococcus pneumoniae, Haemophilus influenzae, nonpneumococcal alpha-hemolytic streptococci, and Staphylococcus aureus in children with acute otitis media. Clin Infect Dis 2002; 34:1301–1309.
64. Block SL, McCarty JM, Hedrick JA, Nemeth MA, Keyserling CH, Tack KJ. Comparative safety and efficacy of cefdinir vs amoxicillin/clavulanate for treatment of suppurative acute otitis media in children. Pediatr Infect Dis J 2000; 19:S159–S165.
65. Adler M, McDonald PJ, Trostmann U, Keyserling C, Tack K. Cefdinir versus amoxicillin/clavulanate acid in the treatment of suppurative acute otitis media in children. Eur J Clin Microbiol Infect Dis 1997; 16:214–219.
66. Adler M, McDonald PJ, Trostmann U, Keyserling C, Tack K. Cefdinir vs. amoxicillin/clavulanic acid in the treatment of suppurative acute otitis media in children. Pediatr Infect Dis J 2000; 19:S166–S170.
67. Hedrick JA, Sher LD, Schwartz RH, Pierce P. Cefprozil versus high-dose amoxicillin/clavulanate in children with acute otitis media. Clin Ther 2001; 23: 193–204.
68. Dowell S. Treatment of otitis media. Pediatr Infect Dis J 2000; 19:1032–1033.
69. Klein JO. In vitro and in vivo antimicrobial activity of topical ofloxacin and other ototopical agents. Pediatr Infect Dis J 2001; 20:102–103; discussion 120-2.
70. Cameron GG, Pomahac AC, Johnston MT. Comparative efficacy of ampicillin and trimethoprim-sulfamethoxazole in otitis media. Can Med Assoc J 1975; 112:87–88.
71. Barnett ED, Teele DW, Klein JO, Cabral HJ, Kharasch SJ. Comparison of ceftriaxone and trimethoprim-sulfamethoxazole for acute otitis media. Greater Boston Otitis Media Study Group. Pediatrics 1997; 99:23–28.
72. Leiberman A, Leibovitz E, Piglansky L, et al. Bacteriologic and clinical efficacy of trimethoprim-sulfamethoxazole for treatment of acute otitis media. Pediatr Infect Dis J 2001; 20:260–264.
73. Hyde TB, Gay K, Stephens DS, et al. Macrolide resistance among invasive Streptococcus pneumoniae isolates. JAMA 2001; 286:1857–1862.
74. Dagan R, Leibovitz E, Fliss DM, et al. Bacteriologic efficacies of oral azithromycin and oral cefaclor in treatment of acute otitis media in infants and young children. Antimicrob Agents Chemother 2000; 44:43–50.
75. Flynn CA, Griffin G, Tudiver F. Decongestants and antihistamines for acute otitis media in children. Cochrane Database Syst Rev 2002; CD001727.

76. Sorum PC, Shim J, Chasseigne G, et al. Do parents and physicians differ in making decisions about acute otitis media? J Fam Pract 2002; 51:51–57.
77. Finkelstein JA, Davis RL, Dowell SF, et al. Reducing antibiotic use in children: a randomized trial in 12 practices. Pediatrics 2001; 108:1–7.
78. Hennessy TW, Petersen KM, Bruden D, et al. Changes in antibiotic-prescribing practices and carriage of penicillin-resistant Streptococcus pneumoniae: a controlled intervention trial in rural Alaska. Clin Infect Dis 2002; 34:1543–1550.
79. Perz JF, Craig AS, Coffey CS, et al. Changes in antibiotic prescribing for children after a community-wide campaign. JAMA 2002; 287:3103–3109.
80. Belongia EA, Sullivan BJ, Chyou PH, Madagame E, Reed KD, Schwartz B. A community intervention trial to promote judicious antibiotic use and reduce penicillin-resistant Streptococcus pneumoniae carriage in children. Pediatrics 2001; 108:575–583.
81. Paradise JL. Managing otitis media: a time for change. Pediatrics 1995; 96:712–715.
82. Dowell SF, Marcy SM, Phillips WR, Gerber MA, Schwartz B. Principles of judicious use of antimicrobial agents for pediatric upper respiratory tract infections. Pediatrics 1998; 101:163–165.
83. McCracken GH. Treatment of acute otitis media in an era of increasing microbial resistance. Pediatr Infect Dis J 1998; 17:576–579.
84. Schwartz B, Bell DM, Hughes JM. Preventing the emergence of antimicrobial resistance: A call for action by clinicians, public health officials, and patients. JAMA 1997; 278:944–945.
85. McCaig L, Besser R, Hughes J. Decline in pediatric antimicrobial drug prescribing among office-based physicians in the United States, 1989–1998. Abstracts of the 2000 IDSA Conference. New Orleans, LA: Infectious Disease Society of America, 2000.
86. Chaput de Saintonge DM, Levine DF, Savage IT, et al. Trial of three-day and ten-day courses of amoxycillin in otitis media. BMJ 1982; 284:1078–1081.
87. Meistrup-Larsen KI, Sorensen H, Johnsen NJ, Thomsen J, Mygind N, Sederberg-Olsen J. Two versus seven days penicillin treatment for acute otitis media. A placebo controlled trial in children. Acta Otolaryngol (Stockh) 1983; 96:99–104.
88. Bain J, Murphy E, Ross F. Acute otitis media: clinical course among children who received a short course of high dose antibiotic. BMJ 1985; 291:1243–1246.
89. Jones R, Bain J. Three-day and seven-day treatment in acute otitis media: a double-blind antibiotic trial. Journal of the Royal College of General Practitioners 1986; 36:356–358.
90. Hendrickse WA, Kusmiesz H, Shelton S, Nelson JD. Five vs. ten days of therapy for acute otitis media. Pediatr Infect Dis J 1988; 7:14–23.
91. Gooch WMR, Blair E, Puopolo A, et al. Effectiveness of five days of therapy with cefuroxime axetil suspension for treatment of acute otitis media. Pediatric Infect Dis J 1996; 15:157–164.
92. Kozyrskyi AL, Hildes-Ripstein GE, Longstaffe SEA, et al. Treatment of acute

otitis media with a shortened course of antibiotics: A meta-analysis. JAMA 1998; 279:1736–1742.
93. Hoberman A, Paradise JL, Burch DJ, et al. Equivalent efficacy and reduced occurrence of diarrhea from a new formulation of amoxicillin/clavulanate potassium (Augmentin) for treatment of acute otitis media in children. Pediatr Infect Dis J 1997; 16:463–470.
94. Cohen R, Levy C, Boucherat M, et al. Five vs. ten days of antibiotic therapy for acute otitis media in young children. Pediatr Infect Dis J 2000; 19:458–463.
95. Paradise JL. Short-course antimicrobial treatment for acute otitis media: not best for infants and young children. JAMA 1997; 278:1640–1642.
96. Schrag SJ, Pena C, Fernandez J, et al. Effect of short-course, high-dose amoxicillin therapy on resistant pneumococcal carriage: a randomized trial. JAMA 2001; 286:49–56.
97. Goldblatt EL. Efficacy of ofloxacin and other otic preparations for acute otitis media in patients with tympanostomy tubes. Pediatr Infect Dis J 2001; 20:116–119; discussion 120-2.
98. Tong MC, Woo JK, van Hasselt CA. A double-blind comparative study of ofloxacin otic drops versus neomycin-polymyxin B-hydrocortisone otic drops in the medical treatment of chronic suppurative otitis media. J Laryngol Otol 1996; 110:309–314.
99. Tutkun A, Ozagar A, Koc A, Batman C, Uneri C, Sehitoglu MA. Treatment of chronic ear disease. Topical ciprofloxacin vs topical gentamicin. Arch Otolaryngol Head Neck Surg 1995; 121:1414–1416.
100. Miro N. Controlled multicenter study on chronic suppurative otitis media treated with topical applications of ciprofloxacin 0.2% solution in single-dose containers or combination of polymyxin B, neomycin and hydrocortisone suspension. Otolaryngol Head Neck Surg 2000; 123:617–623.
101. Goldblatt EL, Dohar J, Nozza RJ, et al. Topical ofloxacin versus systemic amoxicillin/clavulanate in purulent otorrhea in children with tympanostomy tubes. Int J Pediatr Otorhinolaryngol 1998; 46:91–101.
102. Pichichero ME, Pichichero CL. Persistent acute otitis media: I. Causative pathogens. Pediatr Infect Dis J 1995; 14:178–183.
103. Doern GV, Heilmann KP, Huynh HK, Rhomberg PR, Coffman SL, Brueggemann AB. Antimicrobial resistance among clinical isolates of Streptococcus pneumoniae in the United States during 1999–2000, including a comparison of resistance rates since 1994–1995. Antimicrob Agents Chemother 2001; 45:1721–1729.
104. Jones RN, Pfaller MA, Jacobs MR, Appelbaum PC, Fuchs PC. Cefditoren in vitro activity and spectrum: a review of international studies using reference methods. Diagn Microbiol Infect Dis 2001; 41:1–14.

11

Acute Pharyngitis

James S. Tan
Northeastern Ohio Universities College of Medicine, Rootstown
and Summa Health System
Akron, Ohio, U.S.A.

Blaise L. Congeni
Northeastern Ohio Universities College of Medicine, Rootstown
and Children's Hospital Medical Center of Akron
Akron, Ohio, U.S.A.

Acute pharyngitis is among the most frequent illnesses seen in the primary care practice. It is characterized by the presence of increased redness and an exudate or ulceration in the pharynx or tonsil or a membrane that covers the tonsils [1]. Most cases of acute pharyngitis are viral and require only symptomatic treatment. This chapter will emphasize pharyngitis caused by group A beta hemolytic streptococcus (GABHS) because it is the most common bacterial etiology that can be treated with antibiotic therapy and it is associated with suppurative and nonsuppurative complications.

ETIOLOGY AND EPIDEMIOLOGY

Bacterial and viral agents known to be common etiologic agents of pharyngitis are listed in Table 1. GABHS is the most common bacterial agent

TABLE 1 Microbial Causes of Acute Pharyngitis

Pathogens	Syndrome or disease	Estimated percentage of cases
Viral		
Rhinovirus (100 types and 1 subtype)	Common cold	20
Coronavirus (3 or more types)	Common cold	>5
Adenovirus (types 3, 4, 7, 14, and 21)	Pharyngoconjunctival fever, acute respiratory disease	5
Herpes simplex virus (types 1 and 2)	Gingivitis, stomatitis, pharyngitis	4
Parainfluenza virus (type 1–4)	Common cold, croup	2
Influenzavirus (types A and B)	Influenza	2
Coxsackievirus A (types 2, 4–6, 8, and 10)	Herpangina	<1
Epstein-Barr virus	Infectious mononucleosis	<1
Cytomegalovirus	Infectious mononucleosis	<1
Human immunodeficiency virus type 1	Primary human immunodeficiency virus infection	<1
Bacterial		
Streptococcus pyogenes (group A β-hemolytic streptococci)	Pharyngitis and tonsillitis, scarlet fever	15–30
Group C and G β-hemolytic streptococci	Pharyngitis and tonsillitis; scarlatiniform rash	5
Mixed anaerobes	Vincent's angina	<1
Neisseria gonorhoeae	Pharyngitis	<1
Corynebacterium diphtheriae	Diphtheria	<1
Arcanobacterium haemolyticum	Pharyngitis, scarlatiniform rash	<1
Yersinia enterocolitica	Enterocolitis	<1
Yersina pestis	Plague	<1
Franciscella tularensis	Oropharyngeal form of tularemia	<1
Chlamydia		
Chlamydia pneumoniae	Pneumonia, bronchitis, and pharyngitis	Unknown
Chlamydia psittaci	Acute respiratory disease and pneumonia	<1
Mycoplasma		
Mycoplasma pneumoniae	Pneumonia, bronchitis, and pharyngitis	<1

Source: Ref. 2.

causing acute pharyngitis. It accounts for approximately 15–30% of cases in children and 5–10% in adults [2]. Much less common causes of acute pharyngitis are group C and group G streptococci. Both of these groups have been associated with isolated infections, endemic pharyngitis, and community outbreaks, especially among adults [3].

GABHS may occur as outbreaks or endemic infections and is most commonly found in children. Outbreaks are frequently associated with crowding in close quarters. Endemic spread is commonly through contact transmission.

PATHOGENESIS

The extracellular products and toxins produced by GABHS exert damage to the host. These products include streptolysin S and O, streptokinase, DNAase, protease, and pyrogenic exotoxins (erythrogenic toxin responsible for scarlet fever). M protein and M protein–like substances are part of the component of the bacterial cell wall. They contribute to the bacterial virulence by making the bacteria less recognizable by the immune system. There are more than 100 antigen-distinct types of M proteins. One of their functions is to resist destruction by the phagocytes. This resistance can be blocked by M protein–specific antibody.

CLINICAL MANIFESTATIONS

Pharyngitis is an infection that is ubiquitous: it attacks most people at least once a year. Most cases of viral pharyngitis are associated with an upper respiratory tract infection (nasopharyngitis). Nasopharyngitis has a prodrome that may include malaise, diaphoresis, fever, headache, and general aches and pains. Coryza and sore throat follow. Many infections will progress to produce a cough and/or laryngitis. Some viral infections produce predominantly coryza, others more pharyngitis, and others more cough or laryngitis.

In streptococcal pharyngitis, the clinical signs are not unique and are difficult to distinguish from those caused by other infections. The classic manifestations of pharyngitis—significant pharyngeal edema with or without exudates, strawberry tongue, tender cervical lymph nodes, abdominal pain, and rash—are frequently absent. In addition, the clinical findings differ among age groups; hence, young children, school-age children, and adults may have various presentations. Snow et al., in their position paper on the appropriate use of antibiotics in acute pharyngitis, stated that the most reliable predictors of streptococcal pharyngitis include tonsillar exudates, tender anterior cervical lymphadenopathy, history of fever, and absence of cough [4]. They recommended using the Centor criteria [5] in deciding whether to treat empirically without confirmation by culture or rapid antigen testing [4,6]. The sensitivity of the Centor criteria has not been determined. Bisno and Kaplan disagreed with the above recommendations of empiricism by Snow et al. and suggested that 60% of the patients would have no GABHS in the throat culture [7]. Steinhoff et al., in their study of Egyptian children between ages 2 and 13 years of age, showed that symptoms of exudative pharyngitis, tender lymph nodes, and observed temperature greater than 38.0°C each had a high specificity but low sensitivity [8]. Using a positive culture for GABHS as the confirmatory test, the sensitivity was only 12.1% when the combined presence of all of the following criteria were used [9]—namely, fever, pharyngeal exudates, tender enlarged palpable cervical lymph node, and pain on swallowing; however, the specificity was 93.9%. Based on the above findings, it appears that there is not enough information to support empiric treatment based on clinical criteria alone.

It should be emphasized that hoarseness, coughing, runny eyes, or coryza is rarely associated with group A streptococci in any age group [10]. Differentiating clinical features found in viral sore throats are as follows: the presence of fever, sore throat and ulcers in the posterior pharynx is suggestive of Coxsackievirus infection; measles should be considered when the patient has pharyngitis, conjunctivitis, rash, and Koplik spots; parainfluenza and influenza viruses are often associated with a particularly painful pharyngitis accompanied by cough and hoarseness; viral mononucleosis syndrome may also produce pharyngitis with or without exudates—hence, HIV, EBV, herpes simplex, and CMV can produce significant pharyngitis and tend to last longer than other viral causes of pharyngitis, but lymph nodes are generally only mildly tender or not tender at all; in herpes infection, gingivostomatitis may also be observed; rhinovirus, RSV, and coronavirus may present with pharyngitis symptoms but cervical lymphadenopathy and exudative pharyngitis are not found.

Streptococci belonging to Lancefield groups B, C, and G have been reported to cause pharyngitis as well [2,3,11–13]. Generally, the symptoms are milder.

Recurrent or chronic pharyngitis is not uncommon. Approximately 10–25% of patients with GABHS pharyngitis treated with penicillin have bacteriologic failures [14,15]. About half of the patients with GABHS in the pharynx are carriers and do not have active disease and may be misclassified as failures. These streptococcal carriers have no detectable clinical symptoms and no serologic response. Treatment is not necessary, because the carrier state presents no risk for rheumatic fever.

Other bacterial agents have been associated with acute pharyngitis: *Haemophilus influenzae* may cause pharyngitis and epiglottitis; *Corynebacterium diphtheriae* is associated with pharyngitis with membrane formation, also known as diphtheria; *Arcanobacterium haemolyticum*, formerly known as *Corynebacterium haemolyticum*, is also known to cause pharyngitis [16,17]. Some patients may present with scarlet fever–like skin rash. *Neisseria gonorrhoeae* [18] and *Yersinia enterocolitica* have also been associated with acute pharyngitis symptoms [19].

Chlamydia pneumoniae and *Mycoplasma pneumoniae* can cause pharyngitis, but generally will go on to cause cough also, often with wheezing and pneumonia [14,20]. Mixed anaerobic bacterial infections due to spirochetes and fusobacterium (Vincent's angina) cause occasional cases of acute pharyngitis [20].

LABORATORY DIAGNOSIS

Throat culture for the presence of group A streptococci in the throat continues to be the gold standard; however, it does not differentiate infection from the carrier state. False negatives may result from previous antibiotic administration or poor sampling technique such as failure to properly swab the posterior pharynx, tonsils, and tonsillar fossae. Rapid antigen testing using enzyme immunoassay (EIA) in the office provides timely diagnostic information within minutes and has been recommended by various investigators [21,22]. Most of these tests have a reported sensitivity between 60% and 90% and high specificity to indicate the presence of group A streptococcus infection [23]. The sensitivity of the rapid antigen test is proportional to the number of positive clinical criteria devised by Centor [24]. However, this test does not provide the bacteria for susceptibility testing, and similar to the culture, this rapid antigen test may be positive in carriers. In their cost-effective analysis of management of sore throats in children, Tsevat and Kotagal concluded that throat culture is the least costly strategy [25].

Serologic tests such as antistreptolysin O (ASO) and anti-deoxyribonuclease (anti-DNase B), although useful in confirming the presence of recent infection, are not useful in the acute management of sore throat.

For suspected viral causes of pharyngitis, serologic tests for antibody response to EBV and CMV, or rapid antigen tests for adenovirus, RSV, and parainfluenza may be ordered.

MANAGEMENT

Viruses are the most common cause of pharyngitis in the majority of patients. These individuals do not require antimicrobial therapy. GABHS is the most common cause of bacterial pharyngitis. Antimicrobial therapy should be limited to patients with a high probability of GABHS infection. The clinical signs and symptoms are not specific. The desired outcomes in the treatment of pharyngitis due to GABHS are to prevent nonsuppurative complications such as rheumatic fever and post-streptococcal glomerulonephritis, and to prevent suppurative complications (peritonsillar abscess, cervical lymphadenitis, and mastoiditis), to reduce clinical symptoms and discomfort, to allow the rapid resumption of usual activities, to reduce transmission to close contacts, and finally, to minimize the potential adverse effects from the use of inappropriate antimicrobial agents [14].

ANTIMICROBIAL THERAPY

Penicillin, given intramuscularly or orally, remains the drug of choice for streptococcal pharyngitis. Other agents such as macrolides (especially azithromycin) and cephalosporins have been shown to have at least equal efficacy in eradication of the streptococci in the pharynx, and more convenient dosing.

Since 1953, the American Heart Association has recommended, for oral treatment, a regimen of penicillin 3 to 4 times a day for 10 days to maximize eradication of bacteria [26]. Initial attempts to shorten the duration using penicillin V were not successful because of lower rates of microbiologic eradication [27–30]. The Dutch national guidelines appeared to have reached a compromise and advocated the treatment of streptococcal pharyngitis for 7 days [31,32]. The latest guideline from the IDSA and the *Red Book* continue to recommend a 10-day course of oral penicillin as first-line treatment [14,33].

Because compliance is a problem when penicillin is given 3 to 4 times a day, once-daily and twice-daily dosing have been investigated [34,35]. Once-daily dosing of penicillin was not effective, but twice-daily dosing of penicillin was found to be as effective as 3 to 4 doses a day [36]. In addition, once-daily oral amoxicillin appears to be just as effective [36]. The twice-daily regimen using penicillin V is presently recommended in the IDSA guideline and the *Red Book* [14,33].

Cephalosporins have an equal if not better efficacy compared with oral penicillin. Cefdinir, cefixime, cefpodoxime, ceftibuten, and cefuroxime have been shown to be effective [37–41]. For example, Pichichero reported a bacteriologic eradication rate of 90% for a 5-day course of cefpodoxime and 78% for a 10-day course of penicillin V [41]. However, a 10-day course of cefpodoxime had an even better eradication rate of 95%.

Erythromycin is traditionally recommended for a 10-day course. The new macrolides—namely, azithromycin and clarithromycin—have been shown to have equal eradication rate of GABHS with a 5-day course [42,43]. The apparent superiority of cephalosporins and azithromycin in microbiologic eradication compared to penicillins in studies may reflect their greater activity against the carrier state and not necessarily improved clinical activity [44]. However, at present the use of the shorter course has not been endorsed by IDSA or the *Red Book* [14,33].

GABHS has not been reported to have resistance to β-lactam agents; however, resistance to macrolides has been reported worldwide [45–52]. There are two major mechanisms of macrolide resistance, namely, target modification, and active efflux [53]. Interference of the binding of the macrolide to its target on the ribosomal RNA of the bacteria is caused by a ribosomal methylase encoded by an *ermAM* gene. This enzyme causes ribosomal conformation changes resulting in inducible or constitutive cross-resistance to macrolide, and lincomyin and streptogramin B (MLS_B phenotype) resistance. This modification results in high-level macrolide resistance (MIC $\geq$ 64 μg/mL). Active efflux is another mechanism of resistance. It is macrolide specific and is encoded by *mef* gene (M phenotype). Resistance to one macrolide—for example, erythromycin—means resistance to the other macrolides such as azithromycin, clarithromycin, and roxithromycin in either M or MLS_B phenotype. Strains of streptococcus with low-level resistance (MIC = 1–32 μg/mL) are commonly associated with the presence of *mefE* gene. These bacterial cells have an active pump that causes the macrolide to be moved from intracellular to extracellular sites. These bacteria are usually susceptible to clindamycin. Strains of streptococcus that have a high level of macrolide resistance are usually resistant to clindamycin. This resistance is commonly mediated by the *erm* gene. Although the outcome of macrolide treatment in those infected with macrolide-resistant streptococcal pharyngitis is uncertain, it is prudent not to treat these patients with macrolides. With increasing incidence of macrolide resistance worldwide, including the United States, the use of empiric macrolide treatment of pharyngitis should be reconsidered when the incidence of community macrolide resistance is high. Because of the increasing number of publications recommending not to do throat cultures and sensitivity but to rely on clinical presentation or rapid streptococcal scre en [4,54], it will become more difficult for a community to know the true incidence of local antimicrobial resistance pattern including macrolide resistance.

By adding a keto group to C3 of the macrolide molecule, a new group of compounds, ketolides, with better antibacterial activities and less susceptibility to MLS_B resistance has emerged [55]. The first member of this group that has been submitted for Food and Drug Administration approval is telithromycin. This antimicrobial agent has a very similar spectrum of activity as the new macrolides, including coverage of streptococci.

For penicillin-allergic patients, macrolides or clindamycin may be used if the local resistance pattern is known. Pending FDA approval, a ketolide may also be considered. The use of trimethoprim/sulfamethoxazole

TABLE 2 Antimicrobial Therapy for Group A Streptococcal Pharyngitis (Recommendation based mainly on the Practice Guideline from the Infectious Diseases Society [14])

Route	Antimicrobial agent, dosage	Duration	Rating[a]
First-line treatment recommendation for treatment of acute pharyngitis and prevention of acute rheumatic fever			
Oral	Penicillin V	10 days	A-II
	Children: 250 mg b.i.d. or t.i.d.	10 days	A-II
	Adolescents and adults: 250 mg t.i.d. or q.i.d.	10 days	C-III
	Adolescents and adults: 500 mg b.i.d.		
Oral	Amoxicillin	10 days	A-II
	Adolescents and adults: 750 mg once daily		
Oral	First-generation cephalosporins	10 days	See below[b]
	Cephalexin and cephradine		
	Children: 25–50 mg/kg/d in 2 divided doses		
	Adolescents and adults: 500 mg b.i.d.		
	Cefadroxil		
	Children: 30 mg/kg once daily		
	Adolescents and adults: 1 g once daily		
IM	Benzathine penicillin G 1.2 million units	1 dose	A-II
	Benzathine penicillin G 600,000 units (children <27 kg)	1 dose	A-II
	Mixtures of benzathine and procaine penicillin (dose should be based on benzathine penicillin)	1 dose	B-II

For patients allergic to penicillin			
Oral	Erythromycin (dose varies with formulation) Erythromycin ethylsuccinate 40 mg/kg/day (maximum 1.5/day) t.i.d.[c] Erythromycin estolate 20–240 mg/kg/day (maximum 1.5 g/day) t.i.d.[c] Erythromycin stearate 1 g per day in 2 or 4 divided doses[d]	10 days	A-II
Oral	First-generation cephalosporins (should not be used to treat patients with immediate-type hypersensitivity to β-lactam antibiotics)	10 days	A-II
The following shorter course recommendations are not endorsed by IDSA, WHO, and the Redbook [26,54,60]			
Oral	Cefadroxil	5 days	
Oral	Cefixime	5 days	
Oral	Cefdinir	5 days	
Oral	Cefpodoxime	5 days	
Oral	Azithromycin 500 mg first day followed by 250 mg daily for 4 more days	5 days	
Oral	Clarithromycin 500 mg daily	5 days	

[a] Rating based on strength of evidence: A = Good evidence to support a recommendation for use; B = Moderate evidence to support a recommendation for use; C = Poor evidence to support a recommendation; D = Moderate evidence to support a recommendation against use; E = Good evidence to support a recommendation against use. Rating based on quality of evidence: I = Evidence from ≥1 properly randomized controlled trial; II = Evidence from >1 well-designed clinical trial, without randomization; from cohort or case-controlled analytic studies (preferably from >1 center); from multiple time-series; or from dramatic results of uncontrolled experiments.

[b] Not rated by IDSA, however, it stated that amoxicillin has equal efficacy [36].

[c] Based on WHO recommendation [10].

[d] Based on Bisno [2].

and tetracycline is not recommended because of the high percentage of resistance.

Most failure in eradicating streptococci with penicillin may be due to (1) antibiotic noncompliance, (2) reinfection, (3) local bacteria interference, (4) penicillin tolerance, (5) presence of β-lactamase–producing oral microflora, or (6) existence of carrier state [1]. Brook et al. observed that following penicillin therapy, children harbor β-lactamase–producing bacteria in the oropharynx. The β-lactamase produced by these organisms may protect GABHS from the action of penicillin and other β-lactams [56]. Therefore, agents that are not susceptible to β-lactamase action, such as clindamycin or amoxicillin/clavulanate, may be more effective [15,57].

Similarly, in patients with multiple episodes of pharyngitis occurring over months or years, a 10-day course of therapy with clindamycin 20–30 mg/day in three divided doses (in children) or 600 mg/day in two to four divided doses; or amoxicillin/clavulanate 40 mg/kg/day in three divided dose or 500 mg in two divided doses may be advisable because this combination has been shown to yield high rates of eradication of streptococci from the pharynx. For parenteral therapy, single dose of 1.2 million unites of benzathine intramuscularly with or without rifampin 20 mg/kg/day or 300 mg twice daily for 4 days [14].

ANCILLARY MANAGEMENT AND PREVENTION

For a patient with a single episode of streptococcal pharyngitis, a further work-up of the patient or the family is not recommended after antimicrobial therapy unless there is concern about proven recurrent GABHS pharyngitis; routine repeat throat swabs for cultures of the patients or asymptomatic members of the family is not recommended. There is no credible evidence to suggest that the family pet may be the source of GABHS [58]. Children with GABHS pharyngitis should complete a full 24 hours of antibiotic therapy before returning to school or day-care [59].

The IDSA guidelines detailed six indicators of quality of care [14]: (1) obtain microbiologic testing (i.e., throat cultures or rapid antigen detection assay) in patients suspected of having GABHS; (2) patients with positive acute pharyngitis plus a positive test for GABHS should be treated with one of the antimicrobial regimens recommended (see Table 2); (3) antimicrobial therapy should be withheld or discontinued in patients with negative microbiological test results for GABHS; (4) microbiologic testing is not needed in asymptomatic patients who have received an adequate course of antimicrobial therapy; (5) microbiologic testing is not necessary for asymptomatic family contacts of patients of GABHS infection; and (6) avoid prescribing continuous long-term antimicrobial prophylaxis to prevent recurrent episodes of acute pharyngitis except in patients with acute rheumatic fever.

REFERENCES

1. Brook I. Pharyngotonsillitis, peritonsillar, retropharyngeal, and parapharyngeal abscesses, and epiglottitis. In: Tan JS, ed. Expert Guide to Infectious Diseases. Philadelphia: American College of Physicians, 2002:354–375.
2. Bisno AL. Acute pharyngitis. N Engl J Med 2001; 344(3):205–211.
3. Cimolai N, Elford RW, Bryan L, et al. Do the β-hemolytic non-group A streptococci cause pharyngitis? Rev Infect Dis 1988; 10:587–601.
4. Snow V, Mottur-Pilson C, Cooper RJ, Hoffman JR. Principles of appropriate antibiotic use for acute pharyngitis in adults. Ann Intern Med 2001; 134:506–508.
5. Centor RM, Witherspoon JM, Dalton HP, Brody CE, Link K. The diagnosis of strep throat in adults in the emergency room. Med Decis Making 1981; 1:239–246.
6. Cooper RJ, Hoffman JR, Bartlett JG, et al. Principles of appropriate antibiotic use for acute pharyngitis in adults: background. Ann Intern Med 2001; 134:509–517.
7. Bisno AL, Kaplan EL. Appropriate use of antibiotics: pharyngitis. Ann Intern Med 2002; 136:489–490.
8. Steinhoff MC, El Khaleck MKA, Khallaf N, Hamza HS, El Ayadi A, Orabi A. Effectiveness of clinical guidelines for the presumptive treatment of streptococcal pharyngitis in Egyptian children. Lancet 1997; 350:918–921.
9. Memorandum from a Joint/ISFC meetingStrategy for controlling rheumatic fever/ rheumatic heart disease with emphasis on primary prevention. Bull World Health Organ 1995; 73:583–587.
10. Division of Drug Management and Policies. (World Health Organization). WHO Model Prescribing Information. Drugs used in the treatment of streptococcal pharyngitis and prevention of rheumatic fever, 1999.
11. Turner JC, Hayden FG, Lobo MC, et al. Epidemiologic evidence for Lancefield group C β-hemolytic streptococci as a cause of exudative pharyngitis in college students. J Clin Micribiol 1997; 35:1–4.
12. Turner JC, Hayden FG, Kiselica D, et al. Association of group C β-hemolytic streptococci with endemic pharyngitis among college students. JAMA 1990; 264:2644–2647.
13. Gerber MA, Randolph MF, Martin NJ, et al. Community-wide outbreak of group G streptococcal pharyngitis. Pediatrics 1991; 87:598–603.
14. Bisno AL, Gerber MA, Gwaltney JM Jr, Kaplan EL, Schwartz RH. Practice guideline for the diagnosis and management of group A streptococcal pharyngitis. Clin Infect Dis 2002; 35:113–125.
15. Kaplan EL, Johnson DR. Evaluation of group A streptococci from the upper

respiratory tract by amoxicillin with clavulanate after oral penicillin V treatment failure. J Pediatr 1988; 113:400–403.

16. Karpathios T, Drakonaki S, Zervoudaki A, et al. Arcanobacterium haemolyticum in children with presumed streptococcal pharyngotonsillitis or scarlet fever. J Pediatr 1992; 121:735–737.
17. Miller RA, Brancato F, Holmes KK. Corynebacterium hemolyticum as a cause of pharyngitis and scarlatiniform rash in young adults. Ann Intern Med 1986; 105:867–872.
18. Wiesner PJ, Tronca E, Bonin P, Pederson AHB, Holmes KK. Clinical spectrum of pharyngeal gonococcal infection. N Engl J Med 1973; 288:181–185.
19. Cover TL, Aber RC. Yersinia eneterocolitica. N Engl J Med 1989; 321:16–24.
20. Gwaltney JMJ, Bisno AL. Pharyngitis. In: Mandell GL, Bennett JE, Dolin R, eds. Principles and Practice of Infectious Diseases. New York: Churchill Livingstone, 2000:656–662.
21. Webb KH, Needham CA, Kurtz SB. Use of a high-sensitivity rapid strep test without culture confirmation of negative results. J Fam Pract 2000; 49:34–38.
22. Ebell MH, Smith MA, Barry HC, Ives K, Carey M. Does this patient have strep throat? JAMA 2000; 284:1918–2912.
23. Thomson RBJ. Use of microbiology laboratory tests in the diagnosis of infectious diseases. In: Tan JS, ed. Expert Guide to Infectious Diseases. Philadelphia: American College of Physicians, 2002:1–4.
24. Dimatteo LA, Lowenstein SR, Brimhall B, Reiquam W, Gonzales R. The relationship between the clinical features of pharyngitis and the sensitivity of a rapid antigen test: evidence of spectrum bias. Ann Emerg Med 2001; 38:648–652.
25. Tsevat J, Kotagal U. Management of sore throats in children. A cost-effective analysis. Arch Pediatr Adolescent Med 1999; 153:681–688.
26. Bisno AL, Gerber MA, Gwaltney JM Jr, Kaplan EL, Schwartz RH. Diagnosis and management of group A streptococcal pharyngitis: a practice guideline. Infectious Diseases Society of America. Clin Infect Dis 1997; 25:574–583.
27. Gerber MA, Randolph MF, Chanatry J, Wright LL, DeMeo K, Kaplan EL. Five vs ten days of penicillin V therapy for streptococcal pharyngitis. Am J Dis Child 1987; 141:224–227.
28. Schwartz RH, Wientzen RI, Pedreira F, Feroli EJ, Melia GW, Guandolo VL. Penicillin V for group A streptococcal pharyngotonsillitis: a randomized trial of seven vs ten days therapy. JAMA 1981; 246:1790–1795.
29. Stromberg A, Schwan A, Cars O. Five versus ten days treatment of group A streptococcal pharyngotonsillitis: a randomized controlled clinical trial with phenoxymethylpenicillin and cefadroxil. Scand J Infect Dis 1988; 20:37–46.
30. Martin JM, Green M, Barbadora KA, Wald ER. Erythromycin-resistant group A streptococci in schoolchildren in Pittsburgh. N Engl J Med 2002; 346: 1200–1206.
31. De Melker AA, van Balen FAM. Antimicrobial treatment of upper respiratory tract infections from the Dutch perspective. Int J Antimicrob Agents 1997; 9:43–48.
32. Zwart S, Sachs APE, Ruijs GJHM, Gubbels JW, Hoes AW, de Melker RA.

Penicillin for acute sore throat: randomised double blind trial of seven days versus three days treatment or placebo in adults. BMJ 2000; 320:150–154.
33. Committee on Infectious Diseases AAoP. Group A streptococcal infection. 2000 Red Book. 25th ed. Montvale, NJ: Medical Economics, 2001:526–536.
34. Kaufhold A, Pharyngitis Study Group. Randomized evaluation of benzathine penicillin V twice daily versus potassium penicillin V three times daily in the treatment of group A streptococcal pharyngitis. Eur J Clin Microbiol Infect Dis 1995; 14:92–98.
35. Krober M, Weir MR, Themelis NJ, van Hamont JE. Optimal dosing interval for penicillin treatment of streptococcal pharyngitis. Clin Pediatr 1990; 29:646–648.
36. Lan AJ, Colford JM Jr. The impact of dosing frequency on the efficacy of 10-day penicillin or amoxicillin therapy for streptococcal tonsillopharyngitis: a meta-analysis. Pediatrics 2000; 105:e19.
37. Mehra S, van Moerkerke M, Welck J, et al. Short course therapy with cefuroxime axetil for group A streptococcal tonsillopharyngitis in children. Pediatr Infect J Dis 1998; 17:452–457.
38. Adam D, Hostalek U, Troster K. 5-day therapy of bacterial pharyngitis and tonsillitis with cefixime: comparison with 10-day treatment with penicillin V [in German]. Cefixime Study Group. Klin Padiatr 1996; 208:310–313.
39. Boccazzi A, Tonelli P, DeAngelis M, Bellussi L, Passali D, Careddu P. Short course therapy with ceftibuten versus azithromycin in pediatric streptococcal pharyngitis. Pediatr Infect Dis J 2000; 19:963–967.
40. Tack KJ, Henry DC, Gooch WM, Brink DN, Keyserling CH. Five-day cefdinir treatment for streptococcal pharyngitis. Cefdinir Study Group. Antimicrob Agents Chemother 1998; 42:1073–1075.
41. Pichichero ME, Gooch WM, Rodriguez W, et al. Effective short-course treatment of acute group A β-hemolytic streptococcal tonsillopharyngitis. Arch Pediatr Adolescent Med 1994; 148:1053–1060.
42. McCarty JM, Hedrick JA, Gooch WM. Clarithromycin suspension vs. penicillin V suspension in children with streptococcal pharyngitis. Adv Ther 2000; 17: 14–26.
43. Still JG. Management of pediatric patients with group A beta-hemolytic Streptococcus pharyngitis: treatment options. Pediatr Infect J Dis 1995; 14(suppl A): S57–S61.
44. Shulman ST, Gerber MA, Tanz RR. Streptococcal pharyngitis: the case for penicillin therapy. Pediatr Infect J Dis 1994; 13:1–7.
45. Malbruny M, Nagai K, Coquemont M, et al. Resistance to macrolides in clinical isolates of Streptococcus pyogenes due to ribosomal mutations. J Antimicrob Chemother 2002; 49:935–939.
46. Seppala J, Klaukka T, Vuopio-Varkila J, et al. The effect of changes in the consumption of macrolide antibiotics on erythromycin resistance in group A streptococci in Finland. Finnish Study Group for Antimicrobial Resistance. N Engl J Med 1997; 337:441–446.
47. Cornaglia G, Ligozzi M, Mazzariol A, Valentini M, Orefici G, Fontana R.

Rapid increase of resistance to erythromycin and clindamycin in Streptococcus pyogenes in Italy, 1993–1995. The Italian Surveillance Group for Antimicrobial Resistance. Emerging Infect Dis 1996; 2:330–342.
48. Cha S, Lee H, Lee K, Hwang K, Bae S, Lee Y. The emergence of erythromycin-resistant Streptococcus pyogenes in Seoul, Korea. J Infect Chemother 2001; 7:81–86.
49. Alos JI, Aracil B, Oteo J, Torres C, Gomez-Garces JL. High prevalence of erythromycin-resistant, clindamycin/miocamycin-susceptible (M-phenotype) Streptococcus pyogenes; results of a Spanish multicentre study in 1998. Spanish Group for the Study of Infection in the Primary Health Care Setting. J Antimicrob Chemother 2000; 45:605–609.
50. Yan JJ, Wu HM, Huang AH, Fu HM, Lee CT, Wu JJ. Prevalence of polyclonal mefA-containing isolates among erythromycin-resistant group A streptococci in Southern Taiwan. J Clin Microbiol 2000; 38:2475–2479.
51. Perez-Trallero E, Urbieta M, Montes M, Ayestaran I, Marimon JM. Emergence of Streptococcus pyogenes strains resistant to erythromycin in Gipuzkoa, Spain. Eur J Clin Microbiol Infect Dis 1998; 17:25–31.
52. Palavecino EL, Riedel I, Barrios X, et al. Prevalence and mechanisms of macrolide reistance in Streptococcus pyogenes in Santiago, Chile. Antimicrob Agents Chemother 2001; 45:339–341.
53. Johnson NJ, de Azavedo JC, Kellner JD, Low DE. Prevalence and characterization of the mechanisms of macrolide, lincosamide, and streptogramin resistance in isolates of Streptococcus pneumoniae. Antimicrob Agents Chemother 1998; 42:2425–24256.
54. American Academy of Pediatrics. Group A streptococcal infections. In: Pickering, LK, ed. Red Book 2000: Report on the Committee on Infectious Diseases. Elk Grove Village, IL: American Academy of Pediatrics, 2000:526–536.
55. Douthewaite S. Structure-activity relationships of ketolides vs. macrolides. Clin Microbiol Infect 2001; 7(suppl 3):11–17.
56. Brook I, Gober AE. Emergence of β-lactamase-producing aerobic and anaerobic bacteria in the oropharynx of children following penicillin chemotherapy. Clin Pediatr 1984; 23:338–341.
57. Brook I, Hirokawa R. Treatment of patients with a history of recurrent tonsilitis due to group A β-hemolytic streptococci. Clin Pediatr 1985; 24:331–335.
58. Wilson KS, Maroney SA, Gander RM. The family pet as an unlikely source of group A beta-hemolytic streptococcal infection in humans. Pediatr Infect Dis J 1995; 14:372–375.
59. Snellman LW, Stang HJ, Stang JM, Johnson DR, Kaplan EL. Duration of positive throat cultures for group A streptococci after initiation of antibiotic therapy. Pediatrics 1993; 91:1166–1170.

12

Acute Exacerbations of Chronic Obstructive Pulmonary Disease

Antonio Anzueto and Sandra G. Adams
The University of Texas Health Science Center at San Antonio
and The South Texas Veterans Health Care System
San Antonio, Texas, U.S.A.

INTRODUCTION

The diagnosis and treatment of acute exacerbations of chronic obstructive pulmonary disease (AECOPD) is controversial. In this chapter, we will review (1) the epidemiology of this condition; (2) the etiology—many patients with AECOPD are thought to have a combination of viral and bacterial infections, which contribute to their exacerbation; bacterial organisms are isolated more commonly after viral infections in patients with chronic obstructive pulmonary disease (COPD), and the role that bacterial infections play in AECOPD remains a very controversial topic; (3) the use of diagnostic procedures; (4) the efficacy of antibiotics; (5) clinical parameters used to stratify patients' severity; (6) the different groups of antibiotics that can be used; and (7) other therapies, including bronchodilators. We will summarize the current literature with special emphasis on the safety and efficacy of the commonly prescribed drugs.

EPIDEMIOLOGY

Chronic obstructive pulmonary disease (COPD) comprises several clinical conditions, including chronic bronchitis, emphysema, and asthma, that often coexist. Patients are prone to exacerbations under conditions that are usually associated with increased breathlessness; often, there is increase in cough, which may be productive of mucoid or purulent sputum and malaise. These symptoms may produce significant decrement in quality of life. Acute exacerbation of chronic bronchitis (AECOPD) is the classic term that is used in the literature to describe a heterogeneous group of patients, and it involves a wide variety of management recommendations. The interpretation of data in the literature is confusing and difficult to generalize due to the many differences in these populations. The term AECOPD is used throughout this section to describe the typical patient who is over the age of 40 years and has obstructive lung disease by PFTs [1]. Although many of these patients also have chronic bronchitis (as previously defined clinically as presence of persistent productive cough for more than three consecutive months in two consecutive years) [2], they are not required to have a chronic, productive cough to be included in this current definition of AECOPD.

Acute exacerbations are the common cause of morbidity and mortality in this patient population [3,4]. Figure 1A shows the prevalence by age of chronic bronchitis and Figure 1B shows the prevalence by age of emphysema in the United States. COPD currently accounts for approximately 110,00 deaths per year, making it—after heart disease, cancer, and stroke—the fourth leading cause of death (Fig. 1C). It has been estimated that by the year 2020, it will be the third cause of death [5–7]. The cost of treating acute exacerbation COPD is very high, not only because of the economic impact but also because of the increase in morbidity and early mortality. COPD in the United States annually accounts for 16,000,367 office visits, 500,000 hospitalizations, and $18 billion in direct health care cost [5,6,8]. Despite treatment with antibiotics, bronchodilators, and corticosteroids, up to 28% of patients discharged from the emergency department with acute exacerbations have recurrent symptoms within 14 days [9], and 17% relapse and require hospitalization [10]. Significant numbers of hospitalized patients with acute exacerbations have modifiable risk factors, including influenza vaccination, oxygen supplementations, smoking, and occupational exposures. The ability to identify patients who are at risk for relapse should improve decisions about hospital admissions and follow-up appointments. Several investigators have confirmed that relapse is more likely among patients who have lower pretreatment or posttreatment FEV_1, those who receive more bronchodilator treatments or corticosteroids during visits, and those who have higher rates of previous relapse. These factors can provide clinical guidance on the basis of

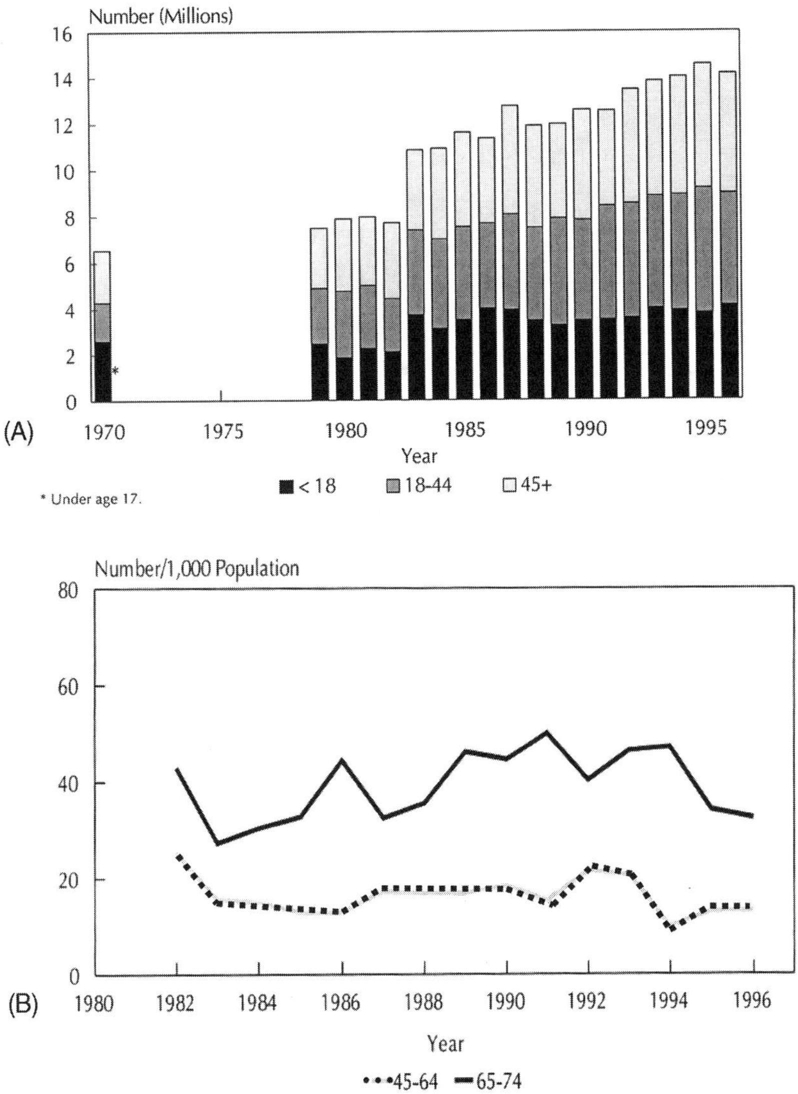

Figure 1 (A) Prevalence of chronic bronchitis by age in the United States from 1970 to 1996; (B) prevalence of emphysema by age in the United States from 1970 to 1996; (C) and death due to COPD 1998. (From Refs. 3 and 5.)

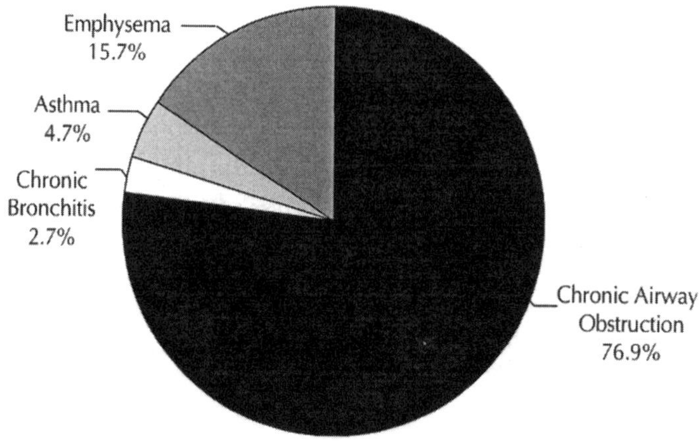

(C) Total Deaths = 114,381 (100%)

FIGURE 1 Continued.

identifying predictors of failure, but it has a very poor sensitivity and specificity. For example, the definition "return to the emergency department of less than 14 days after initial presentation" has a sensitivity of 57% and a specificity of 72% [11].

Several studies have tried to identify the risk factors associated with mortality with acute exacerbation. The Study to Understand Prognosis and Preferences for Outcomes and Rates of Treatment (SUPPORT) enrolled 1016 patients who had severe acute exacerbation of COPD at hospital admission [12] due to respiratory infections, including pneumonia (48%), congestive heart failure (26%), worsening respiratory failure due to lung cancer (3.3%), pulmonary emboli (1.4%), and pneumothorax (1%). The 180-day mortality rate was 33% and the 2-year mortality rate was 49%. Significant predictors of mortality include acute physiology and chronic health evaluation (APACHE III) score [13], body mass index, age, functional status 2 weeks prior to admission, lower ratio of PO_2 to F_IO_2, congestive heart failure, serum albumen level, cor pulmonale, lower activities of daily living scores, and lower scores on the Duke Activity Status Index. This study also reported that only 25% of patients were both alive and able to report a good, very good, or excellent quality of life 6 months after discharge.

In another large prospective cohort study of patients who were admitted to intensive care units with COPD-related respiratory failure [14], the in-hospital mortality rate, 23.8%, was predicted by number of hospital days before transfer to intensive care unit, and the non/respiratory component of the APACHE III score. A separate analysis to identify true predictors of 180-day mortality included acute physiological score, age, and hospital days before transfer to intensive care unit. A separate analysis to identify true predictors of 180-day mortality included acute physiological score, old age, and more hospital days before transfer to intensive care unit. Activities of daily living were also significant predictors of univariate analysis [14].

In a recent report, a cohort of 101 patients with moderate to severe COPD (mean FEV_1 41.9% predicted), which was closely followed up for 2.5 years, increased dyspnea and colds at onset of exacerbation were associated with prolonged recovery times. Recovery was incomplete in a significant proportion of COPD exacerbations [15]. Patients with frequent exacerbations (median 3 to 8/year) experience significantly worse quality of life, as measured by the St George's Respiratory Questionnaire. Factors that predict frequent exacerbations were the number of exacerbations in the previous year and a history of bronchitic symptoms (cough and sputum production), though lung function was not related [16].

ETIOLOGY

Although respiratory infections are assumed to be the main risk factors for exacerbation of COPD, other factors are also involved [17]. Health education of patients, smoking cessation, pulmonary rehabilitation, good nutritional status, and early medical intervention are all considered helpful in preventing exacerbations [18,19]. Table 1 summarizes other known risk factors for exacerbation of COPD.

During bacterial infection in AECOPD, a variety of microorganisms have been shown to be associated with these exacerbations, including *Haemophilus influenzae, Haemophilus parainfluenzae, Moraxella catarrhalis,* and *Streptococcus pneumoniae* [20]. It has been described that a minority of these patients have atypical pathogens such as *Mycoplasma pneumoniae* and *Chlamydia pneumoniae*, but because of limitations with the diagnosis, the true prevalence of these organisms is not known (Fig. 2).

There have been several recent studies demonstrating that patients with the most severe obstructive lung disease have a significantly higher prevalence of gram-negative organisms such as Enterobacteriaceae and *Pseudomonas* species [21–23]. One of the first groups of investigators to report these findings was Eller et al. [21], who evaluated sputum cultures from 112 inpatients with AECOPD. Sixty-four percent of patients with an FEV_1 of 35% of less predicted versus only 30% of those with FEV_1 of 50% or more (P = 0.016) had evidence of gram-negative organisms. The most commonly isolated organisms (from these patients with severe obstructive lung disease) included Enterobacteriaceae and *Pseudomonas* species, *Proteus vulgaris,*

TABLE 1 Differences in Characteristics Based on Antibiotic Selection

	First-line	Second-line	Third-line
Days of therapy	8.9 ± 3.3	8.3 ± 2.3	7.5 ± 2.5[a]
Weeks between AECOPD	17.1 ± 22	22.7 ± 30	34.3 ± 35.5[a]
14-day failure rate (N = 36)	19%	16%	7%[a]
Hospitalizations (% of total failures)	53%	14%	8%[a]
Cost per episode (US $)	942 ± 2173	563 ± 2296	542 ± 1946

Data are presented in percentages (as indicated) and otherwise in mean ± standard deviation.
[a] $P \leq 0.05$ third-line versus first-line.
Source: Ref. 48.

Serratia marcescens, *Stenotrophomonas maltophilia*, and *Escherichia coli*. Miravitlles et al. [22] recently published a study with similar results that also supported these findings. These investigators evaluated the relationship between FEV_1 and the isolation of diverse pathogens in the sputum of 91 patients with COPD who presented with type 1 (severe) or type 2 (moderate) symptoms of AECOPD. Patients were separated into groups by FEV_1 ($\geq$50% versus <50% predicted). There were significantly larger numbers of *H. influenzae* and *P. aeruginosa* in the group with FEV_1 less than 50% predicted ($P < 0.05$). In contrast, there were significantly larger numbers of non–potentially pathogenic microorganisms in the group with FEV_1 of 50% or more ($P < 0.05$). These authors also performed a multivariate analysis with logistic regression and found that *H. influenzae* was cultured significantly

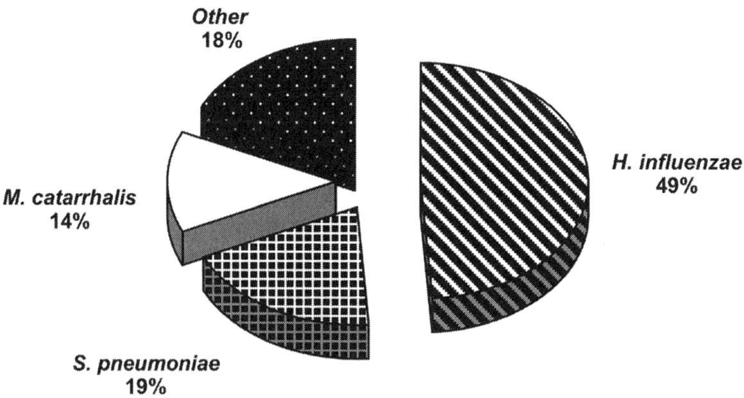

FIGURE 2 Most frequent microorganisms isolated in acute exacerbation of COPD.

more commonly in patients who were actively smoking (odds ratio [OR] 8.2, confidence interval [CI] 1.9–43) and whose FEV_1 was less than 50% predicted (OR 6.85, CI 1.6–52). *P. aeruginosa* was also cultured significantly more frequently in those with poor lung function, FEV_1 less than 50% (OR 6.6, CI 1.2–124) (Fig. 3).

Pathogenesis

Although the role of smoking in COPD is well established, tobacco smoking is not the sole factor responsible. Airway infection has been suggested as an important cause for the worsening of this disease. COPD is an inflammatory disease and exacerbations are associated with an additional increase in airway inflammation (measured in sputum), especially in exacerbations associated with bacterial infection [24]. Murphy and Sethi [25] proposed the vicious cycle hypothesis (Fig. 4). This hypothesis proposes that airway damage from chronic infection or colonization occurs in these patients when the bacteria cause the host to continuously release inflammatory mediators. Persistent infection results in lung inflammation and, as a consequence, lung function progressively decreases. The host response to infection is inflammatory cells that are found in sputum both in stable COPD and during acute exacerbations. These cells are primarily neutrophils and macrophages. Inflammatory mediators that are of significance in attracting these inflammatory cells to the airway are interleukin-6 (IL-6), interleukin-8 (IL-8), tumor necrosis factor–α (TNF-α) and leukotrine B4 (LTB4). End products of these inflammatory cells that mediate airway damage are neutrophil elastase (NE) and matrix

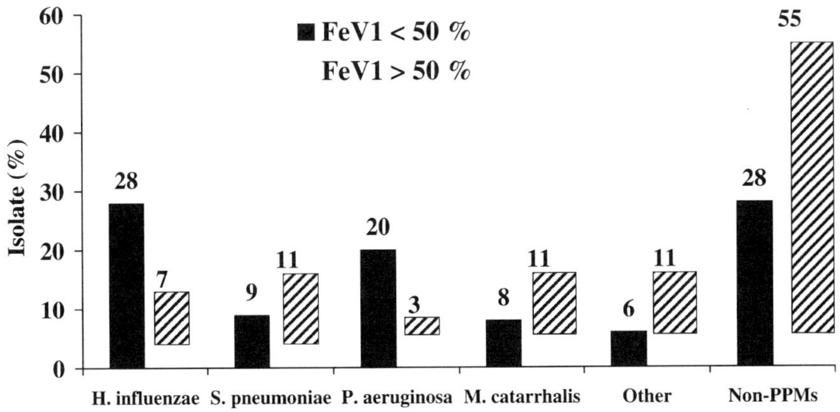

FIGURE 3 The relation of pathogens isolated in patients with COPD and the severity of lung function (FeV_1). (From Ref. 22.)

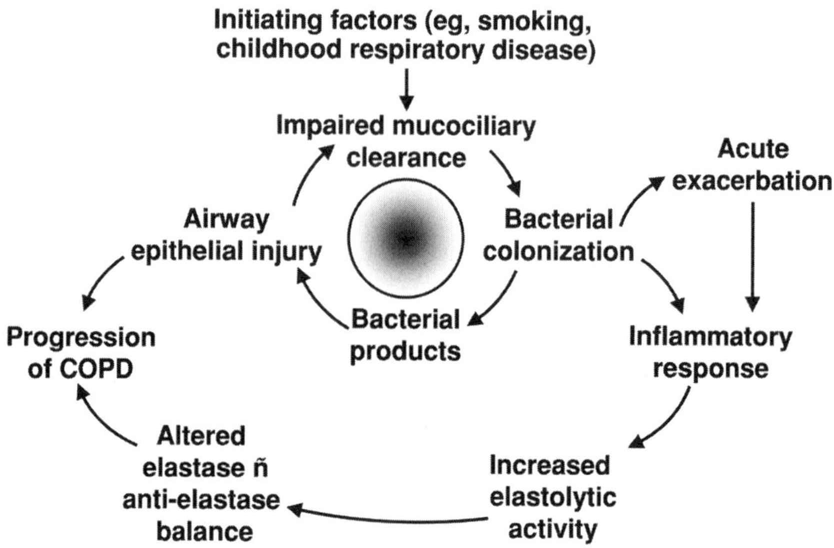

FIGURE 4 Vicious cycle hypothesis—relationship of lung injury and persistent infection. (From Ref. 25.)

metalloproteinases (MMPs). Sputum inflammatory markers increase substantially with during AECOPD and therefore could represent useful objective indicators of response to treatment [26]. Recent observations have shown that the inflammation in COPD extends beyond the lung, and increased inflammatory markers are measurable in the serum, and further increase with exacerbations [27,28].

Patients with recurrent AECOPD suffer with significant morbidity associated with their condition. Kanner et al. [29] evaluated the loss of lung function of 5887 smokers with obstruction to airflow by PFTs (FEV_1/FVC <70%, with FEV_1 of 55%–90%) in the Lung Health Study. These investigators grouped all of the self-reported illnesses that occurred in this population together as lower respiratory infections (LRI), which included episodes of bronchitis, pneumonia, influenza, and chest colds. Several important findings were reported in this study: (1) continuous smokers had significantly more LRI than sustained quitters ($P = 0.0003$), which was due to an increased number of LRI with time in continuous smokers, but not in sustained quitters, (2) continuous smokers with chronic bronchitis had LRI rates that were 158–189% of those without chronic bronchitis ($P < 0.001$), (3) LRI rates increased with time in continuous smokers whether or not they reported chronic bronchitis ($P = 0.008$), and (4) in continuous smokers with 1.5 LRI or more per year, over 44% of the mean predicted loss in lung function (measured by FEV_1) per year was attributed to these acute exacerbations. Therefore, evaluation of the participants of this study with mild COPD demonstrated that self-reported LRI were associated with significant long-term adverse effects on lung function in those who continued to smoke cigarettes. This study provides further evidence supporting the "vicious cycle hypothesis."

Diagnostic Procedures

A recent evidence-base analysis has summarized the best available information related to the use of diagnostic tests in AECOPD [30,31]. These reviews concluded that data on the utility of most diagnostic tests are limited. However, chest radiography and arterial blood gas sampling seem useful, whereas acute spirometry does not. On the basis of observational studies of patients with AECOPD treated in emergency departments or hospitals, chest radiographs are a useful diagnostic test. One study evaluated 685 patients: chest radiographs showed a 16% abnormality rate, mainly the presence of infiltrates consistent with pneumonia [32]. In another prospective cohort study of 128 hospital admissions for asthma or COPD, 21% of patients had a change in management that was prompted by the chest radiograph. Most patients had new pulmonary infiltrate or evidence of congestive heart failure [33]. We recommend that in patients with AECOPD, if they are evaluated in an emergency room and/or require hospitalization, a chest radiograph be obtained in order to rule out any other abnormalities. Although the CT scan is more sensitive, and therefore potentially valuable in evaluation of the acute exacerbation, there are no randomized, controlled trials on which to base a recommendation.

Spirometric assessment at presentation or during treatment of acute exacerbation is not useful in judging the severity or guiding the management of the patient. Peak expiratory flow rate and FEV_1 are correlated ($r = 0.84$; $P < 0.001$), but the FEV_1 showed no significant correlation with PO_2 and only weak correlation with PCO_2 [10]. At this time, there are no data to support the routine use of peak flow meters or FEV_1 assessment as useful in the management of COPD exacerbations; therefore, we do not recommend it.

TREATMENT WITH ANTIBIOTICS

The specific etiology of AECOPD is difficult to determine in an outpatient office setting on the basis of symptoms and signs. Sputum studies, although they can be potentially useful, have significant limitations in routine use mainly related to the delay in obtaining the results, cost, and lack of sensitivity and specificity. Recent treatment guidelines for AECOPD reflect the lack of evidence-base data to provide specific recommendations for the use of antibiotics [30,31]. The GOLD guideline, which was a NHLBI/WHO initiative for COPD recommend antibiotic choices on the basis of local sensitivity patterns of the most common pathogens associated with AECOPD, but did not provide any specific guidelines [1].

There have been a number of clinical trials examining the use of antibiotics in the treatment of AECOPD [17–20]. Many of the earlier studies showed either no benefit, or minimal benefit, when antibiotics were prescribed. Some of the more recent publications, including a recent meta-analysis [34], demonstrated a benefit of antibiotics during an acute exacerbation, but not in preventing exacerbations. In 1987, Anthonisen et al. [35] reported the results of a large-scale placebo-controlled trial designed to determine the effectiveness of antibiotics in the treatment of AECOPD. In this study, 173 patients with chronic bronchitis were followed for 3.5 years, during which time they had 362 exacerbations. This study finally brought some conformity to the definition of AECOPD and was the first widely accepted classification for the severity of presenting symptoms. Patients who are classified in the severe range of "AECOPD" include those with all three clinical symptoms (of increased shortness of breath, increased sputum production, and a change in sputum purulence) at initial presentation. The patients were randomized to either antibiotics or placebo in a double-blind, crossover fashion. Three oral antibiotics were used (chosen by the primary physician) for 10 days: amoxicillin, trimethoprim-sulfamethoxazole (co-trimoxazole), and doxycycline. Approximately 40% of all exacerbations were type 1 (severe), 40% were type 2 (moderate), and only 20% were type 3 (mild). Patients with the most severe exacerbations (type 1) received a significant benefit from antibiotics, whereas there was no significant difference between antibiotic and placebo in patients who had only one of the defined symptoms (type 3). Overall, the antibiotic-treated patients showed a more rapid improvement in peak flow, a greater percentage of clinical successes, and a smaller percentage of clinical failures than those who received placebo. In addition, the length of illness was 2 days shorter for the antibiotic-treated group. The major criticisms of this study were that no microbiology test was performed and that all antibiotics were assumed to be equivalent.

Allegra et al. [36] found significant benefit with the use of amoxicillin-clavulanate acid (Augmentin®) therapy compared with placebo in patients with severe disease. Patients who received this antibiotic exhibited a higher success rate (86.4% vs. 50.3% in the placebo group, $P < 0.01$) and a lower frequency of recurrent exacerbations. In 1995, Saint et al. [34] published the results of a meta-analysis examining the role of antibiotics in the treatment of AECOPD (Fig. 5). These investigators analyzed nine randomized, placebo-

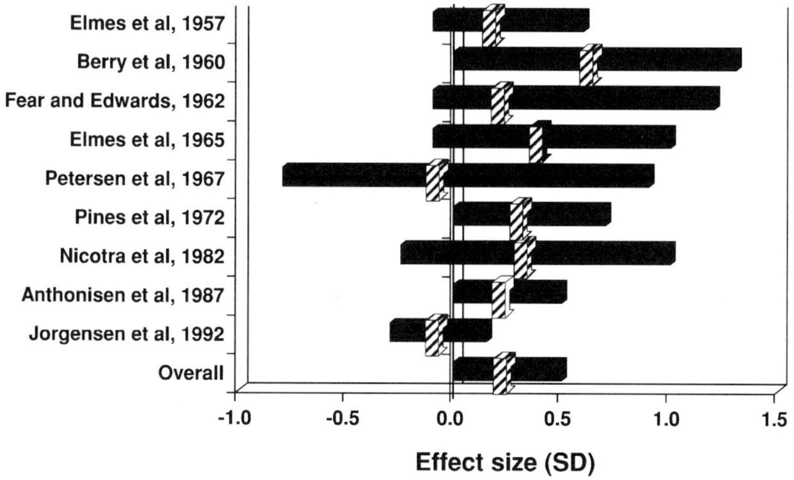

FIGURE 5 Effect sizes (mean differences in outcome divided by the pooled standard deviation) in nine studies of the use of antibiotics for exacerbations of COPD. Horizontal lines denote 95% confidence intervals. The data indicate a significant improvement due to antibiotic therapy. (From Ref. 34.)

controlled trials published between 1957 and 1992. Unfortunately, there was not a single common outcome reported in each of the studies included in this analysis. However, some outcomes that were available for analysis and comparison in many of the studies include (1) the mean number of days of illness, (2) the overall symptom score, and (3) the changes in peak expiratory flow rate. Using this form of analysis, there was an overall, statistically significant benefit for the antibiotic-treated patients. Analysis of the studies that provided data on expiratory flow rates, noted an improvement of 10.75 L/min in the antibiotic-treated groups. The authors conclude that this antibiotic-associated improvement is likely to be clinically significant; particularly in patients with low baseline peak flow rates and limited respiratory reserve.

There are additional potential benefits of antibiotic therapy for patients with AECOPD. Antibiotics can reduce the burden of bacteria in the airway [37]. Bronchoscopic studies, using sterile protected specimen brush, have demonstrated that approximately 25% of stable COPD patients are colonized (usually $\leq 10^3$ organisms) with potentially pathogenic bacteria [38,39]. However, a much larger percentage (50–75%) [39–42] of patients with acute exacerbations have potentially pathogenic microorganisms in addition to significantly higher concentrations (frequently $\geq 10^4$ organisms) of bacteria in the large airways. Because treatment with appropriate antibiotics significantly decreases the bacterial burden (and frequently eradicates the organisms that are sensitive) at the 72-hour follow-up bronchoscopy, it is speculated that the proper choice of antibiotic reduces the risk of progression to more severe infections, such as pneumonia [42]. The eradication of bacteria by antibiotics is thought to break the vicious circle of infection (i.e., lung destruction leading to progression of the lung disease). Another study that reports similar findings of gram-negative pathogens is a prospective, randomized, double-blind, placebo-controlled trial evaluating the use of ofloxacin in 90 consecutive patients with AECOPD who required mechanical ventilation, which was recently published by Nouira et al. [43]. These authors demonstrated a significant number of gram-negative organisms (including *E. coli*, *P. mirabilis*, and *P. aeruginosa*) in their study population of patients with severe AECOPD. In addition to supporting the findings of the previously reported studies, this trial demonstrated that treating these pathogens is important for improving outcomes in this high-risk population. The antibiotic-treated group had a significantly lower in-hospital mortality rate (4% vs. 22%, $P = 0.01$) and significantly reduced length of stay in the hospital (14.9 vs. 24.5, $P = 0.01$) compared with the placebo group. In addition, the patients receiving ofloxacin were less likely to develop pneumonia than those on placebo, especially during the first week of mechanical ventilation (mean $\pm$ standard deviation: 7.2 ± 2.2 days [range 4–11] vs. 10.6 ± 2.9 days [range 9–14], $P = 0.04$ by log-rank test).

If the use of antibiotics to treat AECOPD has all the potential benefits discussed, does it matter which agent is chosen? In the Anthonisen et al. study [35], the assumption was made that all of the antibiotics were equivalent; thus, the specific agent prescribed was not considered important. Moreover, most of the recently published antibiotic trials were designed to compare a new antibiotic with an established compound for the purpose of new product registration and licensing. Equivalence is the desired outcome of such trials, and therefore the agent chosen for comparison is not considered important. In addition, these trials frequently include patients with poorly defined disease severity (often without any obstructive lung disease) and acute illness of minor severity. Another problem with interpreting the literature on AECOPD is the large variation in time frame (48 hours to 28 days) that is used to assess patients for relapse (or the resolution of symptoms) [43–46]. "Relapse" can most clearly be defined as treatment failure resulting in a return visit due to persistent or worsening symptoms [44]. However, many of these patients do not seek medical care, despite persistent symptoms. The published relapse rates for patients with AECOPD range from 17% to 32%. Despite the problems with many of the published antibiotic trials, there are some retrospective trials that emphasize the importance of choosing the correct antibiotic for treatment of patients with AECOPD. A recent retrospective study of outpatients with documented COPD, conducted at our institution, evaluated the risk factors for therapy failure at 14 days after an acute exacerbation [47]. The participating patients had a total of 362 exacerbations over an 18-month period. One group received antibiotics (270 visits) and the second group (92 visits) did not. Both groups had similar demographics and severity of underlying COPD. The patients' mean age was 67 ± 10 years ($\pm$SD), 100% of patients had a greater than 50 pack-per-year smoking history, and 45% were active smokers. Based on the American Thoracic Society's COPD classification, 39% had mild disease, 47% moderate disease, and 14% severe disease. The majority (95%) with severe symptoms at presentation (type 1) received antibiotics, versus only 40% with mild symptoms. The overall relapse rate (defined as a return visit with persistent or worsening symptoms within 14 days) was 22%. After an extensive multivariate analysis, the major risk factor for relapse was lack of antibiotic therapy (32% vs. 19%, $P < 0.001$ compared to the antibiotic-treated group). The type of antibiotic used was also an important variable associated with the 14-day treatment failure. Patients treated with amoxicillin had a 54% relapse rate compared with only 13% for the other antibiotics ($P < 0.01$). Furthermore, treatment with amoxicillin resulted in a higher incidence of failure, even when compared with those who did not receive antibiotics ($P = 0.006$) (Fig. 6). Other variables, such as COPD severity, types of exacerbation, prior or concomitant use of corticosteroids, and current use of chronic oxygen therapy were not significantly associated with the 14-day relapse. This study

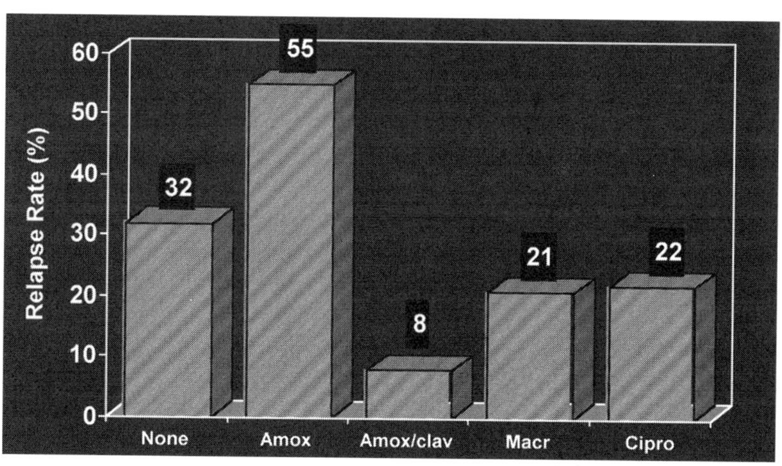

FIGURE 6 Acute exacerbations of chronic obstructive pulmonary disease: 14-day relapse rates after treatment with or without antibiotics. (From Ref. 47.)

showed that the use of antibiotics was associated with a significantly lower rate of therapy failure. In contrast to Anthonisen's data [27], our data show that antibiotics are beneficial regardless of the severity of AECOPD (i.e., those with mild AECOPD still gained benefit from treatment with antibiotics). Furthermore, the patients who received antibiotics and whose treatment failed within 14 days had a significantly higher rate of hospital admissions than those who did not receive antibiotics. Although there may be many explanations for these treatment failures, the most likely is that the pathogens were resistant to amoxicillin.

Recently Destache et al. reported the impact of antibiotic selection, antimicrobial efficacy, and related cost in AECOPD [48]. This study was a retrospective review of 60 outpatients from a pulmonary clinic of a teaching institution who had the diagnoses of COPD and chronic bronchitis. The participating patients had a total of 224 episodes of AECOPD requiring antibiotic treatment. The antibiotics were arbitrarily divided into three groups: first-line (amoxicillin, co-trimoxazole, erythromycin, and tetracycline), second-line (cephradine, cefuroxime, cefaclor, cefprozil), and third-line (amoxicillin-clavulanate, azithromycin, and ciprofloxacin) agents. The failure rates were significantly higher (at 14 days) for the first-line compared with the third-line agents (19% vs. 7%, $P < 0.05$). When compared with those who received the first-line agents, the patients treated with the third-line agents had significantly longer time between exacerbations (34 weeks vs. 17 weeks $P < 0.02$), overall fewer hospitalizations (3/26 [12%] vs. 18/26 [69%] patients, $P < 0.02$), and considerably lower total cost ($542 vs. $942, $P < 0.0001$) (Table 1).

Based on the results of these studies, in addition to widespread reports of increasing antimicrobial resistance to the common pathogens isolated in patients with AECOPD, appropriate antibiotic selection is extremely important. Therefore, it is not only essential to treat these patients with antibiotics, it is actually critical to choose the appropriate one.

END POINT FOR THE TREATMENT OF AECOPD

Conventional end points for efficacy of antibiotics treatment in AECOPD include symptom and bacteriological resolution measured at 2 to 3 weeks after the treatment was started. Most of these end points rely solely on the subjective report of symptom improvement. These end points have been used for drug registration purposes but lack clinical relevance [49]. It has been suggested by several reports that the infection-free interval (i.e., the time to next episode of AECOPD) may be a more suitable end point in this patient population [50–52]. Recently, Wilson et al. [53] showed a significant increase in the infection-free interval in patients with AECOPD treated with gemifloxacin as compared with clarithromycin. This end point may reflect the ability of the antibiotic to achieve adequate bacteriologic eradication of the airway. This study showed that this end point was associated with decreased hospitalization rates, so this can be translated into cost savings, improved quality of life, and potentially slower progression of the underlying airway obstruction.

CLINICAL PARAMETERS FOR STRATIFYING PATIENTS INTO RISK GROUPS

Since the morbidity and mortality rates of AECOPD are high, many investigators have attempted to describe characteristics that could be used to risk-stratify patients with AECOPD. Some studies have validated a few of the following risk factors for treatment failure; others show different factors associated with increased risk of relapse. Despite these conflicting studies [43–46], the clinical parameters that are implicated as possible risk factors for treatment failure in AECOPD include (1) older age (>65 years old), (2) severe underlying COPD ($FEV_1 < 35\%$ predicted), (3) frequent exacerbations (≥ 4/year), (4) more severe symptoms at presentation (Anthonisen et al. [27] types 1 [severe] and 2 [moderate]), (5) comorbidities (especially cardio/pulmonary disease, but also congestive heart failure, diabetes mellitus, chronic renal failure, and chronic liver disease), and (6) prolonged history of COPD (>10 years).

Some authors state that many infections in AECOPD are noninvasive and will eventually resolve spontaneously [30,31]. However, because the costs of failed treatment remain high, better strategies are needed for the treatment of these exacerbations. Niederman et al. recently reported that age older than 65 years and inpatient treatment are the major determinants contributing to the overall cost of AECOPD [54]. The cost was estimated at $1.2 billion for the 207,540 inpatients 65 years of age and older versus only $452 million for 5.8 million outpatients in the same age group. The mean length of stay was longer, and the in-hospital mortality rate was significantly higher for those older than 65 years of age (Table 2).

Based on the concept of risk-stratification of patients by clinical parameters, a target approach for the treatment of AECOPD has been proposed by the Canadian Respiratory Society [20]. This group developed a classification for patients presenting with symptoms of acute bronchitis using the following factors: (1) number and severity of acute symptoms, (2) age, (3) severity of airflow obstruction (measured by FEV_1), (4) frequency of exacerbations, and (5) history of comorbid conditions. This symposium suggested that patients could be adequately profiled into different categories. Acute bronchitis (group 1) includes healthy people without previous respira-

TABLE 2 Cost of Treatment of Acute Exacerbation of Chronic Bronchitis

Age group	Hospital costs (millions of dollars)	Outpatient costs (millions of dollars)
≥65 years	1141	34
<65 years	408	14
All ages	1549	48

Source: Ref. 54.

tory problems. "Simple" AECOPD (group 2) includes those patients whose age is less than 65 years, those who have had 4 or fewer exacerbations per year, those with minimal or no impairment in lung function (by pulmonary function tests), *and* those without any comorbid conditions. "Complicated" AECOPD (group 3) includes patients older than 65 years, those with FEV_1 less than 50% predicted, *or* those with 4 or more exacerbations per year.

TABLE 3 Patient Profiles from the Canadian Chronic Bronchitis Guidelines

Acute bronchitis (group 1)
- Healthy people without previous respiratory problems

"Simple" chronic bronchitis (group 2)
- Age ≤65 years old *and*
- <4 exacerbations per year *and*
- Minimal or no impairment in pulmonary function *and*
- No co-morbid conditions

"Complicated" chronic bronchitis (group 3)
- Age >65 years old *or*
- FEV_1 <50% predicted *or*
- ≥4 exacerbations per year

"Complicated" chronic bronchitis with co-morbid illness (group 4)
- Above criteria for group 3, plus:
  - Congestive heart failure *or*
  - Diabetes *or*
  - Chronic renal failure *or*
  - Chronic liver disease *or*
  - Other chronic disease

Source: Ref. 20.

Finally, "complicated" AECOPD with associated comorbid illnesses (group 4) includes patients with congestive heart failure, liver disease, diabetes, or chronic renal failure (Table 3).

CHARACTERISTICS OF THE "IDEAL" ANTIBIOTIC FOR THE TREATMENT OF AECOPD

Characteristics of the "ideal" antibiotic that are important to consider when choosing these agents for patients with AECOPD include:

1. Significant activity against the most common pathogens isolated in patients with AECOPD and whether there are substantial gaps in the coverage of these organisms.

2. Adequate coverage of the most likely pathogens in patients with AECOPD based on patient profiles that define the most likely spectrum of etiologic pathogens. As previously described, this is especially important in patients with severe underlying obstructive lung disease, who are more commonly infected with gram-negative organisms than those with mild COPD. In addition, patients with risk factors for a more complicated course (those in group 3 ["complicated"] and group 4 ["complicated" with comorbid conditions]) should be prescribed antibiotics with adequate coverage for the usual pathogens in AECOPD, as well as for gram-negative organisms. Our recommendations from patient stratification and treatment are summarized in Table 4.

3. Susceptibility of the antimicrobial agent to the likely pathogens in AECOPD. There is an increasing prevalence of *H. influenzae* and *M. catarrhalis* that produce bacterial enzymes that inactivate traditional β-lactam antibiotics [55,56]. In addition, a growing number of these organisms are resistant to many of the antibiotics that are currently available [57]. It is important to know which of the mechanisms of resistance of these agents are clinically important for the treatment of AECOPD. It is also critical to know the local resistance rates of these microorganisms prior to prescribing a specific antibiotic for therapy. Please see Chapter 2 for a thorough discussion on resistance of these organisms to many of the antibiotics that are commonly used to treat AECOPD.

4. Good penetration into sputum, bronchial mucosa, and epithelial lining. The goal of antimicrobial therapy is to deliver the appropriate drug to the specific site of infection. In AECOPD, the bacteria are predominantly found in the airway lumens, along the mucosal cell surfaces, and within the mucosal tissue. Various antibiotic classes exhibit markedly different degrees of penetration into the tissues and secretions of the respiratory tract (Table 5) [58,59]. Although there are no studies that demonstrate the concentration

TABLE 4 Our Recommendations for Antibiotic Therapy

Category	Probable pathogen	Oral therapy
Acute bronchitis (group 1)	Viral	Symptomatic
"Simple" AECOPD (group 2)	*Haemophilus* spp. (*H. influenzae*), *M. catarrhalis*, *S. pneumoniae*, Atypical organisms (possibly)	Doxycycline *or* newer macrolide (azithromycin/clarithromycin) *or* newer cephalosporins
"Complicated" AECOPD (groups 3 & 4)	As above, with the possible addition of *Pseudomonas* spp, Enterobacteriaceae, and other gram-negative organisms	Fluoroquinolones[a] Amoxicillin-Clavulanate

[a] If at risk for *Pseudomonas* infection, use ciprofloxacin.
Source: Refs. 20 and 126.

of antibiotics at one particular intrapulmonary site is better than any other site, the concentrations of antibiotics in sputum, bronchial mucosa, epithelial lining fluid, and macrophages are thought to be predictive of clinical efficacy (Table 5). These antibiotics exhibit a concentration-effect relationship.

5. Easy to take with minimal side effects. In a recent survey, patient compliance was demonstrated to be significantly improved when medications were given once or twice a day, rather than three or more times [60]. In addition, shorter courses of therapy (<14 days) were associated with better compliance. Of the patients interviewed, more than 80% stated a preference for once- or twice-daily dosing and more than 54% admitted to noncompliance with the prescribed regimen (taking the antibiotic sporadically or not completing the full course).

6. Cost-effective, considering more than acquisition cost of antibiotics. It is clear that multiple factors should be considered when selecting an antibiotic for the treatment of AECOPD, in addition to just the acquisition cost. These other economic end points are important when defining the cost-effectiveness of any particular antibiotic, such as: (1) the cost of treatment failures (including the need for further antibiotics and the days of lost work), (2) the amount saved by preventing hospitalization, (3) the duration of disease-free intervals, and (4) the development of antimicrobial resistance. Although there is not adequate cost-effectiveness data currently available to support the use of any particular antibiotic, the importance of these factors is

TABLE 5 Percentage of Serum Concentrations of Antibiotic Achieved in Sputum, Epithelial Lining Fluid (ELF), and Bronchial Mucosa

Antibiotic	Sputum	ELF	Bronchial mucosa
PCN			
Amoxicillin		13%	40%
Piperacillin	10–14%		27–40%
Ceph			
Cefixime			34–36%
Ceftazidime	2–15%		51%
Cefuroxime	14%		
Doxycycline	18%		
Macrolides			
Erythromycin	5%	114%	
Azithromycin		3200–5700%	
Clarithromycin		3900–10,300%	
Quinolones			
Ciprofloxacin	200%	140–185%	240%
Gatifloxacin	125%	170%	170%
Sparfloxacin		1250%	360%
Moxifloxacin		870%	170%
Aminoglyc			
Amikacin	10%		
Gentamicin	20%		
Tobramycin		50%	

PCN = Penicillin. Ceph = Cephalosporins. Aminoglyc = Aminoglycosides.
Source: Refs. 58 and 59.

supported by the retrospective studies (previously discussed) by Destache et al. [48] and Niederman et al. [54].

INDIVIDUAL ANTIBIOTIC AGENTS

The six characteristics described above for selecting the "ideal" antibiotic are outlined below for each of the major classes of antibiotics prescribed for the treatment of AECOPD.

Penicillins

This group of antibiotics was one of the first classes used for treatment of patients with AECOPD. The medications in this class include amoxicillin and amoxicillin/clavulanate (Augmentin®). Amoxicillin was previously one of the most commonly prescribed antibiotics for AECOPD, but the development of β-lactamase by *H. influenzae* and *M. catarrhalis* currently limits their usefulness. Amoxicillin has been shown to be effective therapy (in early studies) for those with mild AECOPD; however, it is not currently recommended unless the local resistance rates are monitored closely and are very low. Dosing of this agent is t.i.d. or q.i.d., which also decreases its usefulness due to compliance issues. In contrast, Augmentin is dosed b.i.d. or t.i.d., has a much wider spectrum of activity (including gram-negative organisms), and is effective against β-lactamase–producing organisms. Despite limited data available regarding the activity of this antibiotic on penicillin-resistant *S. pneumoniae* [57], Augmentin is most useful for patients with AECOPD in Groups 3 and 4 [20]. The pharmacokinetically enhanced formulation of amoxicillin/clavulanate (2000/125 mg) was designed to achieve high levels of amoxicillin over the dosing duration to eradicate isolates of *S. pneumoniae* with amoxicillin MICs of 4 μg/ml or less. A recent study showed that this combination was at least as effective clinically and bacteriologically and was as well tolerated as levofloxacin in the treatment of AECOPD [61]. The side effects of these two agents are similar and primarily involve gastrointestinal symptoms (especially diarrhea). The acquisition cost of amoxicillin is very low; however, the overall cost is probably much higher in some institutions due to the significant numbers of treatment failures [47]. The currently approved FDA drugs include amoxicillin 500–750 mg t.i.d. or q.i.d. and Augmentin® 125/500 mg t.i.d. or 500/875 mg b.i.d. × 10 days; the 125/2000 formulation is pending approval by the FDA.

Cephalosporins

Despite their relatively poor activity and suboptimal respiratory pharmacokinetics, the first-generation cephalosporins have been used extensively in the management of AECOPD [17]. Two antibiotics from this group (cephalexin and cefaclor) have been shown to be ineffective in severe infections and are probably not the best choice for the treatment of AECOPD. The newer cephalosporins (especially third-generation) may have some advantages of improved efficacy and safety and may be used as an option for the treatment of patients in group 2 [20]. FDA-approved drugs from this group include a 10-day course of cefprozil (Cefzil®) 250/500mg b.i.d., cefuroxime axetil (Ceftin®) 250/500 mg b.i.d., loracarbef (Lorabid®) 400 mg b.i.d., cefixime (Suprax®) 200/400 mg b.i.d. or q.d., cefpodoxime proxetil (Vantin®) 100/200 mg b.i.d., and ceftibuten (Cedex®) 400 mg q.d.

Trimethoprim-Sulfamethoxazole

This antibiotic became very popular in the late 1970s, most likely due to enhanced compliance with the b.i.d. regimen. Many of the early comparison studies against cephalosporins and amoxicillin did not demonstrate any significant differences; however, these trials were performed prior to the marked increases in antimicrobial resistance [17]. Currently, the penicillin-resistant strains of *S. pneumoniae* and other common pathogens are highly resistant to these drugs [20,56]. There have also been concerns about the toxicities of trimethoprim-sulfamethoxazole, including acute renal insufficiency and the risk of severe skin reactions (particularly in elderly patients). Because many of the new agents available today have fewer side effects as well as potentially enhanced activity, there has been a dramatic decline in the usefulness of this compound.

Tetracycline

This group of antibiotics includes a naturally occurring molecule (tetracycline) and semi-synthetic molecules (doxycycline and minocycline). Several of the early studies with tetracycline (performed in the 1960s and 1970s) concluded that these antibiotics were effective in the treatment of AECOPD. However, the more recent studies have shown that tetracycline has poor activity against *H. influenzae* as well as many of the other commonly isolated organisms in these patients. In contrast, doxycycline (Vibramycin®/Doryx®) has been found to be especially active against *M. catarrhalis*, and minocycline is more active against *H. influenzae* and *S. pneumoniae*. Other advantages of these semisynthetic antibiotics include better oral absorption and a prolonged half-life, which allows for twice-daily dosing [62]. The sputum concentrations are lower for doxycycline than for minocycline. Despite these differences in the pharmacokinetic properties, Maesen et al. [63], in a randomized, double-blind prospective study, demonstrated that there were no significant differences in the response rates between doxycycline and minocycline in the treatment of AECOPD. The most important limitation to the widespread use of this class of drugs is the increasing emergence of microbial resistance. This class of antibiotics is useful in patients who have allergies to other medications and for treatment of patients in group 2 ("simple" AECOPD).

Macrolides

Erythromycin, a macrolide derived from *Streptomyces,* inhibits RNA-dependent protein synthesis by reversibly binding to the 50S ribosomal subunit of susceptible microorganisms. Azithromycin, clarithromycin, and dirithromycin are semisynthetic derivatives of erythromycin (Table 6). These "advanced" macrolides have significantly better tissue penetration and pharmacokinetics as a result of structural modifications [64,65]. The in vitro activity of macrolides against respiratory pathogens is shown in Table 7 [64,66]. Of the macrolides, erythromycin has the lowest in vitro activity

TABLE 6 Pharmacokinetic Comparison of Macrolides

Variable	Erythromycin	Clarithromycin	Azithromycin	Dirithromycin
Intravenous form	Yes	No	Yes	No
Gastrointestinal intolerance	Yes	No	No	No
Feeding affects absorption	Yes	No	No	No
Drug interactions (hepatic c P450)	Yes	Yes	No	No
Prolonged tissue level	No	Yes	Yes	Yes

c P450 = cytochrome P450 system.
Source: Ref. 64.

against *H. influenzae*, whereas azithromycin has the highest. Due to the predominance of this organism in AECOPD, erythromycin should not be used to treat this condition.

As previously discussed, the rates of antimicrobial resistance have increased significantly over the past few years. The patterns of macrolide resistance are complex and involve at least two mechanisms [67]. One involves an alteration in ribosomal targets (ribosomal methylase [*ermAM*]) of the bacteria, which is known to result in true clinical resistance. The second mechanism is more prevalent (>75%) and involves the organism actively pumping the macrolide out of the cell (macrolide efflux [*mefE*] mutant strains). Waites et al. found that resistance of *S. pneumoniae* strains to clindamycin predicted a high level of resistance to clarithromycin, mediated

TABLE 7 Microbiology: In Vitro Activity of Respiratory Pathogens to Macrolides (MIC_{90})

	Erythromycin	Clarithromycin	Azithromycin	Dirithromycin
Streptococcus pneumoniae				
PCN S	0.016–0.25	≤0.008–0.12	0.016–0.06	N/A
PCN R	>32	>8	>32	N/A
H. influenzae	2–32	2–16	0.5–4.0	8–16
Moraxella catarrhalis	0.06–2.0	0.03–1.0	≤0.016–0.05	0.25–1.0
Chlamydia pneumoniae	0.25	<0.1	0.25–2	0.5

PCN S = Penicillin-sensitive strains. PCN R = Penicillin-resistant strains.
Data: MIC_{90} = minimum concentration to inhibit 90% of isolates. Ranges are due to the different values reported.
Source: Refs. 64 and 66.

by *ermAM* (true resistance) [68]. However susceptibility to clindamycin in the strains that were resistant to clarithromycin indicated a lower level of efflux-based resistance, mediated by *mefE*. It is not known if these *mefE* strains actually result in clinical resistance, because treatment failures are uncommon in patients treated with these "advanced" macrolides [69,70]. Gotfried et al. [69] found no significant differences in the clinical outcomes of patients at their institution who were infected with macrolide-resistant *S. pneumoniae* compared with macrolide-sensitive strains. In another publication, Gottfried [70] examined several studies involving the eradication rate of *S. pneumoniae* in patients treated for AECOPD. Although approximately 15% of the pneumococcal isolates were resistant to clarithromycin in vitro, the bacteriologic eradication rate was between 91% and 93% for the clarithromycin-treated patients. Therefore, the reported increases in the prevalence of in vitro resistance of *S. pneumoniae* to the "advanced" macrolides do not appear to be associated with a proportional rise in the rate of clinical failures.

The dosing of the macrolides varies among the different antibiotics. Erythromycin must be given every 6–8 hr (usually for a 10-day course). Both azithromycin and dirithromycin are given only once a day and are effective with dosing regimens of 3 to 5 days [64,70]. Direct comparison of azithromycin (3-day course) and clarithromycin (10-day course) showed no difference in response rate or adverse reactions [71]. A recent study with the new extended-release preparation of clarithromycin has been shown to be effective when given once a day for 5 to 7 days [72]. In general, macrolides are safe antibiotics. Treatment with erythromycin often results in significant gastrointestinal symptoms, including nausea, vomiting, abdominal cramps, and diarrhea. This drug also has significant interaction with drugs that are metabolized in the liver via the P450 enzyme system [64]. The newer-generation macrolides are better tolerated, have minimal gastrointestinal symptoms, and fewer drug interactions. However, clarithromycin has a distinctive taste perversion that is less common with the extended-release preparation.

FDA-approved macrolides to treat AECOPD include erythromycin 250/500 mg every 6–8 hr × 10 days; clarithromycin (Biaxin®) 250/500 mg b.i.d. × 10 days, or two 500 mg tablets once daily for 7 days; azithromycin (Zithromax®) 500 mg on day 1, then 250 mg q.d. on days 2–5; and dirithromycin (Dynabac®) 500 mg a day × 5 days.

Fluoroquinolones

The fluoroquinolones are extremely potent and offer broad-spectrum coverage against the most common organisms in patients with AECOPD (Table 8). Some of the more recently developed quinolones have enhanced activities against many gram-positive species (i.e., *S. pneumonia*), atypical pathogens

TABLE 8 Fluoroquinolone Activity Against Common Respiratory Pathogens (MIC_{90})

Pathogen	Ciprofloxacin	Levofloxacin	Gatifloxacin	Moxifloxacin
S. pneumoniae	0.5–3.13	1.0–3.13	0.06–1	0.03–0.25
PCN S	2	1–2	0.06–0.25	0.06–0.12
PCN R	2	1–2	0.06–0.25	0.06–0.12
H. influenzae	0.015–4.0	0.03	0.004–0.016	0.008–0.06
M. catarrhalis	0.015–0.1	0.06–0.12	0.004–0.03	0.004–0.03
C. pneumoniae	2–4	0.25	0.06–0.5	0.06

PCN S = Penicillin-sensitive strains. PCN R = Penicillin-resistant strains.
Data: MIC_{90} = minimum concentration required to inhibit 90% of isolates. Ranges are due to the different values reported.
Source: Refs. 56,57,78, and 79.

(i.e., *Chlamydia pneumoniae, Mycoplasma pneumoniae,* and *Legionella pneumophila*), and anaerobes [73]. The quinolones have a unique mechanism of action in that they interfere with bacterial replication by inhibiting enzymes (called topoisomerases) that are responsible for maintaining bacterial DNA supercoiling [74]. Although four types of topoisomerases exist, only two of these are targeted by the quinolones: (1) topoisomerase IV and (2) DNA gyrase. The bactericidal activity against gram-positive bacteria is primarily a result of the quinolones targeting topoisomerase IV, whereas the activity against gram-negative organisms involves DNA gyrase [75]. The overall resistance rates of the quinolones have remained low among community-acquired respiratory pathogens but have increased among nosocomial pathogens. The three known mechanisms involved in the development of quinolone resistance include (1) mutational changes in microbial DNA topoisomerases, (2) selected alterations in bacterial outer membrane proteins, and (3) the development of a highly active efflux system (that pumps the antibiotic out of the cell) [76].

As a group, the quinolones are concentrated intracellularly in most tissues, including the sputum, the epithelium lining fluid, and the bronchial mucosa (Table 5). They also have favorable clinical pharmacokinetics including low serum protein binding (which allows the majority of the drug to diffuse freely into the extravascular space), high oral bioavailability (>90%), and a prolonged half-life (>8–12 hours) [77–79]. Another important characteristic of the quinolones is the significant post-antibiotic effect (PAE), which results in continued suppression of an organism's growth after short exposure to the antimicrobial agent [80]. Most of the newer quinolones exhibit PAEs of 1–6 hours and may be important in preventing the emergence of resistance.

The efficacy of the quinolones in the treatment of AECOPD has been demonstrated in multiple clinical trials. Ball et al. [76] summarized the early clinical trials comparing individual quinolones with other antibiotics that are frequently used for these lower respiratory tract infections. The majority of these studies demonstrated clinical efficacy rates (as well as bacterial eradication rates) of greater than 90%. The studies involving the most recently approved agents in this class of antibiotics (gatifloxacin and moxifloxacin) also demonstrate similar rates of clinical success [74,81]. Recent reports have shown the efficacy of shorter course of therapy (5 days) with the new fluoroquinolones [82]. A useful classification of the quinolones is by "generations," which allows for differentiation of their antibacterial spectrums of activity [76,83]. Modifications of the side chains of the quinolone rings are responsible for these different clinical spectrums and adverse side effects. The new generation quinolones (gatifloxacin, moxifloxacin) are the more potent agents against *S. pneumoniae* and anaerobe organisms [74].

In general, the quinolones are well tolerated and have an adverse event rate of approximately 4–5% [81]. These adverse effects, which are generally mild and transient, include rash, dizziness, headache, gastrointestinal disturbances (usually nausea, vomiting, dyspepsia, diarrhea, abdominal pain, etc.), and minor hematological abnormalities. The gastrointestinal side effects of the quinolones are usually not as severe and frequent as those associated with macrolides or with amoxicillin/clavulanate. Some drugs that are not available were associated with severe phototoxic reactions, disturbing metallic taste and liver toxicity. Quinolones have also been associated with a prolonged QTc interval but thus far have not resulted in adverse clinical outcomes [84].

The FDA recommends that all quinolones be avoided in patients receiving class IA or class III antiarrhythmic agents, in patients with known prolongation of the QTc interval, and in those with uncorrected hypokalemia.

The two major types of drug interactions involving this group of antibiotics include a reduction in gastrointestinal absorption of the quinolones and alterations in the metabolism of other drugs. Many medications that contain multivalent cations (such as antacids containing magnesium or aluminum, sucralfate, iron, zinc, and calcium) appear to significantly reduce the absorption of all the quinolones. Therefore, these agents should be dosed at least 2–4 hours before or after the administration of these antibiotics [85]. Many of the quinolones cause alterations in other medications via the hepatic cytochrome P450 system. When administered concomitantly, these agents may lead to an increase in the concentration of theophylline, warfarin, and caffeine.

FDA-approved and currently available drugs from this group include ciprofloxacin (Cipro®) 500/750 mg b.i.d. × 10 days, gatifloxacin (Tequin®) 400 mg q.d. × 10 days, levofloxacin (Levaquin®) 500 mg b.i.d. × 10 days, moxifloxacin (Avelox®) 400 mg q.d. × 5 days, and ofloxacin 400 mg b.i.d. × 10 days.

BRONCHODILATOR THERAPY

Bronchodilator drugs are the primary therapeutic interventions in patients with AECOPD (Table 9). Unfortunately there are no clearly defined objective end points that can routinely be use to assess the patient's improvement. The end point that most investigators use is improvement in symptoms. Other parameters, such as improvement in physical findings or pulmonary functions tests, are more variable. Evidence does not support online measurement of FEV_1 during an exacerbation [12,86–88]. The bronchodilators used to treat acute exacerbations of chronic obstructive lung disease are short-acting β-2 agonists, long-acting β-2 agonists, and anticholinergic agents [88–94].

The clinical studies available have shown that short-acting β-2 agonists and ipratropium bromide are equally efficacious during acute exacerbations. While some studies suggest that adding ipratropium bromide to a short- or long-acting β-2 agonist improves the patient's spirometry and clinical response [94,95], other studies do not show an improvement in spirometry or clinical symptoms [88,92,95]. The current clinical practice is to use first a short-acting β-2 agonist and then ipratropium bromide if the patient's symptoms do not improve. These agents may be used concomitantly.

The inhaled route for delivering these drugs has been shown to result in fewer adverse events and maximum efficacy. Patients can receive metered-dose inhalers (MDI) in combination with devices such as large-volume attachments (spacers), breath-attenuated MDI, and dry-powdered inhalers.

TABLE 9 Pharmacotherapy for Acute Exacerbations of Chronic Lung Disease

Bronchodilator therapy	Short-acting β-2 agonists, by MDI with spacer	Ipratropium bromide, MDI alone or in combination with short-acting β-2 agonist	Long-acting β-2 agonist. Salmeterol → AECOPD
Corticosteroids	Oral prednisone therapy, 40 mg p.o. q.d., for 7–10 days	If the patient cannot tolerate p.o. therapy, short course of I.V. Solu-Medrol	
Theophylline	Due to poor safety profile, its use is not recommended		

Source: Refs. 90–95, 111, and 113.

The techniques for using MDI and their attachments must be taught to the patients and reinforced [96]. Drug deposition may vary among delivery systems. Nebulization has been a preferred mode to deliver bronchodilators during acute exacerbation mainly because patients may have difficulty using MDI devices. The safety and value of continued drug nebulization delivery has not been established in COPD [97]. Randomized controlled trials comparing MDI with nebulization have not shown the superiority of continuous nebulization therapy [98]. In mechanically ventilated patients, bronchodilator delivery via MDI with a spacer has a higher particle deposition as compared to nebulized [99,100]. The dose scheduled for the β-2 agonists and ipratropium bromide during an acute exacerbation has not been established.

There is no evidence that oral or intravenous β-2 agonists improve bronchodilator response; therefore these routes of administration are not recommended. High doses of β-2 agonists are known to be associated with increased side effects, including tachyrhythmias, tremor, and morbidity. Recent studies have described the increased rate of cardiac events associated with β-2 agonists in patients with COPD [101], and failed to show a benefit of regular use of albuterol in stable patients [102]. Short-acting β-2 agonists may be associated with an idiosyncratic bronchoconstriction response and tachyphylaxis with a decrease in the patient's clinical response [103].

Ipratropium bromide has been demonstrated to have minimal side effects, mainly unpleasant taste and cough. There is no evidence that patients on ipratropium bromide can develop tolerance to chronic therapy [93,103].

Methylxanthines, theophylline, and/or aminophylline have been shown to have comparable or less bronchodilator effect than β-2 agonists or anticholinergic agents [104,105]. The major limitation of these drugs is the need for continuous blood level monitoring [106,107], and their side effects include cardiac arrhythmias, electrolyte imbalances, and extensive drug interactions [106]. Because of the potential for fatal adverse side effects and the need for continuous serum level monitoring, we do not recommend the use of methylxanthines in the treatment of acute exacerbations [106,108].

TREATMENT WITH CORTICOSTEROIDS

Corticosteroids are recommended in most cases of AECOPD. There is a consensus that patients with significant bronchodilator response are more likely to benefit from this therapy [109], but the precise role or corticosteroids is not well established. Corticosteroids can be administered intravenously, orally, and by inhalation (Table 9). The use of inhaled corticosteroids during acute exacerbations has not been studied.

Albert et al. [110] published thc first randomized, double-blind, placebo-controlled trial of systemic corticosteroids in the treatment of AECOPD.

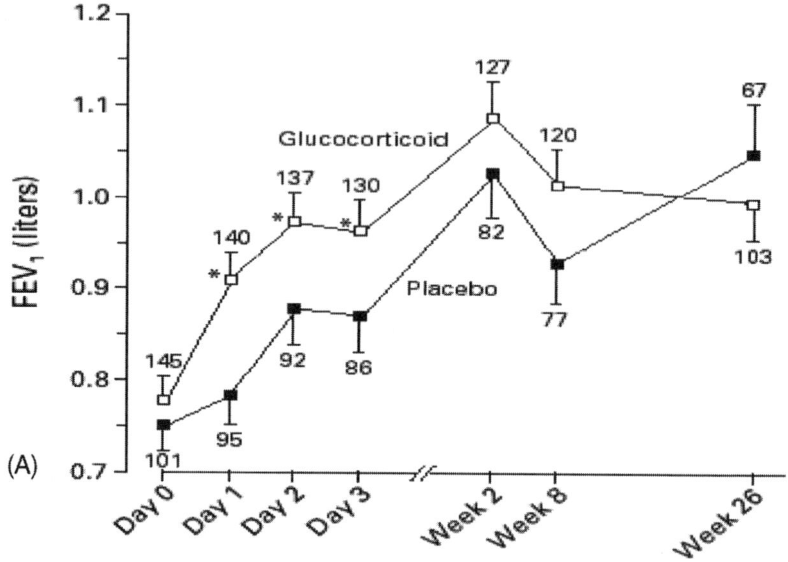

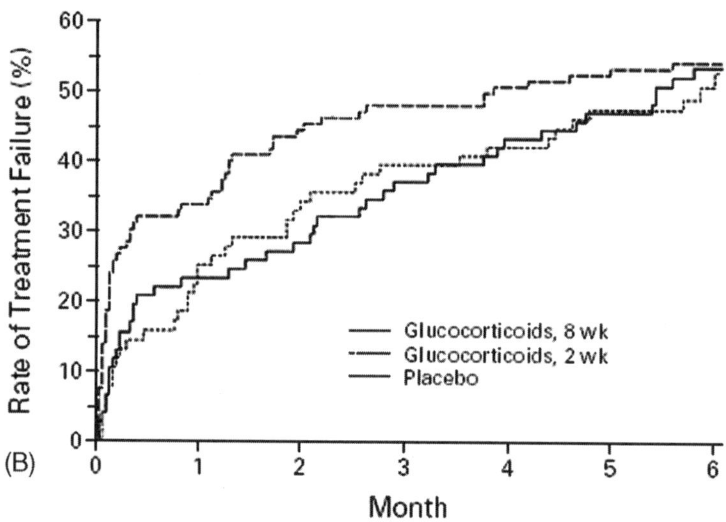

FIGURE 7 (A) FEV_1 response to corticosteroids and placebo and (B) long-term effect of two doses of corticosteroids and placebos. (From Ref. 113.)

A regimen of I.V. methylprednisolone four times daily for 3 days produced an early improvement in FEV_1 that was observed during the treatment period [110]. Recent studies have suggested that a short course of oral prednisone therapy can be useful [111,112]. A 2-week course of 30 mg daily oral prednisone in patients with severe airflow obstruction resulted in a significantly lower rate of treatment failure, a decreased length of hospital stay, and a more rapid improvement in FEV_1 [111]. In the largest study published to date—the Systemic Corticosteroids in Chronic Obstructive Pulmonary Disease Exacerbations (SCCOPE) study—271 patients with an acute exacerbation of COPD were enrolled [113]. Patients received placebo or a two-dose regimen of corticosteroids therapy for 2 or 8 weeks. For the combined glucocorticoid group, the risk of treatment failure as compared to placebo was reduced by 10 percentage points (33% vs. 23%, respectively), and FEV_1 improved statistically significantly during the first 3 days of therapy. There was no difference in FEV_1 after 2 weeks. The SCCOPE trial demonstrated equivalent outcome between 2-week and 8-week corticosteroid regimens (Fig. 7).

Because all the published studies have excluded patients who received systemic corticosteroids within the preceding month, it is not known if corticosteroid treatment is also efficacious in these patients. Inhaled nebulized corticosteroids (budesonide) also improve post-bronchodilator FEV_1. Regular use of inhaled corticosteroids may reduce the numbers of yearly exacerbations. The appropriate duration of therapy is in the range of 5 days to 2 weeks. The 10-day course has been studied best.

Well-known side effects of systemic corticosteroids are the major limiting factors of this therapy. The SCCOPE trial showed that hyperglycemia was significantly more frequent in patients who received corticosteroids compared with placebo [113]. In patients with COPD, corticosteroid-induced myopathy may be more common than was initially appreciated. Histologically, both myopathic changes and generalized muscle fiber atrophy have been reported [114]. In one study, survival of patients with steroid-induced myopathy was significantly lower compared to those without myopathy, but with similar airflow obstruction [114,115].

MUCUS-CLEARING STRATEGIES: EXPECTORANTS, MUCOLYTICS, AND MUCOKINETIC AGENTS

In COPD, mucus is generally copious and tenacious and is a major symptom in patients during both stable condition and exacerbations. Current data suggest that pharmacologic mucus-clearing strategies do not shorten the disease course of patients with acute exacerbation or improve FEV_1 [116,117].

We cannot recommend the use of any currently available mucolytic agents during acute exacerbations of AECOPD.

PREVENTION

The two most important prevention measures are smoking cessation and active immunizations, including influenza and pneumococcal vaccinations.

Active smoking cessation should be included in the therapy of these patients. The annual rate of decline of the forced expiratory volume in 1 second (FEV_1) of a smoker is approximately 80 cc/per year. In contrast, the rate decline in FEV_1 in nonsmokers is 25 to 30 cc per year [2]. The Lung Health Study showed that in middle-aged patients with normal or mild decrease in lung function, smoking cessation resulted in an improvement in FEV_1 after one year. In this study, 35% of patients who stopped smoking after the first annual visit registered an increase in mean post bronchodilator FEV_1 of 57 mL, whereas patients who continue to smoke experienced a decline in FEV_1 mean—38 mL [118].

Cigarettes are among the most addicting products known, and the vast majority of patients who quit smoking relapse within months. Nicotine is the main addictive substance in cigarettes; thus, most patients experience severe withdrawal symptoms when they abruptly stop smoking [119]. The U.S. Department of Health and Human Services has published extensive clinical practice guidelines on smoking cessation [120]. Nicotine replacement therapy is widely used to overcome the patient's withdrawal symptoms. The use of nicotine replacement therapy should always include behavior modification programs to increase the likelihood of success. Recently, it has being demonstrated that some antidepressants, especially bupropion (Zyban®) can be an effective antismoking product [121].

Influenza is an important cause of lower respiratory tract infections. Influenza A and B often reach epidemic proportions during the winter months. The impact of influenza is critical to the development of other lower respiratory tract infections including AECOPD and pneumonia. Epidemiological studies have shown that the frequency of lower respiratory tract infections and their morbidity and mortality are markedly reduced with influenza vaccination [122] In order to define the effects of influenza, and the benefits of influenza vaccination in elderly persons with chronic lung disease, Nichol et al. [123] conducted a retrospective, multiseason cohort study in a large managed care organization. The outcomes in vaccinated and unvaccinated individuals were compared after adjustment for baseline demographics and health characteristics. This study showed that vaccination rates were greater than 70%. In patients that were not vaccinated, the hospitalization rates for pneumonia and influenza were twice as high in the influ-

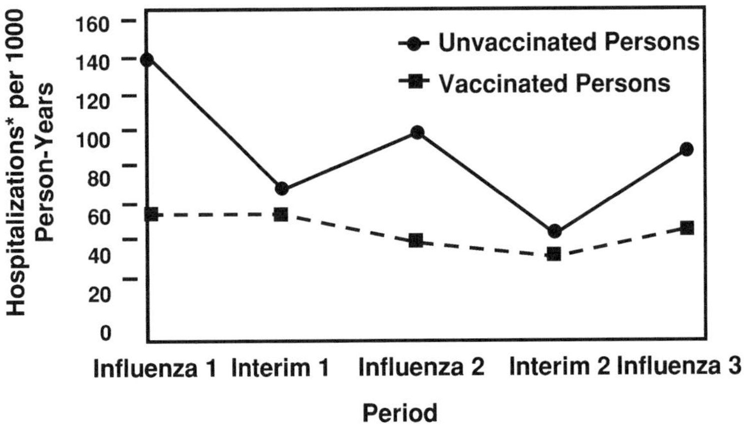

FIGURE 8 Observed annualized rates of hospitalization for pneumonia and influenza among vaccinated and unvaccinated persons for each study period. (From Ref. 123.)

enza season as they were in the interim (non-influenza) periods (Fig. 8). The Vaccinated patient group had fewer outpatient visits, fewer hospitalizations, and fewer deaths. Consequently, the influenza vaccine should be given to patients with COPD.

The polyvalent vaccine based on pneumococcal capsule serotypes has been shown to be effective in preventing pneumococcal bacteremia and pneumonia [124]. The available 23-serotype vaccine has been shown to have an aggregate efficacy of more than 60%. Its efficacy tends to decline with age and with worsening of patient immune state [125]. The vaccine is also recommended in patients with COPD. There are no contraindications for use of either pneumococcal or influenza vaccine immediately after an episode of pneumonia or AECOPD. Vaccines can be given simultaneously without affecting their potency. There are no other vaccines available in adults to prevent lower respiratory tract infections. Vaccines intended to prevent infectious due to nontypable *Haemophilus* sp. or *Pseudomonas* sp. are being developed but are not yet available.

SUMMARY

The cost, morbidity, and mortality related to AECOPD remain unacceptably high, especially in patients with significant underlying obstructive lung disease. Because those with AECOPD are a heterogeneous group, it is important to risk-stratify them based on clinical parameters and patient demographics. As described in detail in this chapter, the use of antibiotics, bronchodilators, and corticosteroids are important components in the management of these patients. In particular, it is essential to administer an appropriate antimicrobial agent from the start of therapy, so that the risks of treatment failure and the morbidity of AECOPD may be minimized [126].

REFERENCES

1. Pauwels RA, Buist S, Calvery PMA, Jenkins CR, Hurd SS, on behalf of the GOLD Scientific Committee. Global Strategy for the diagnosis, management, and prevention of Chronic Obstructive Pulmonary Disease. NHLBI/WHO Global Initiative for Chronic Obstructive Pulmonary Disease (GOLD) Workshop Summary. Am J Respir Crit Care Med 2001; 163:1256–1276.
2. American Thoracic Society. Standards for the diagnosis and care of patients with chronic obstructive pulmonary disease. Am J Respir Crit Care Med 1995; 152:S77–S121.
3. Peters DK, Kochanek DK, Murphy SL. Deaths: final data for 1996. Natl Vital Stat Rep 1998; 47:1–100.
4. Higgins MW, Thom T. Incidence, prevalence and mortality: Intra- and intercountry difference. In: Hensley MJ, Saunders NA, eds. Clinical Epidemiology of Chronic Obstructive Pulmonary Disease. New York: Marcel Dekker, 1990:23–43.
5. Statistical Abstract of the United States 1997. US Department of Commerce, Bureau of the Census. Washington, DC US Department of Commerce, 1997.
6. Healthcare Cost and Utilization Project. 1997 Nationwide Inpatient Sample. Agency for Healthcare Research and Policy. Available at: www.ahcpr.gov/data/hcup/hcupnet.htm.
7. Murray CJ, Lopez AD. Alternative projections of mortality and disability by cause 1990-2020: Global Burden of Disease Study. Lancet 1997; 349:1498–1504.
8. Feinleib M, Rosenberg HM, Collins JG, et al. Trends in COPD morbidity and mortality in the United States. Am Rev Respir Dis 1989; 140:S9–S18.
9. Ball P, Tillotson G, Wilson R. Chemotherapy for chronic bronchitis. Controversies. Presse Med 1995; 24:189–194.
10. Emerman CL, Effron D, Lukens TW. Spirometric criteria for hospital admission of patients with acute exacerbations of COPD. Chest 1991; 99:595–599.
11. Murata GH, Gorby MS, Kapsner CO, et al. A multivariate model for the prediction of relapse after outpatient treatment of decompensated chronic obstructive pulmonary disease. Arch Intern Med 1992; 152:73–77.
12. Connors AF Jr, Dawson NV, Tomas C, et al. Outcomes following acute exacerbation of severe chronic obstructive lung disease. The SUPPORT investigators (Study to Understand Prognoses and Preferences for Outcomes and Risks of Treatment). Am J Respir Crit Care Med 1996; 154:959–967.

13. Knaus WA, Wagner DP, Draper EA, et al. The APACHE III prognostic system. Risk prediction of hospital mortality for critically ill hospitalized adults. Chest 1991; 100:1619–1636.
14. Seneff MG, Wagner DP, Wagner RP, et al. Hospital and 1-year survival of patients admitted to intensive care units with acute exacerbation of chronic obstructive pulmonary disease. JAMA 1995; 274:1852–1857.
15. Seemungal TAR, Donaldson GC, et al. Time course and recovery of exacerbations in patients with chronic obstructive pulmonary disease. AJRCCM 2000; 161:1608–1613.
16. Seemungal TAR, Donaldson GC, et al. Effect of exacerbation on quality of life in patients with chronic obstructive pulmonary disease. AJRCCM 1998; 157:1418–1422.
17. Ball P. Epidemiology and treatment of chronic bronchitis and its exacerbations. Chest 1995; 108(suppl 2):S43–S52.
18. Ball P, Tillotson G, Wilson R. Chemotherapy for chronic bronchitis controversies. Presse Med 1995; 24:189–194.
19. Ball P, Harris JM, Lowson D, et al. Acute infective exacerbations of chronic bronchitis. QJ Med 1995; 88:61–68.
20. Balter MS, Hyland RH, Low DE, et al. Recommendations on the management of chronic bronchitis: a practical guide for Canadian physicians. Can Med Assoc J 1994; 151(suppl 10):5–23.
21. Eller J, Ede A, Schaberg T, et al. Infective exacerbations of chronic bronchitis. Relation between bacteriologic etiology and lung function. Chest 1998; 13: 1542–1548.
22. Miravitlles M, Espinosa C, Fernandez-Laso E, et al. Relationship between bacterial flora in sputum and functional impairment in patients with acute exacerbations of COPD. Chest 1999; 116:40–46.
23. Soler N, Torres A, Ewig S, et al. Bronchial microbial patterns in severe exacerbations of chronic obstructive pulmonary disease (COPD) requiring mechanical ventilation. Am J Respir Crit Care Med 1998; 157:1498–1505.
24. Sethi S, Muscarella K, Evans N, Klingman KL, Grant BJB, Murphy TF. Airway inflammation and etiology of acute exacerbations of chronic bronchitis. Chest 2000; 118:1557–1565.
25. Murphy TF, Sethi S. Bacterial infections in chronic obstructive pulmonary disease. Am Rev Respir Dis 1992; 146:1067–1083.
26. Gompertz S, O'Brien C, Bayley DL, Hill SL, Stockley RA. Changes in bronchial inflammation during acute exacerbations of chronic bronchitis. Eur Respir J 2001; 17:1112–1119.
27. Seemugal T, Harper-Owen R, Bhowmik A, Moric I, Sanderson G, Message S, et al. Respiratory viruses, symptoms and inflammatory markers in acute exacerbations and stable chronic obstructive pulmonary disease. Am J Respir Crit Care Med 2001; 164:1618–1623.
28. Malo O, Sauleda J, Busquets X, Miralles C, Augusti A, Noguera A. Systemic inflammation during exacerbations of chronic obstructive pulmonary disease. Arch Bronconeumol 2002; 38:172–176.

29. Kanner RE, Anthonisen NR, Connett JE. Lower respiratory illnesses promote FEV_1 decline in current smokers but not ex-smokers with mild chronic obstructive pulmonary disease. Am J Respir Crit Care Med 2001; 164:358–364.
30. Snow V, Lascher S, Mottur-Pilson for the Joint Expert Panel of Chronic Obstructive Pulmonary Disease of the American College of Chest Physicians and the American College of Physicians-American Society of Internal Medicine. Evidence base for management of acute exacerbations of chronic obstructive pulmonary disease. Ann Intern Med 2001; 134:595–599.
31. Bach BB, Brown C, Gelfand SE, McCrory DC. Management of acute exacerbations of chronic obstructive pulmonary disease: a summary and appraisal of published evidence. Ann Intern Med 2001; 134:600–620.
32. Emerman CL, Cydulka RK. Evaluation of high-yield criteria for chest radiography in acute exacerbation of chronic obstructive pulmonary disease. Ann Emerg Med 1993; 22:680–684.
33. Tsay TW, Gallagher EJ, Lombardi G, et al. Guidelines for the selective ordering of admission chest radiography in adult obstructive airway disease. Ann Emerg Med 1993; 22:1854–1858.
34. Saint S, Bent S, Vittinghoff E, et al. Antibiotics in chronic obstructive pulmonary disease exacerbations: a meta-analysis. JAMA 1995; 273:957–960.
35. Anthonisen NR, Manfreda J, Warren CP, et al. Antibiotic therapy in acute exacerbation of chronic obstructive pulmonary disease. Ann Intern Med 1987; 106:196–204.
36. Allegra L, Grassi C. Ruolo degli antibiotici nel trattamento delle riacutizza della bronchite cronica. Ital J Chest Dis 1991; 45:138–148.
37. Sonnesyn SW, Gerdin DN. Antimicrobials for the treatment of respiratory infection. In: Niederman MS, Sarosi GA, Glassroth J, eds. Respiratory infections: a scientific basis for management. Philadelphia, PA: WB Saunders, 1994:511–537.
38. Cabello H, Torres A, Celis R, et al. Bacterial colonization of distal airways in healthy subjects and chronic lung disease: a bronchoscopic study. Eur Respir J 1997; 10:1137–1144.
39. Mansó JR, Rosell A, Manterola J, et al. Bacterial infection in chronic obstructive pulmonary disease. Study of stable and exacerbated outpatients using the protected specimen brush. Am J Respir Crit Care Med 1995; 152: 1316–1320.
40. Fagon JY, Chastre J, Trouillet JL, et al. Characterization of distal bronchial microflora during acute exacerbation of chronic bronchitis. Am Rev Respir Dis 1990; 142:1004–1008.
41. Martinez JA, Rodriguez E, Bastida T, et al. Quantitative study of the bronchial bacterial flora in acute exacerbations of chronic bronchitis. Chest 1994:105:976.
42. Soler N, Torres A, Ewig S, et al. Bronchial microbial patterns in severe exacerbations of chronic obstructive pulmonary disease (COPD) requiring mechanical ventilation. Am J Respir Crit Care Med 1998; 147:1498–1505.
43. Nouira S, Marghli S, Belghith M, et al. Once daily oral ofloxacin in chronic

obstructive pulmonary disease exacerbation requiring mechanical ventilation: a randomized placebo-controlled trial. Lancet 2001; 358:2020–2025.

44. Murata GH, Gorby MS, Chick TW, et al. Use of emergency medical services by patients with decompensated obstructive lung disease. Ann Emerg Med 1989; 18:501–506.
45. Murata GH, Gorby MS, Chick TW, et al. Treatment of decompensated chronic obstructive pulmonary disease in the emergency department–correlation between clinical features and prognosis. Ann Emerg Med 1991; 20:125–129.
46. Murata GH, Gorby MS, Kapsner CO, et al. A multivariate model for the prediction of relapse after outpatient treatment of decompensated chronic obstructive pulmonary disease. Arch Intern Med 1992; 152:73–77.
47. Adams S, Melo J, Luther M, et al. Antibiotics are associated with lower relapse rates in outpatients with acute exacerbations of chronic obstructive pulmonary disease. Chest 2000; 117:1345–1352.
48. Destache CJ, Dewan N, O'Donohue WJ, et al. Clinical and economic considerations in the treatment of acute exacerbations of chronic bronchitis. J Antimicrob Chemother 1999; 43(suppl A):107–113.
49. Ball P. Future antibiotic trials. Semin Respir Infect 2000; 15:82–89.
50. Anzueto A, Rizzo JA, Grossman RF. The infection-free interval: its use in evaluating antimicrobial treatment in acute exacerbations of chronic bronchitis. Clin Infect Dis 1999; 28:1344–1345.
51. Chodosh S, McCarthy J, Farkas S, Drehobl M, Tosiello R, Shan M, et al. Randomized, double-blind study of ciprofloxacin and cefuroxime axetil for treatment of acute exacerbations of chronic bronchitis. Clin Inf Dis 1998; 27:722–729.
52. Chodosh S, Schreurs JM, Siami G, Barkman HW Jr, Anzueto A, Shan M, et al. Efficacy of oral ciprofloxacin vs. clarithromycin for treatment of acute exacerbations of chronic bronchitis. Clin Infect Dis 1998; 27:730–738.
53. Wilson R, Schentag JJ, Ball P, Mandell L for the 068 Study Group. A comparison of gemifloxacin and clarithromycin in acute exacerbations of chronic bronchitis and long-term clinical outcomes. Clin Ther 2002; 4:639–652.
54. Niederman MS, McCombs JS, Unger AN, et al. Treatment cost of acute exacerbations of chronic bronchitis. Clin Ther 1999; 21:576–592.
55. De Groot R, Dzoljic-Danilovic G, van Klingeren B, et al. Antibiotic resistance in *Haemophilus influenzae*: mechanisms, clinical importance, and consequences of therapy. Eur J Pediatr 1991; 150:534–546.
56. Doern GV, Brueggemann A, Holley HP Jr, et al. Antimicrobial resistance of *Streptococcus pneumoniae* recovered from outpatients in the United States during the winter months of 1994 to 1995: results of a 30-center national surveillance study. Antimicrob Agents Chemother 1996; 40(5):1208–1213.
57. Doern GV. Antimicrobial resistance with *Streptococcus pneumoniae* in the United States. Seminars in Respiratory and Critical Care Medicine 2000; 21:273–284.
58. Nix DE. Intrapulmonary concentrations of antimicrobial agents. Infect Dis Clin North Am 1998; 12:631–646.

59. Fick RB, Stillwell PC. Controversies in the management of pulmonary disease due to cystic fibrosis. Chest 1989; 95:1319–1327.
60. Gallup organization. Consumer attitudes toward antibiotic use. New York: American Lung Association, 1995.
61. Anzueto A, File T, Sethi S, et al. Comparative efficacy and safety of pharmacokinetically enhanced amoxicillin/clavulanate vs. levofloxacin in AECB. Am J Respir Crit Care 2002; 165:A270.
62. Chopra I, Howkey PM, Hinton M. Review: tetracyclines, molecular and clinical aspects. J Antimicrob Chemother 1992; 27:245–277.
63. Maesen PFV, Davies BI, Van Den Bergh JJ. Doxycycline and minocycline in the treatment of respiratory infections: a double-blind comparative clinical, microbiological and pharmacokinetic study. J Antimicrob Chemother 1989; 23:123–129.
64. Alvarez-Elcoro S, Enzler MJ. The macrolides: erythromycin, clarithromycin, and azithromycin. Mayo Clin Proc 1999; 74:613–634.
65. Patel KB, Xuan D, Tessier PR, et al. Comparison of bronchopulmonary pharmacokinetics of clarithromycin and azithromycin. Antimicrob Agents Chemother 1996; 40:2375–2379.
66. Boswell FJ, Wise R. Advances in the macrolides and quinolones. Infect Dis Clin North Am 1998; 12:647–670.
67. Waites K, Johnson C, Banks S, et al. Use of clindamycin disks to predict high-level macrolide resistance in *Streptococcus pneumoniae*. 9th ECCMID Berlin, Germany (poster P0878), 1999.
68. Gotfried MH. Comparison of bacteriologic eradication of *Streptococcus pneumoniae* by clarithromycin and reports of increased antimicrobial resistance. Clin Ther 2000; 22:2–14.
69. Gotfried MG, Neuhauser MM, Garey KW, et al. In vitro *Streptococcus pneumoniae* (SP) resistance: correlation with outcomes in patients with respiratory infections. J Antimicrob Chemother 1999; 44(suppl A):83.
70. Swanson RN, Lainez-Ventosilla A, De Salvo MC, et al. 3-day azithromycin 500 mg qd vs. 10-day clarithromycin 500 mg bid for acute exacerbation of chronic bronchitis in adults. Am J Respir Crit Care Med 2002; 165: A269.
71. Bradbury F. Comparison of azithromycin versus clarithromycin in the treatment of lower respiratory tract infections. J Antimicrob Chemother 1993; 31(suppl E):153–162.
72. Anzueto A, Fisher CL, Busman T, et al. Comparison of the efficacy of extended-release clarithromycin tablets and amoxicillin/clavulanate tablets in the treatment of acute exacerbations of chronic bronchitis. Clin Ther 2001; 23:72–86.
73. Blondeau JM. A review of the comparative in-vitro activities of 12 antimicrobial agents, with a focus on five now 'respiratory quinolones. J Antimicrob Chemother 1999; 43(suppl B):1–11.
74. Walker RC. Symposium on antimicrobial agents—part XIII: the fluoroquinolones. Mayo Clin Proc 1999; 74:1030–1037.
75. Ng EY, Trucksis M, Hooper DC. Quinolone resistance mutations in topo-

isomerase IV: relationship to the flqA locus and genetic evidence that topoisomerase IV is the primary target and DNA gyrase is the secondary target of fluoroquinolones in *Staphylococcus aureus*. Antimicrob Agents Chemother 1996; 40:1881–1888.
76. Ball P, Fernald A, Tillotson G. Therapeutic advances of new fluoroquinolones. Exp Opin Invest Drugs 1998; 7(5):1–23.
77. Blondeau JM. Expanded activity and utility of the new fluoroquinolones: a review. Clin Ther 1999; 21:3–40.
78. Bauernfeind A. Comparison of the antimicrobial activities of the quinolones Bay 12-8039, gatifloxacin (AM 1155), trovafloxacin, clinafloxacin, levofloxacin, and ciprofloxacin. J Antimicrob Chemother 1997; 40:39–51.
79. Brueggemann AB, Kugler KC, Doern GV. In vitro activity of BAY 12-8039, a novel 8-methoxyquinolone, compared to activities of six fluoroquinolones against *Streptococcus pneumoniae*, *Haemophilus influenzae*, and *Moraxella catarrhalis*. Antimicrob Agents Chemother 1997; 41:1594–1597.
80. Boswell F, Andrews JM, Wise R. Pharmacodynamic properties of Bay 12-8939 on gram-positive and gram-negative organisms as demonstrated by studies of time-kill kinetics and post-antibiotic effect. Antimicrob Agents Chemother 1997; 41:1377–1379.
81. Rodvold KA. Clinical safety profile of newer fluoroquinolones. Infect Med 1999; 16(suppl F):41–53.
82. Gotfried MH, De Abate A, Fogarty C, et al. Comparison of 5-day, short course gatifloxacin therapy with 7-day gatifloxacin therapy and 10-day clarithromycin therapy for acute exacerbation of chronic bronchitis. Clin Ther 2001; 23:97–107.
83. Trautner I, Rodriguez-Barradas MC. New antibiotics against resistant Gram-positive organisms: quinupristin/dalfopristin, linezolid, and newer fluoroquinolones. BioMedicina 2000; 3:113–117.
84. Owens RC, Ambrose PG. Torsades de Pointes associated with fluoroquinolones. Pharmacotherapy 2002; 22:663–672.
85. Radandt JM, Marchbanks CR, Dudley MN. Interactions of fluoroquinolones with other drugs: mechanisms, variability, clinical significance, and management. Clin Infect Dis 1992; 14:272–284.
86. Emerman CL, Connors AF, Lukens TW, et al. Relationship between arterial blood gases and spirometry in acute exacerbations of chronic obstructive pulmonary disease. Ann Emerg Med 1989; 22:1854–1858.
87. Emerman CT, Cydulka RK. Use of peak expiratory flow rate in emergency department evaluation of acute exacerbation of chronic obstructive pulmonary disease. Ann Emerg Med 1996; 27:159–163.
88. O'Driscoll BR, Taylor RJ, Horsley MG, et al. Nebulised salbutamol with and without ipratropium with and without ipratropium bromide in acute airflow obstruction. Lancet 1989; 1:1418–1420.
89. Backman R, Hellström PE. Fenoterol and ipratropium bromide for treatment of patients with chronic bronchitis. Curr Ther Res 1985; 38:135–140.
90. Emerman CL, Cydulka RK. Effect of different albuterol dosing regimens in

the treatment of acute exacerbation of chronic obstructive pulmonary disease. Ann Emerg Med 1997; 29:474–478.

91. Shretha M, O'Brien T, Haddox R, et al. Decreased duration of emergency department treatment of chronic obstructive pulmonary disease exacerbations with the addition of ipratropium bromide to beta-agonist therapy. Ann Emerg Med 1991; 20:1206–1209.
92. Moayyedi P, Congleton J, Page RI, et al. Comparison of nebulized salbutamol and ipratropium bromide with salbutamol alone in the treatment of chronic obstructive pulmonary disease. Thorax 1995; 50:834–837.
93. Karpel JF. Bronchodilator response to anticholinergic and beta-adrenergic agents in acute and stable COPD. Chest 1991; 99:871–876.
94. Brown IG, Chan CS, Kelly CA, et al. Assessment of the clinical usefulness of nebulized ipratropium bromide in patients with chronic airflow limitation. Thorax 1984; 39:272–276.
95. Cydulka RK, Emerman CL. Effects of combined treatment with glycopyrrolate and albuterol in acute exacerbation of chronic obstructive pulmonary disease. Ann Emerg Med 1995; 25:470–473.
96. Turner MO, Patel A, Ginsburg S, et al. Bronchodilator delivery in acute airflow obstruction. A meta-analysis. Arch Intern Med 1997; 157:1736–1744.
97. Mestitz H, Copland JM, McDonald CF. Comparison of outpatient nebulized vs. metered dose inhaler terbutaline in chronic airflow obstruction. Chest 1989; 96:1017–1020.
98. Turner JR, Corkery KJ, Eckman D, et al. Equivalence of continuous flow nebulizer and metered-dose inhaler with reservoir bag for treatment of acute airflow obstruction. Chest 1988; 93:476–481.
99. Dhand R, Jubran A, Tobin MJ. Bronchodilator delivery by metered-dose inhaler in ventilator-supported patients. Am J Respir Crit Care Med 1995; 151:1827–1833.
100. Duarte AG, Dhand R, Reid R, et al. Serum albuterol levels in mechanically ventilated patients and healthy subjects after metered-dose inhaler administration. Am J Respir Crit Care Med 1996; 154:1658–1663.
101. Au DH, Crutis JR, et al. Inhaled beta-agonists and risk of myocardial ischemia. Am J Respir Crit Care Med, 2000, A489.
102. Cook D, et al. Regular versus as-needed short-acting inhaled β-agonist therapy for chronic obstructive pulmonary disease. Am J Respir Crit Care Med 2001; 163:85–90.
103. Tashkin DP, Ashutosh K, Bleeker ER, et al. Comparison of the anticholinergic bronchodilator ipratropium bromide with metaproterenol in chronic obstructive pulmonary disease: a 90 day multicenter study. Am J Med 1986; 8(suppl 5A):81–89.
104. Rice KL, Leatherman JW, Duane PG, et al. Aminophylline for acute exacerbations of chronic obstructive pulmonary disease. A controlled trial. Ann Intern Med 1987; 107:305–309.
105. Jenne JW. What role for theophylline therapy? Thorax 1994; 49:97–100.
106. Emerman CL, Devlin C, Connors AF. Risk of toxicity in patients with elevated theophylline levels. Ann Emerg Med 1990; 19:643–648.

107. Emerman CL, Connors AF, Lukens TW, et al. Theophylline concentrations in patients with acute exacerbations of COPD. Am J Emerg Med 1990; 8:289–292.
108. Mahon JL, Laupacis A, Hodder RV, et al. Theophylline for irreversible chronic airflow limitation: a randomized study comparing n of 1 trials to standard practice. Chest 1999; 115:38–48.
109. Hudson LD, Monti CM. Rationale and use of corticosteroids in chronic obstructive pulmonary disease. Med Clin North Am 1990; 74:661–690.
110. Albert RK, Martin TR, Lewis SW. Controlled clinical trial of methylprednisolone in patients with chronic bronchitis and acute respiratory insufficiency. Ann Intern Med 1980; 92:753–758.
111. Davies L, Angus RM, Calverley PM. Oral corticosteroids in patients admitted to hospital with exacerbations of chronic obstructive pulmonary disease: a prospective randomized controlled trial. Lancet 1999; 354:456–460.
112. Thompson WH, Nielson CP, Carvalho P, et al. Controlled trial of oral prednisone I outpatients with acute COPD exacerbation. Am J Respir Crit Care Med 1996; 154:407–412.
113. Niewoehner DE, Erbland ML, Deupree RH, et al. Effect of systemic glucocorticoids on exacerbations of chronic obstructive pulmonary disease. Department of Veterans Affairs Cooperative Study Group. N Engl J Med 1999; 340: 1941–1947.
114. Decramer M, de Bock V, Dom R. Functional and histologic picture of steroid-induced myopathy in chronic obstructive pulmonary disease. Am J Respir Crit Care Med 1996; 153:1958–1964.
115. Decramer M, Lacquet LM, Fagard R, et al. Corticosteroids contribute to muscle weakness in chronic airflow obstruction. Am J Respir Crit Care Med 1994; 150:11–16.
116. Langlands JH. Double-blind clinical trial of bromhexine as a mucolytic drug in chronic bronchitis. Lancet 1970; 1:448–450.
117. Peralta J, Poderoso JJ, Corazza C, et al. Ambroxol plus amoxicillin in the treatment of exacerbations of chronic bronchitis. Arzneimittelforschung 1987; 37:969–971.
118. Anthonisen NR, Connett JE, Kiley JP, et al. Effect of smoking intervention and the use of an inhaled anticholinergic bronchodilator on the rate of decline of FeV1. JAMA 1994; 272:1497–1505.
119. Fiore MC, Jorenby DE, Baker TB. Tobacco dependence and the nicotine patch. Clinical guidelines for effective use. JAMA 1992; 268:2687–2694.
120. Fiose MC, Bailey WC, Cohen SJ, et al. Smoking cessation: clinical practice guidelines. No. 18. MD Rockville: USD Department of Health and Human Services, (Publication No. 96-0692, 1996).
121. Jorenby DE, Leischow SJ, Nides MA, et al. A controlled trial of sustained-release bupropion, a nicotine patch, or both for smoking cessation. N Engl J Med 1999; 340:685–691.
122. Centers for Disease Control and Prevention. Prevention and control of influenza: recommendations for the Advisory Committee on Immunization practices. MMWR Morb Mortal Wkly Rep 1995; 44(RR-31):1–22.

123. Nichol KL, Baken L, Nelson A. Relation between influenza vaccination and outpatient visits, hospitalization, and mortality in elderly persons with chronic lung disease. Ann Intern Med 1999; 130:397–403.
124. Centers for Disease Control and Prevention. Update on adult immunization: recommendations of the Immunization Advisory Committee Pneumococcal Disease. MMWR Morb Mortal Wkly Rep 1191; 40(RR-12):42–44.
125. Butler JC, Breiman RF, Campbell JF, et al. Pneumococcal polysaccharide vaccine efficacy. An evaluation of current recommendations. JAMA 1993; 270:1826–1831.
126. Adams SG, Anzueto A. Treatment of acute exacerbations of chronic bronchitis. In: Anzueto A, ed. Antibiotics in Respiratory Infections. Seminar Respir Infect 2000; 15:234–247.

13

Treatment of Pneumonia in Nonhospitalized Patients

Thomas M. File, Jr.
Northeastern Ohio Universities College of Medicine, Rootstown
and Summa Health System
Akron, Ohio, U.S.A.

INTRODUCTION

Community-acquired pneumonia (CAP) is a common disorder that is potentially life-threatening, especially in older adults and those with comorbid disease. However, the majority of patients with CAP have an illness of relatively mild severity and can be safely treated in the ambulatory setting.

Clinicians are constantly challenged to treat CAP appropriately and cost-effectively. Although most patients have only mild disease, many clinicians feel uneasy about whether they can be safely treated as outpatients. Over the past decade, numerous guidelines for management of CAP have been published that provide guidance for the stratification of patients as well as appropriate processes of care. Recommendations within these guidelines provide direction regarding appropriate management of patients treated as outpatients.

EPIDEMIOLOGY

In the United States, approximately 4–5 million cases of community-acquired pneumonia (CAP) occur each year, accounting for 10 million physician visits, approximately 500,000 hospitalizations, and approximately 45,000 deaths [1]. Although mortality has ranged from 2% to 30% among hospitalized patients, mortality is less than 1% for patients who are not hospitalized—which is the large majority of patients.

CAP occurs more commonly in children under the age of 5 years and in adults over the age of 65 years. The incidence of CAP for persons between the ages of 5 and 60 years has been reported to be between 100 and 500 per 100,000 population [2]. In a series of studies, Foy and coworkers examined the attack rate of pneumonia by age in a prepaid medical care group that had a population of 180,000 when the study ended in February 1975 [3]. The overall annual rate of pneumonia was 12 per 1,000 population per year. Rates were highest in the 0–4 years of age group at 12 to 18 per 1,000 population. Between the ages of 5 and 60 years, the rate ranged from 1 to 5 per 1,000 population. In 1987, Houston et al. restrospectively evaluated the incidence of pneumonia (nursing home and community-associated) in elderly patients and residents 65 years of age or older in Homestead County, Minneapolis, Minnesota [4]. The overall incidence rate for an initial episode of pneumonia was 3032 per 100,000 population; this rate rose to 7923 per 100,000 population among residents aged 85 or above. In a prospective study of all adult patients (≥18 years of age) hospitalized for CAP in two counties in Ohio during 1991 (Ohio Community Based Pneumonia Incidence Study), Marston et al, reported an incidence rate of 280 cases per 100,00 population [5]. The rate was 962 cases per 100,000 for persons older than 65 years of age. In this study, the incidence was higher among blacks than whites and higher among males than females. The incidence of CAP is highest in the winter months and during influenza epidemics.

PATHOGENESIS OF CAP

In a healthy individual, the lower respiratory tract is kept essentially sterile by very effective pulmonary defense mechanisms that include anatomic barriers as well as humoral, cell-mediated, and phagocytic immunity. Although normal individuals commonly aspirate their upper respiratory tract flora, pneumonia develops when there is a breakdown in the pulmonary host defenses, when the invading organisms are virulent, or when a large inoculum size of the microorganism is introduced. Aspiration remains the most common route of acquiring pneumonia. Less commonly, organisms enter the lungs by inhalation, or by a hematogenous or contiguous route.

The phagocytes play an important role in protecting the host against most pathogens causing CAP. Cell-mediated immunity plays an important role against viruses and intracellular infectious agents such as *Mycobacterium*, *Legionella*, and *Chlamydia* species.

Several studies have evaluated risk factors for pneumonia [6–10]. Documented conditions associated with increased risk for pneumonia include increasing age, smoking, alcoholism, asthma, immunosuppression, institutionalization, dementia, seizure disorder, congestive heart failure, peripheral vascular disease, and chronic obstructive pulmonary disease. The elderly appear at increased risk related to a variety of factors such as increased number of underlying conditions, increase hospitalizations, age-related impairments and host-defense mechanisms, and decreased immune response. Several of these risk factors increase the likelihood of aspiration, which is a key factor in the pathogenesis of pneumonia. A common factor that predisposes to CAP is smoking. Cigarette smoke not only causes chronic bronchitis but also impairs local defense mechanisms, thus contributing to damage of the airway. Subsequently, the patient is at an increased risk of experiencing an acute lower respiratory tract infection such as CAP. Overcrowding in institutions is a risk factor for outbreaks of pneumococcal pneumonia. Outbreaks have occurred in jails and nursing homes.

When recurrent episodes of bacterial pneumonia occur, the presence of underlying predisposition (i.e., congenital defects, immunoglobulin [IgG] deficiency, acquired immunodeficiency syndrome) should be considered.

CLINICAL MANIFESTATIONS

Adult patients who are immunocompetent should be evaluated for pneumonia if they present with symptoms that include cough, sputum production, labored breathing (including altered breath sounds and rales), and/or fever. Other symptoms can include chest pain, myalgia, headache, dyspnea, and fatigue. Many of these symptoms may also be present in patients with upper respiratory tract infections, other lower respiratory tract infections (i.e., acute bronchitis, chronic bronchitis) as well as noninfectious diseases (i.e., reactive airways disease, atelectasis, CHF, vasculitis, pulmonary embolism, and malignancy). An accurate diagnosis of CAP is important because antibiotic therapy is usually indicated for pneumonia but is usually not indicated for most upper respiratory tract infections or acute bronchitis, because most are viral in etiology. Given the potential danger associated with antibiotic overuse (increased bacterial resistance and unnecessary side effects) and the cost of inappropriate therapy, recent guidelines recommend that a chest x-ray be obtained for the routine evaluation of patients with suspected CAP [1,11,12]. The rationale is to appropriately establish the diagnosis of pneumonia and differentiate respiratory illnesses such as acute bronchitis.

While it is generally considered that the chest x-ray is necessary to establish a diagnosis of CAP, I acknowledge that in the "real world" many health care providers treat patients on the basis of clinical manifestations only. It is very important to point out, however, that distinguishing CAP from other respiratory illnesses such as acute bronchitis is very difficult on clinical grounds alone. A review of published studies of pneumonia indicates no combination of clinical findings can reliably define the presence of pneumonia [13]. Moreover the absence of any vital sign abnormality or any abnormalities on chest auscultation substantially reduces the likelihood of pneumonia. Because pneumonia is therefore very unlikely in the absence of these abnormalities, I recommend a strategy of assigning a diagnosis of CAP without chest x-ray confirmation be considered only if there are significant clinical manifestations (i.e., new cough with abnormal vital signs and localized auscultatory findings). To treat with antibiotics in the absence of these findings is likely to be associated with the use of these agents for nonbacterial respiratory illnesses (i.e., viral or noninfectious) and contribute to the already high risk of antimicrobial resistance.

The clinical course of CAP is variable among patients. In a study of patients with ambulatory CAP, the median time to resolution for fever was 3 days; for myalgia, 5 days, for dyspnea, 6 days; and for both cough and fatigue, 14 days [14]. Symptoms can be expected to last even longer in more seriously ill patients. In another study, Fine et al. found that 86% of paticnts had one or more persisting pneumonia-related symptom at 30 days [15]. Such information should be imparted to patients for better awareness of their illness and anticipated clinical course.

SITE-OF-CARE DECISION: DEFINING LOW-RISK PATIENTS FOR AMBULATORY CARE

A key decision facing the clinician is whether to hospitalize the patient with CAP. A general consensus is that approximately 75% of patients can be appropriately treated as outpatients [1]. The initial site-of-care decision has an impact on the extent of diagnostic testing as well as the choice of empirical antimicrobial therapy. The advantages of not hospitalizing patients for CAP are considerable. The cost of inpatient care is up to 20 times higher than that of outpatient care [16]. In addition, most patients indicate a preference for home care if it is considered as safe. In a study conducted by Coley et al. 80% of patients with CAP said they would prefer home care and would be willing to pay an average of 24% of their monthly income to make sure of it [17]. Ambulatory care also avoids many of the iatrogenic complications associated with hospitalization. For elder patients, particularly, a reduction in immobilization (i.e., time in a hospital bed) time can facilitate better convalescence.

The decision to hospitalize a patient with CAP or to treat as an outpatient depends on many variables, including the severity of illness, associated disease, adequacy of home support, and probability of compliance. Recognized risk factors for increased mortality of patients with CAP include extreme of age, comorbid illnesses (i.e., malignancy, congestive heart failure, coronary artery disease, alcoholism, abnormality of vital signs), and several laboratory and radiographic findings [10]. The admission decision remains a judgmental one; however, prognostic scoring rules have been developed that provide support for this decision [18,19].

A pneumonia severity of index score, the "pneumonia prediction rule," has been developed from studies of the pneumonia Patient Outcomes Research Team (PORT), and it can assist clinicians in making the site-of-care

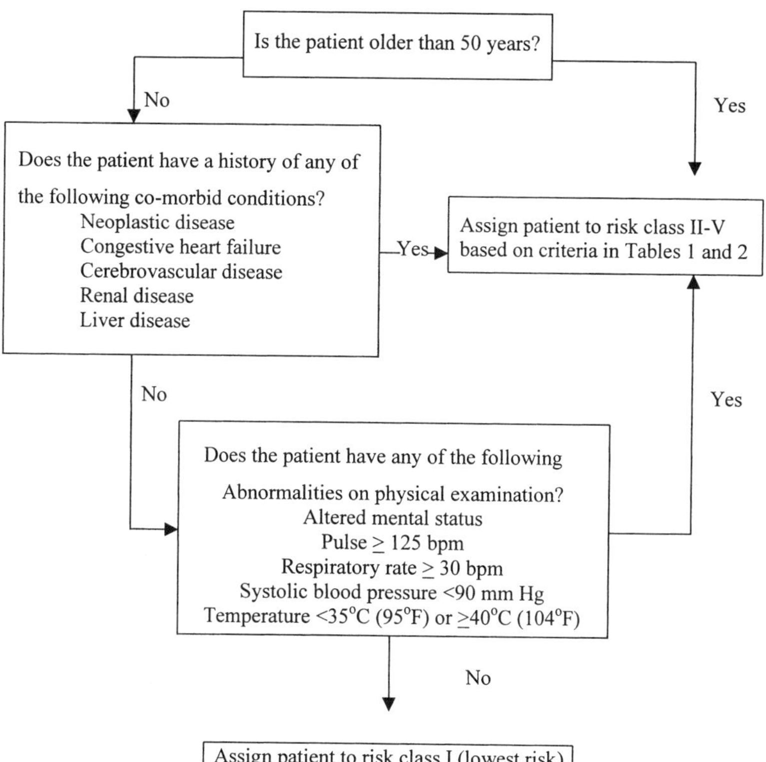

FIGURE 1 Assessing risk in patients with community-acquired pneumonia.

TABLE 1 Scoring System of the Prediction Rule for Patients Assigned to Risk Classes II through V

Patient characteristic	Points assigned[a]
Demographic factor	
Age (male)	No. of years of age
Age (female)	No. of years of age–10
Nursing home resident	+10
Comorbid illnesses	
Neoplastic disease[b]	+30
Liver disease[c]	+20
Congestive heart failure[d]	+10
Cerebrovascular disease[e]	+10
Renal disease[f]	+10
Physical examination finding	
Altered mental status[g]	+20
Respiratory rate ≥30 breaths/min	+20
Systolic blood pressure <90 mmHg	+20
Temperature <35°C or >40°C	+15
Pulse >125 beats/min	+10
Laboratory or radiographic finding	
Arterial pH<7.35	+30
Blood urea nitrogen >30mg/dL	+20
Sodium <130 mEq/L	+20
Glucose >250 mg/dL	+10
Hematocrit <30%	+10
Arterial partial pressure of oxygen <60 mm Hg[h]	+10
Pleural effusion	+10

[a] A total point score for a given patient is obtained by adding the patient's age in years (age-10, for females) and the points for each applicable patient characteristic. Points assigned to each predictor variable were based on coefficients obtained from the logistic regression model used.
[b] Any cancer except basal or squamous cell cancer of the skin that was active at the time of presentation or diagnosed within 1 year of presentation.
[c] A clinical or histologic diagnosis of cirrhosis or other form of chronic liver disease such as chronic active hepatitis.
[d] Systolic or diastolic ventricular dysfunction documented by history and physical examination as well as chest radiography, echocardiography, Muga scanning, or left ventriculography.
[e] A clinical diagnosis of stroke, transient ischemic attack, or stroke documented by MRI or computed axial tomography.
[f] A history of chronic renal disease or abnormal blood urea nitrogen and creatinine value documented in the medical record.
[g] Disorientation (to person, place, or time, not known to be chronic), stupor, or coma.
[h] In Pneumonia Patient Outcome Research Team cohort study, an oxygen saturation value <90% on pulse oximetry or intubation before admission was also considered abnormal.
Source: Ref. 18.

decision [18]. The prediction rule stratifies patients to one of five categories by using a point system based on several variables. Most of the information needed for scoring is easily available from the history and physical examination. The prediction rule is a two-step process and first considers age (over 50), the presence of comorbid conditions, and the presence of abnormal vital signs. If any of these are present, then points are assigned to each condition for which a total score and classification can be determined (Fig. 1) (Tables 1,2). This process has been validated as a method for identifying patients at risk for death, and it has been shown to be an effective method for triaging patients and particularly for identifying "low risk" patients who can be safely treated away from the hospital [20–24].

In contrast, the British Thoracic Society guidelines recommend an assessment of severity based on the presence of "adverse prognostic features" [19]. These adverse features include age greater than 50 years; coexisting disease; and four additional specific "core" features: mental confusion, elevated urea nitrogen, respiratory rate > 30/minute, and low blood pressure, hence CURB. "Additional" adverse prognostic features include hypoxemia and bilateral or multilobe pulmonary infiltrates on chest radiograph. Patients who display none of the features listed are at low risk for death and do not normally require hospitalization, whereas those who display two or more "core" adverse prognostic features should be hospitalized. This rule was studied in prospective trial in the United Kingdom and found to correlate well with mortality [25].

Prediction rules may oversimplify the way physicians interpret important variables, and therefore these approaches are meant to contribute to, rather than supersede, physicians' judgment. Because hypoxemia is an important factor, clinicians are encouraged to use pulse oximetry for assessment of severity and oxygen requirement. In addition, support system outside the hospital, substance abuse, and other factors that may interfere with com-

TABLE 2 Mortality Rates Based on Risk Class as Determined by Prediction Rule

		Validation cohort		
Risk class	No. of points	No. of patients	Mortality, %	Recommended site of care
I	—[a]	3034	0.1	Outpatient
II	≤70	5778	0.6	Outpatient
III	71–90	6790	2.8	Outpatient or brief inpatient
IV	91–130	13,104	8.2	Inpatient
V	>130	9333	29.2	Inpatient

[a] Absence of predictors.
Source: Ref. 18.

pliance should be considered whenever home treatment is contemplated. (For further discussion of CAP severity of illness evaluation, refer to Chapter 14).

ETIOLOGY

The etiologic pathogens of CAP have changed in prevalence over time. While *S. pneumoniae* remains the most common causative pathogen, a number of newer pathogens, such as *C. pneumoniae* and sin nombre virus (hantavirus), have been recognized in recent years (Table 3). However, prospective studies for evaluating the cause of CAP in adults have failed to identify the cause of 40–60% of cases, and two or more etiologies have been identified in 2%–5% of cases [26]. The most common etiologic agent identified in virtually all studies of CAP is *Streptococcus pneumoniae*. Based on a review of more than 15 published reports from North America that covers more than two decades and from mostly hospitalized patients, the ranges for prevalence of specific bacterial pathogens as causes of pneumonia are reported as follows: *S. pneumoniae* 20–60%; *H. influenzae* 3–10%; *M. pneumoniae* 1–6%; *C. pneumoniae* 4–6%; *Legionella* species 2–8%; viruses 2–13%; aspiration 6–10%; *S. aureus* 3–5%; gram-negative bacilli 3–5%; and miscellaneous 10–20% [27]. Few of these studies used techniques to isolate anaerobic bacteria, which may have been identified in studies using transtracheal aspirates and may account for 20–30% of all cases of CAP. The frequency of other etiologies—for example, *Chlamydia psittaci* (psittacosis), *Coxiella burnetii* (Q fever), *Francisella tularensis* (tularemia), and endemic fungi (histoplasmosis, coccidioidomycosis, blastomycosis)—varies with location.

The relative proportion rates for studies evaluating specific etiologic causes vary depending on the strictness of criteria for diagnosis, age group, geographic location, and whether an epidemic is occurring at the time of evaluation. Therefore, an attempt to compare various studies can be problematic.

Specific Etiology and Epidemiological Setting

No convincing association has been demonstrated between individual symptoms, physical findings or laboratory test results, and specific etiology. However, and although not absolute, certain pathogens cause CAP more commonly among persons with specific risk factors.

The pneumococcus is classically a pathogen of the elderly and patients with a variety of medical conditions, including chronic obstructive lung disease, congestive heart failure, asplenia, immunoglobulin deficiency, hematological malignancy, and HIV infection. The incidence of pneumococcal bacteremia is extremely high in newborns and infants up to 2 years of age, low in teenage children and young adults, then increases in elderly adults. Recent

TABLE 3 Pathogens Associated With Community-Acquired Pneumonia

Traditional pathogens
Streptococcus pneumoniae
Haemophilus influenzae
Mycoplasma pneumoniae
Oral anaerobes
Gram-negative bacilli (less common)
Staphylococcus aureus (less common)
Influenza
More recently recognized pathogens
Legionella species
Chlamydia pneumoniae (strain TWAR)
Moraxella (*Branhamella*) *catarrhalis*
Sin nombre virus (hantavirus)
Parainfluenza
Respiratory syncytial
Pathogens with increasing prevalence or epidemiologic factors
Mycobacterium tuberculosis
Pneumocystis carinii (associated with HIV infection)
Less Common pathogens in immunocompetent host
Bacteria
Neisseria meningitidis
Streptococcus pyogenes
Alpha-hemolytic streptococci (i.e., S. milleri)
Coxiella burnetti (Q fever)
Chlamydia psittaci
Fungi
Histoplasma capsulatum
Coccidioides immitis
Blastomyces dermatitidis
Viruses
Influenza
Parainfluenza
Adenovirus
Respiratory syncytial
Varicella
Less common pathogens in immunocompromised host
Bacteria
Nocardia species
Mycobacterium species (i.e., avium complex)
Fungi
Aspergillus species
Candida species
Cryptococcus species
Rhizopus species
Viruses
Herpes simplex
Cytomegalovirus
Toxoplasma species

studies continue to document the emergence of drug-resistant *S. pneumoniae* (DRSP). The emergence and rapid accumulation of DRSP isolates has posed a new challenge for practitioners.

Legionella infection has a varied epidemiological picture. Cases can occur in clusters or sporadically from the community or in the hospital setting. It appears there is geographic variance of incidence, because more cases are reported from the north central and northeastern regions of the United States; however, some of this variation may depend on the extent of diagnostic testing [28]. There also may be local environmental factors that are important and still not well defined. In a controlled study of risk factors associated with *Legionella* pneumonia, Straus et al. observed the following as predisposing conditions: recent travel with an overnight stay, stay outside the home, recent domestic plumbing, renal or liver failure, smoking, diabetes, systemic malignancy, and other immunosuppressive states [29]. Water is the major reservoir; organisms can be found in freshwater environments worldwide. *Legionella* can also be isolated from moist soil. Transmission to humans occurs when water containing the organism is aerosolized in respiratory droplets (1–5 μm in diameter) and inhaled or aspirated. Aerosol-producing devices that have been associated with outbreaks include cooling towers, evaporative condensers, respiratory therapy equipment, showers and faucets, whirlpool spas, decorative fountains, and an ultrasonic mist machine in a supermarket.

While it has historically been believed that *M. pneumoniae* primarily involves adolescents or young adults, recent studies suggest that this organism causes pneumonia among healthy adults of any age [30]. In the Ohio Community Based Pneumonia Incidence Study, this pathogen was an important cause of CAP both in persons under 50 years of age as well as in older age groups [5]. *M. pneumoniae* infections are ubiquitous and occur in both urban and rural settings. In urban areas, infection tends to be endemic, usually occurring year round; and epidemics often occur in cyclical 4-to 7-year intervals. Risk factors such as smoking or the presence of comorbid conditions are not as significant for *M. pneumoniae* as for other respiratory pathogens.

Geographic and Epidemiological Associations

The prevalence of pneumonia due to specific pathogens would be expected to vary along differences in environmental conditions and other predisposing conditions. The geographic and epidemiological associations that likely influence causes of CAP may explain differences in prevalence rates for specific pathogens observed in studies from different locations. Pathogens of geographic association include *Legionella*, sin nombre virus, endemic fungi, *Coxiella burnetii*, *Francisella tularensis*, and tuberculosis. Epidemiological

TABLE 4 Epidemiological and Underlying Conditions Related to Specific Pathogens in Selected Patients with Community-Acquired Pneumonia

Condition	Commonly encountered pathogens
Alcoholism	*Streptococcus pneumoniae*, anaerobes, gram-negative bacilli
COPD/smoker	*S. pneumoniae*, *Haemophilus influenzae*, *Moraxella catarrhalis*, *Legionella* species
Nursing-home residency	*S. pneumoniae*, gram-negative bacilli, *H. influenzae*, *Staphylococcus aureus*, anaerobes, *Chlamydia pneumoniae*
Poor dental hygiene	Anaerobes
Epidemic Legionnaire's disease	*Legionella* species
Exposure to bats or soil enriched with bird droppings	*Histoplasma capsulatum*
Exposure to bird	*Chlamydia psittaci*
Exposure to rabbits	*Francisella tularensis*
HIV infection (early stage)	*S. pneumoniae*, *H. influenzae*, *Mycobacterium tuberculosis*
Travel to the Southwestern United States	*Coccidioides immitis*
Exposure to farm animals or parturient cats	*Coxiella burnetii*[a]
Influenza active in community	Influenza, *S. pneumoniae*, *S. aureus*, *Streptococcus pyogenes*, *H. influenzae*
Suspected large-volume aspiration	Anaerobes, chemical pneumonitis
Structural disease of the lung (bronchiectasis or cystic fibrosis)	*Pseudomonas aeruginosa*, *Burkholderia* (*Pseudomonas*) *cepacia*, or *S. aureus*
Injection drug use	*S. aureus*, anaerobes, *M. tuberculosis*
Airway obstruction	Anaerobes

Note. COPD = chronic obstructive pulmonary disease.
[a] Agent of Q fever.
Source: Ref. 1.

conditions associated with specific pathogens in selected patients with CAP are listed in Table 4.

Etiology Correlated with Site of Care

An awareness of the likely etiology and different settings is important for the appropriate formulation of guidelines relevant to CAP patients. Thus, there is practical importance in characterizing the etiology of CAP based on the severity of disease as judged by the site of care (outpatient vs. inpatient vs. ICU admission). Table 5 lists the most common pathogens associated with CAP based on the collective results of recent studies and based on relative severity of illness.

In several studies that evaluated the etiology of CAP in ambulatory patients, the percent of cases due to *M. pneumoniae* ranged from 17 to 37% [26]. The cause of CAP treated in an ambulatory setting was evaluated by Marrie et al., who found that nearly half of the cases were due to atypical agents. The study population consisted of patients presenting to an emergency department or to practitioner offices. An etiologic diagnosis was made in 50% of 149 patients using serologic methods. Sputum culture was not part of the routine protocol, which in part accounts for the finding of only one case of *S. pneumoniae* [31]. Etiologic agents included *M. pneumoniae* (22.8%), *C. pneumoniae* (10.7%), *M. pneumoniae* combined with *C. pneumoniae* (3.4%), and *Coxiella burnetii* (2.7%). The cause of the pneumonia was undetermined in 48.3%. The outcome of patients was similar, whether they had an atypical agent identified or the cause was unknown. A study of 170 patients with CAP treated as outpatients from a single center in Switzerland

TABLE 5 Etiology of Community-Acquired Pneumonia

Most Common Causes[a]		
Ambulatory patients	Hospitalized (Non-ICU)[b]	Severe (ICU)
S. pneumoniae	*S. pneumoniae*	*S. pneumoniae*
M. pneumoniae	*M. pneumoniae*	*H. influenzae*
H. influenzae	*C. pneumoniae*	*Legionella* spp.
C. pneumoniae	*H. influenzae*	Gram-negative bacilli
Viruses	*Legionella* spp.	*S. aureus*
	Aspiration	

ICU = Intensive care unit.
[a] Based on collective data from recent studies.
[b] Excluding *Pneumocystis* spp.
Source: Ref. 31.

TABLE 6 Etiology of Nonsevere Community-Acquired Pneumonia: Correlation with Severity

	Percentage of Cases by Fine Score		
	Fine I(58)	Fine II(47)	Fine III(70)
Conventional organisms	31	55	51
S. pneumoniae	28	45	46
H. influenzae	3	4	1
O	0	4	3
Atypical organisms	69	45	49
M. pneumoniae	40	15	14
C. pneumoniae	14	9	23
Legionella spp	0	9	4
Coxiella burnetti	14	11	6

( ) = number of patients.
Source: Ref. 33.
Fine Class-refer to Ref. 18.

found 14% and 6% of cases, respectively, with *M. pneumoniae* and *C. pneumoniae* as the likely pathogen (21.8% were attributed to *S. pneumoniae*) [32]. Another study evaluating patients with nonsevere CAP (mostly ambulatory) from Spain found the most commonly identified organism in patients younger than 50 years of age and without significant comorbid conditions or abnormality of vital signs (Fine class I) was *Mycoplasma* (40% of cases), whereas *S. pneumoniae* was the most common pathogen in the older patients or those with underlying disease or abnormality of vital signs (Fine class II and III), Table 6 [33].

MICROBIOLOGICAL DIAGNOSIS

The utility of diagnostic studies to determine the etiologic agents of CAP is controversial. There should be a balance between reasonable diagnostic procedures and empirical therapy. At present, there are no rapid, easily performed, accurate, cost-effective methods that allow immediate results at the point of service (i.e., the initial evaluation by a clinician in an office or acute care setting). There is no routine diagnostic test that can consistently identify the etiologic agent. The recent guidelines for the management of CAP from the American Thoracic Society (ATS) advocate an empirical approach, whereas those from the Infectious Disease Society of America (IDSA) places a somewhat increased emphasis on diagnostic testing for the possibility of pathogen-directed antimicrobial therapy when the pathogen is identified [1,12]. The IDSA rationale is summarized as follows:

To permit optimal antibiotic selection in terms of activity against a specific pathogen (this especially applies to drug-resistant *S. pneumoniae*);
To permit antibiotic selection that limits the consequences of antibiotic abuse in terms of cost, resistance, and adverse drug effects;
To identify pathogens of potential epidemiological significance such as *Legionella*, TB

Nevertheless, it is recognized that most patients are treated empirically, especially outpatients for whom little diagnostic testing is utilized or recommended. Although no studies have clearly demonstrated a cost-effective advantage of establishing an etiologic diagnosis, there really have been no specific studies designed to address this issue. An obvious concern regarding empirical therapy without pathogen identification is the possible overuse of certain agents, which could lead to more resistance. Theoretically, one could be able to lessen the emergence of resistance, and therefore focus therapy, if one could identify the pathogen.

A detailed history can be important in the evaluation of CAP and may be helpful in alerting one to the possibility of an etiologic diagnosis. Epidemiological clues that may lead to diagnosis considerations are listed in Table 4.

For patients who are not seriously ill and do not require hospitalization, it is questionable whether any diagnostic tests are of benefit. The IDSA guidelines state that it is desirable, but optional, to perform a sputum gram stain with or without culture; the Canadian statement suggests that sputum examination possibly could be helpful in settings where pneumococcal resistance is common; the ATS statement indicates that sputum culture and gram stain for outpatients are not required unless a drug-resistant pathogen or an organism not covered by usual empirical therapy is suspected [1,11,12].

Of all the potential diagnostic studies, the most controversial is the study of expectorated sputum for gram stain and culture. It is acknowledged that this test is limited by the fact that many patients cannot produce a good specimen, patients often receive antimicrobial agents prior to evaluation, and many specimens show inconclusive results. In addition, the results of these tests will not be available for the prescriber to direct antimicrobial therapy. Nevertheless, results of good sputum cultures may prove useful for patients who clinically fail initial treatment (i.e., if a culture reveals isolation of macrolide-resistant *S. pneumoniae* in a patient treated empirically with a macrolide); and such information will add to the collective data regarding the predominant strains within a local setting. (The reader is referred to more comprehensive discussions in each of the guideline statements.) However, *antimicrobial therapy should be initiated promptly and should not be delayed in an attempt to obtain pretreatment specimens for microbiologic studies from acutely ill patients* [it is my experience that if patients are able to produce a good sputum sample, they are able to expectorate such specimens readily. If patients are unable to produce expectorated sputum in an expeditious manner, appropriate empirical antimicrobial therapy should be initiated without delay].

MANAGEMENT

Antimicrobial agents are the mainstays of treatment for patients with CAP. Decisions concerning specific therapy are guided by several considerations such as spectrum of activity, pharmacokinetics, efficacy, safety profile, cost, and whether a specific pathogen is identified.

The emergence of resistant respiratory pathogens, particularly drug-resistant strains of *S. pneumoniae* (DRSP), is becoming a significant concern that has complicated initial empirical management of CAP. Despite the rapid increase in DRSP, the clinical relevance for the outcome of CAP remains controversial, depending on the class of antimicrobial agent considered. Nevertheless, awareness of this resistance has had a significant impact on empirical therapy for patients treated for CAP because this can be a significant disease even for those treated as outpatients. The reader is referred to Chapter 3 for further discussion of the clinical relevance of DRSP for CAP.

Because patients treated for CAP in the ambulatory setting are for the most part treated empirically, the selection of specific antimicrobial regimens is based largely on the most likely pathogen. The most common (key) pathogens associated with nonsevere CAP are *S. pneumoniae*, *M. pneumoniae*, *C. pneumoniae*, and *H. influenzae*. Antimicrobial agents generally considered effective for these pathogens include the macrolides, newer fluoroquinolones, and doxycycline. While the β-lactam antibiotics (such as penicillins and cephalosporins) are effective against most isolates of *S. pneumoniae* and *H. influenzae*, they are not clinically effective for the "atypical pathogens."

Recent recommendations for empirical antimicrobial therapy from representative guidelines (i.e., North America and Britain) are summarized in Table 7 [1,11,12,19,34]. There is clearly a variation in health-care practices and policies in these different geographic locations as well as in local antimicrobial susceptibilities that influence specific recommendations. Although the different guidelines vary in their emphasis of the importance of defining the etiologic agents so that directed-therapy can be implemented, it is acknowledged that the majority of patients will be treated empirically. This

TABLE 7 Comparison of Recommendations of Recently Published Guidelines for Empirical Antimicrobial Therapy of Community-Acquired Pneumonia in Adults (from North America and United Kingdom)

Guideline	Empiric therapy for outpatients[a]
Centers for Disease Control-Drug Resistant *S. pneumoniae* Therapeutic Working Group (2000) [34]	Macrolide[b]; or doxycycline; or beta-lactam[c] or antipneumococcal fluoroquinolone[d] [Not 1st-line because of concerns for emerging resistance]
Canadian Infectious Disease Society/Canadian Thoracic Society (2000) [11]	Without modifying factors 1. Macrolide 2. Doxycycline With modifying factors COLD[e] (no recent Antibiotics or steroids) 1. New Macrolide[f] 2. Doxycycline COLD[e] (Recent Antibiotics or steroids) 1. Antipneum fluoroquin[d] 2. [Amox/Clav or 2-G Ceph] and Macrolide

Infectious Diseases Society of America (2000) [1]	Doxycycline; or macrolide; or antipneum Fluoroquin[d] Selection considerations: choice should be influenced by regional antibiotic susceptibility patterns for *S. pneumoniae* and the presence of risk factors for PRSP[g]. For older patients or those with underlying disease, antipneum fluoroquin may be preferred; some authorities prefer to reserve fluoroquin for such patients
American Thoracic Society (2001) [12]	No cardiopulmonary disease, no modifying factors[b]: azithromycin or clarithromyicn (doxycycline if allergic or intolerant to macrolides)
	Modifying factors[h]. β-lactam (cefpodoxime, cefuroxime, high-dose amoxicillin, amoxicillin/clavulanate; or parenteral ceftriaxone followed by p.o. cefpodxoime) *plus* [Macrolide or doxycycline]; or antipneum fluoroquin[d]
British Thoracic Society (2001) [19]	Amoxicillin 500–1000 mg t.i.d. (Alternative—erythromycin or clarithromycin)

[a] Site of care.
[b] Erythromycin, clarithromycin, or azithromycin.
[c] Cefuroxime axetil, amoxicillin, amoxicillin-clavulane, cefpodoxime, cefprozil; does not cover atypical pathogens.
[d] Antipneumococcal fluoroquionlone=levofloxacin, sparfloxacin, gatifloxacin, moxifloxacin.
[e] Chronic obstructive lung disease.
[f] Clarithromycin, azithromycin.
[g] PRSP=penicillin-resistant *S. pneumoniae*.
[h] Risks for drug-resistant *S. pneumoniae* (includes antimicrobial therapy within past 3 months, recent hospitalization, multiple comorbidities, elderly, exposure to day-care center) or cardiopulmonary disease.

is particularly the case for outpatients for whom diagnostic testing is not cost efficient and is not emphasized. Moreover, even at tertiary-level university centers where multiple diagnostic testing methods are used for patients who require hospitalization, an etiologic agent is found in only 50% (approximately) of cases [27].

The selection of specific antimicrobial regimens for empirical therapy in the guidelines is based largely on the most likely pathogens (aided by knowledge of commonly encountered pathogens in one's own geographic area and an appreciation of their usual susceptibilities patterns), and clinical studies. Other factors for consideration of specific antimicrobials that are mentioned in some of the guidelines include tolerance (adverse effects), ease of administration, and cost. Epidemiological information that may indicate the likelihood of a particular pathogen (such as recent epidemics of influenza, recent travel, and recent exposure to animals or other patients with specific infections) and disease severity (i.e., outpatient vs. inpatient) also significantly influences therapeutic choices.

Recommendations from Recent Guidelines for Empirical Therapy of Outpatient CAP

All the new North American guidelines variably recommend macrolides, doxycycline, or an antipneumococal fluoroquinolone (i.e., levofloxacin, gatifloxacin, and moxifloxacin) as treatment options for patients who are mildly ill and can be treated as outpatients. In general, the North American guidelines recommend a macrolide as first-line treatment for outpatients with no comorbidity or risk factors for DRSP.

In the Canadian statement, outpatients are stratified into those without modifying factors, for whom a macrolide may be used, and those with modifying factors (such as chronic obstructive lung disease or use of recent antibiotics or steroids —for which there may be a greater likelihood of DRSP) for whom fluoroquinolones are considered more appropriate as first-line empirical therapy. The IDSA statement indicates that the selection considerations among the three options should be influenced by regional antibiotic susceptibility patterns for *S. pneumoniae* and the presence of risk factors for drug-resistant *S. pneumoniae* (such as the use of antimicrobial agents within the previous 3 months). The statement further indicates that "for older patients or those with underlying disease, a fluoroquinolone may be a preferred choice; some authorities prefer to reserve fluoroquinolones for such patients"—thus, implying macrolide as first-line therapy for those patients without comorbidity or risk factors for DRSP. The CDC statement is similar but stresses that macrolides should be used first-line and fluoroquinolones should be reserved for cases associated with failure to or because of allergy to other agents or cases due to documented DRSP. The rationale is that fear of widespread use may lead to the development of fluoroquinolone resistance among the respiratory pathogens (as well as other pathogens colonizing the treated patients). Similar to the Canadian statement, the revised ATS guidelines recommends stratifying outpatients into two categories (Table 7) with macrolides being recommended as first-line therapy for patients with no cardiopulmonary disease, and no risks for DRSP, aspiration, or enteric gram-negatives. Doxycycline is a second choice (because of less reliable activity against *S. pneumoniae*) if patients are intolerant of or allergic to macrolides. The statement indicates that if *H. influenzae* is not likely, any macrolide could be used, including erythromycin. For more complex outpatients, the ATS statement recommends either a β-lactam/macrolide combination or monotherapy with an antipneumococcal fluoroquinolone. The rationale is the concern for likely DRSP and the possibility of clinical failure if the macrolides are used alone.

One difference between the North American guidelines and the British Thoracic Society (BTS) guidelines is the positioning of the macrolides as first-line options for empirical therapy of "low-risk" outpatients. All the North American statements include the macrolides as preferred first-line or as an equal option for patients with low risk for drug-resistant strains, whereas the primary agent recommended in the BTS statement is β-lactam (i.e., amoxicillin) and not macrolides (the macrolides are positioned as alternative agents). The difference in the emphasis placed on the importance of the "atypical" pathogens as well as the expression of macrolide-resistant *S. pneumoniae* in North America compared with Europe partly explains this variance. Because *M. pneumoniae* and *C. pneumoniae* are common causes of outpatient CAP (including older patients) and it is not possible to reliably predict the etiology solely on clinical manifestations, the North American statements include coverage of these common pathogens for empirical therapy. On the other hand, the British guidelines state that because *M. pneumoniae* exhibits epidemic periodicity every 4–5 years and largely affects younger persons, a policy for initial empirical therapy that aims always to cover this pathogen is unnecessary. Furthermore, in the United States most macrolide resistance is a result of increased drug efflux encoded by *mef* gene and with MICs < 16 mg/ml. It is possible that achievable levels of the newer macrolides (azithromycin, clarithromycin) may overcome this resistance. In Europe, most macrolide resistance is caused by ribosomal methylase encoded by *erm* gene; this results in high-level resistance to macrolides that cannot be overcome. In addition, at the time of the development of the North American guidelines, cases of macrolide failure for outpatients, particularly for cases not associated with risks for DRSP, had been infrequent. Of note, however, the continuing increasing frequency of macrolide resistance among pneumococci in North America is of concern and will require treatment recommendations for empirical therapy of CAP in the United States to be periodically reevaluated.

New Drugs

While managing CAP according to the empirical principles outlined before has led to measurable benefits in patient outcomes, the morbidity and mortality associated with this disease remain generally unchanged over the past few decades. This is due, in part, to the increasing prevalence of patients at risk (i.e., elderly, increased underlying conditions) as well as the limitations of current antibiotics in the face of growing antibacterial resistance. These issues highlight the need for antibacterial agents with activity against resistant strains of *S. pneumoniae* as well as with a low potential to induce resistance.

Until recently, therapeutic options for managing CAP due to known or suspected cases of drug-resistant pneumococcal infections were primarily limited to the fluoroquinolones. Although vancomycin is nearly certain to provide antibiotic coverage for DRSP, it is not active against other key respiratory pathogens (i.e., atypicals, *H. influenzae*) and there is a strong reason not to use this drug until it is needed because of fear of emergence of other resistant organisms (i.e., VRE, VRSA). Other agents effective against DRSP include quinupristin/dalfopristin, linezolid and the ketolides. However, the focus of therapy of quinupristin/dalfopristin and linezolid is more for nosocomial infections (and particularly for VRE or MRSA). Telithromycin is the first of a new class of macrolide-type antibiotic, the ketolides [35]. It is a novel addition to the macrolide–lincosamide–streptogramin-B (MLS_B) group of antibacterials specifically designed to treat community-acquired RTIs. In vitro studies have demonstrated the efficacy of telithromycin against such common respiratory pathogens as *S. pneumoniae* (including penicillin- and erythromycin-resistant strains), *H. influenzae*, *M. catarrhalis*, *Streptococcus pyogenes*, and *S. aureus* and against *Legionella*, *Chlamydia*, and *Mycoplasma* species. Furthermore, its structure confers a low potential to select for resistance or induce cross-resistance among other MLS_B antibacterials.

Length and Route of Antimicrobial Treatment

There is a lack of controlled trials that can specifically address the question as to length of therapy. The decision is usually based on the pathogen isolated, response to treatment, comorbid illness, and complications. Until further data are forthcoming, it seems reasonable to treat bacterial infections such as those caused by *S. pneumoniae* until a patient is afebrile for 72 hours. Most randomized clinical trials for the new fluoroquinolones or newer macrolides have shown good outcomes with 7–10 days of therapy (azithromycin may be used for shorter courses of treatment in ambulatory patients because of its longer half-life in tissue). Pneumonia caused by *Legionella* should be treated longer (i.e., 14–21 days), depending on the clinical response.

For many pathogens, there is no clear advantage of intravenous therapy over oral therapy, and the panel endorses use of oral antimicrobial agents for patients who tolerate these drugs if oral bioavailability and activity are adequate. However, for most patients admitted to the hospital, the common practice is to at least begin therapy with intravenous drugs. Changing from intravenous to oral therapy is associated with a number of economic, health care, and social benefits. Conditions for changing from intravenous to oral include stable or improving condition, ability to ingest drugs, and a functional gastrointestinal tract. In most cases these conditions are met within 2–3 days. Ideally the parenteral drugs should be given in an oral formulation with adequate bioavailability; if no oral formulation is available, then an oral agent with a similar spectrum of activity should be selected on the basis of in vitro or predicted susceptibility patterns of established or probable pathogen.

PREVENTION OF CAP

Despite controversies over efficacy of the polysaccharide pneumococcal vaccine (PPV), both PPV and the influenza vaccines are recommended according to current guidelines by the Centers for Disease Control and Prevention (at ages 65 and 50 respectively for immunocompetent adults without other risk factors) [36,37]. In a recent meta-anaylysis of 14 trials totaling more than 48,000 patients, PPV prevented definite pneumonia by 71% and mortality by 32% (but not all-cause death) [38]. However, there was no benefit seen for patients 55 years of age or older. A significant advance has been the development and licensure of the pneumococcal conjugate vaccine in infants. The benefits of this vaccine over the PPV have yet to be demonstrated in adults [39].

Smoking-cessation counseling for all smokers is an important effort for reduction of the burden of all respiratory tract infections.

CONCLUSION

Timeliness and appropriateness of antimicrobial therapy constitute the hallmarks of CAP treatment. The mortality rate is relatively low in the mild to moderate cases (Classes I through III). These patients may be treated in the ambulatory setting. CAP will continue to represent a significant threat to patients in the future as the number of patients at risk (the elderly and those with comorbid conditions) increase. Better, rapid diagnostic methods to define the etiologic pathogens are needed to allow more specific, directed therapy. It seems reasonable that patients will respond better and antibiotics can be used more appropriately if the specific pathogen is known, but good studies in support of this approach are needed. Although not discussed in this review, a greater understanding of the pathogenesis and host response should lead to new approaches of therapy. As the complexities of the host response are revealed, it is likely therapeutic benefits may be realized. The optimal approach to management continually will need to be reassessed as new information is generated.

REFERENCES

1. Bartlett JG, Dowell SF, Mandell LA, File TM Jr, Musher DM, Fine MJ. Guidelines from the Infectious Diseases Society of America. Practice guidelines for the management of community-acquired pneumonia in adults. Clin Infect Dis 2000; 31:347–382.
2. Mandell LA. Community-acquired pneumonia: etiology, epidemiology, and treatment. Chest 1995; 108(suppl):35S–42S.
3. Foy HM, Cooney MK, Allan I, et al. Rates of pneumonia during influenza epidemics in Seattle, 1964 to 1975. JAMA 1979; 241:253.
4. Houston MS, Silverstein MD, Suman VJ. Community-acquired lower respiratory tract infection in the elderly: A community-based study of incidence and outcome. J Am Board Fam Pract 1995; 8(5):347–356.
5. Marston BJ, Plouffe JF, File TM Jr, and the CBPIS Study Group. Incidence of community-acquired pneumonia requiring hospitalization: Results of a population-based active surveillance study in Ohio. Arch Intern Med 1997; 157: 1709–1718.
6. European Study on Community-Acquired Pneumonia (ESOCAP) committee, Huchon G, Woodhead M, et al. Management of adult community-acquired lower respiratory tract infections. Eur Respir Rev 1998; 8(61):391–426.
7. Marrie TJ. Community-acquired pneumonia: epidemiology, etiology, treatment. Infect Dis Clin North Am 1998; 12(3):723–739.
8. Koivula I, Sten M, Makela PH. Risk factors for pneumonia in the elderly. Am J Med 1994; 96:313–320.
9. Saitz R, Ghali WA, Moskowitz MA. The impact of alcohol-related diagnoses on pneumonia outcomes. Arch Intern Med 1997; 157:1446–1452.
10. Fine MJ, Smith MA, Carson CA, et al. Prognosis and outcomes of patients with community-acquired pneumonia. JAMA 1996; 275:134–141.
11. Mandell LA, Marrie TJ, Grossman RE, et al. Canadian guidelines for the initial management of community-acquired pneumonia: an evidence-based update by the Canadian Infectious Diseases Society and the Canadian Thoracic Society. Clin Infect Dis 2000; 31:383–421.
12. Niederman MS, Mandell LA, Anzueto A, et al. Guidelines for the management

of adults with community-acquired pneumonia (American Thoracic Society). Am J Respir Crit Care Med 2001; 163:1730–1754.
13. Metlay JP, Kapoor WN, Fine MJ. Does this patient have community-acquired pneumonia? JAMA 1997; 278:1440–1445.
14. Metlay JP, Atlas SJ, Borowsky LH, Singer DE. Time course of symptom resolution in patients with community-acquired pneumonia. Resp Med 1998; 92: 1137–1142.
15. Fine MJ, Stone RA, Singer DE, et al. Processes and outcomes of care for patients with community-acquired pneumonia: results from the Pneumonia Patient Outcomes Research Team (PORT) cohort study. Arch Intern Med 1999; 159:970–980.
16. Niederman MS, McCombs JS, Unger AN, Kumar A, Popovian R. The cost of treating community-acquired pneumonia. Clin Ther 1998; 20:820–837.
17. Coley CM, Yi-Hwei L, Medsger AR, et al. Preference for home vs. hospital care among low-risk patients with community-acquired pneumonia. Arch Intern Med 1996; 156:1565–1571.
18. Fine MJ, Auble TE, Yealy DM, et al. A prediction rule to identify low-risk patients with community-acquired pneumonia. N Engl J Med 1997; 336:243–250.
19. British Thoracic Society. Guidelines for the management of community-acquired pneumonia in adults. Thorax 2001; 56(suppl IV):iv1–iv64.
20. Atlas SJ, Benzer TI, Borowsky LH, et al. Safely increasing the proportion of patients with community-acquired pneumonia treated as outpatients: an interventional trial. Arch Intern Med 1998; 158:1350–1356.
21. Flanders WD, Tuckter G, Krishnadasan A, Martin D, Honig E, McClellan WM. Validation of the pneumonia severity index. Importance of study-specific recalibration. J Gen Intern Med 1999; 14:333–340.
22. Marras TK, Gutierrez C, Chan CK. Applying a prediction rule to identify low-risk patients with community-acquired pneumonia. Chest 2000; 118:1339–1343.
23. Chan SS, Yuen EH, Kew J, Cheung WL, Cocks RA. Community-acquired pneumonia—implementation of a prediction rule to guide selection of patients for outpatient treatment. Eur J Emerg Med 2001; 8:279–286.
24. Stauble SP, Reichlin S, Dieterle T, Leimenstoll B, Schoenenberger R, Martina B. Community-acquired pneumonia—which patients are hospitalized? Swiss Med Weekly 2001; 131:188–192.
25. Lim WS, Lewis S, MacFarlane JT. Severity prediction rules in community-acquired pneumonia: a validation study. Thorax 2000; 55:219–223.
26. File TM Jr, Tan JS. Incidence, etiologic pathogens and diagnostic testing of community-acquired pneumonia. Current Opinion Pulm Med 1997; 3:89–97.
27. Bartlett JG, Mundy LM. Current concepts: Community-acquired pneumonia. N Engl J Med 1995; 333(24):1618–1624.
28. File TM Jr, Plouffe JF. Legionella. Curr Infect Dis Reports 1999; 1:65–72.
29. Straus WL, Plouffe JF, File TM Jr, et al. Risk factors for domestic acquisition of Legionnaires' disease. Arch Intern Med 1996; 156:1685–1692.
30. File TM Jr, Tan JS, Plouffe JF. The role of atypical pathogens: *Mycoplasma*

pneumoniae, *Chlamydia pneumoniae*, and *Legionella pneumophila* in respiratory infection. Infect Dis Clin North Am 1998; 12(3):569–592.

31. Marrie TJ, Peeling RW, Fine MJ, et al. Ambulatory patients with community-acquired pneumonia: the frequency of atypical agents and clinical course. Am J Med 1996; 101:508–515.
32. Bochud PY, Moser F, Erard P, et al. Community-acquired pneumonia. A prospective outpatient study. Medicine 2001; 80(2):75–87.
33. Falguera M, Sacristan O, Nogues A, et al. Non-severe community-acquired pneumonia: correlation between cause and severity or comorbidity. Arch Intern Med 2001; 161(15):1866–1870.
34. Heffelfinger JD, Dowell SF, Jorgensen JH, et al. Management of community-acquired pneumonia in the era of pneumococcal resistance: a report from the drug-resistant Streptococcus pneumoniae Therapeutic Working Group. Arch Intern Med 2000; 160:1399–1408.
35. Leclercq R. Overcoming antimicrobial resistance: profile of a new ketolide antibacterial, telithromycin. J Antimicrob Chemother 2001; 48(suppl B):9–23.
36. Centers for Disease Control and Prevention. General recommendations on immunization. Recommendations of the Advisory Committee on Immunization Practices (ACIP) and the American Academy of Family Practice Physicians. MMWR Morbi Mortal Wkly Rep 2002; 51:No.RR-2.
37. Gardner P, Pickering LK, Orenstein WA, Gershon AA, Nichol K. Guidelines for quality standards for immunization. Clin Infect Dis 2002; 35:503–511.
38. Cornu C, Yzebe D, Leophonte P, Gaillt J, Boissel JP, Cucherat M. Efficacy of pneumococcal polysaccharide vaccine in immunocompetent adults: a meta-analysis of randomized trials. Vaccine 2001; 19:4780–4790.
39. Klugman KP. Efficacy of pneumococcal conjugate vaccines and their effect on carriage and antimicrobial resistance. Lancet Inf Dis 2001; 1:85–91.

14

Treatment of Hospitalized Patients with Community-Acquired Pneumonia

Michael S. Niederman
Winthrop University Hospital
Mineola
and SUNY at Stony Brook
Stony Brook, New York, U.S.A.

Pneumonia is the sixth leading cause of death in the United States and the number-one cause of death from infectious diseases [1]. The infection can occur in patients who are living in the community (community-acquired pneumonia, CAP) or in those who are already hospitalized (nosocomial pneumonia, NP), but today the distinction between community and nosocomial infection is less clear because the "community" includes complex patients such as those who have recently been hospitalized, those in nursing homes, and those with chronic diseases who are commonly managed in such facilities as dialysis centers or nursing homes. Although patients with varying degrees of immune function can be affected by CAP, this discussion is confined to patients with CAP admitted to the hospital who are immune competent individuals, and excludes discussion of patients with HIV infection or traditional immune suppression (cancer chemotherapy, immune suppressive medications).

Of the 5.6 million patients with CAP treated in 1994, only 1.1 million were admitted to the hospital, yet this minority of patients accounted for the majority of cost in managing this illness [2]. In fact, a total of $8.4 billion was spent on the care of CAP patients, and only $0.4 billion was spent on the care of the 4.5 million outpatients [2]. Among those who are hospitalized, the elderly account for a disproportionate amount of expense: they make up only about a third of all pneumonia patients, yet are responsible for more than half of the dollars spent on this illness. This in turn is a reflection of the fact that the elderly are more often hospitalized than a younger population and have a higher frequency of comorbid illness [2].

From these data, it is clear that one of the major management issues in CAP is deciding who gets admitted to the hospital. In addition, once patients are hospitalized, the key management decisions hinge on deciding the appropriate site of care (medical floor or ICU), initiating the correct therapy as soon as possible, and recognizing the patient's response to therapy. If a patient responds appropriately, then the hospital stay can be abbreviated, especially with a timely switch to oral antibiotic therapy. If the patient is not responding as expected, then it is necessary to do a thorough evaluation to recognize unusual or unexpected pathogens (tuberculosis, fungal disease), to treat drug-resistant organisms, to diagnose pneumonia complications (empyema, pulmonary embolus), and to rule out mimics of pneumonia (malignancy, inflammatory lung disease). This chapter focuses on the management of inpatients with CAP and emphasizes the approach to management, including algorithms for therapy and the management of this illness in an era of increasingly common rates of infection with antibiotic-resistant organisms.

CLINICAL FEATURES OF CAP

Symptoms (Table 1)

The classic symptoms of CAP, including cough, sputum production, dyspnea, and fever, are common in patients with an intact immune response, but less frequent in the elderly and chronically ill. Although cough is present in up to 80% of all patients, it is less frequent in those who are elderly, in those with serious comorbidity, or in individuals coming from nursing homes [3,4]. Elderly patients with CAP may have nonrespiratory presentations of illness and may be afebrile, and these findings have been identified as predictors of mortality [5]. This may be the consequence of the fact that a nonrespiratory presentation is usually a reflection of an impaired immune response, but it may also be a reason for the patient to have a delayed presentation to medical attention, and the physician in turn may delay the diagnosis of pneumonia in this setting. In keeping with these observations, the absence of pleuritic chest pain, which is generally a common symptom in patients with certain forms of pneumonia, was identified in one study to be a poor prognostic finding [6].

In an elderly patient, the nonrespiratory presentations of CAP can include symptoms of confusion, falling, failure to thrive, altered functional

TABLE 1 Clinical Features of CAP

Finding	Comment
Fever, chills	More likely with intact immune system, but can be absent in the elderly and immune suppressed (including steroid therapy)
Dyspnea	Present in only 70%
Worsening of chronic underlying illness	May be the only clue to pneumonia in the elderly
Cough and purulent sputum	Cough in up to 80%; 50% with purulence. Appearance of sputum cannot always identify bacterial infection.
Duration of symptoms	Tend to be longer in the elderly
Absence of respiratory symptoms	Associated with increased mortality, especially the absence of pleuritic chest pain
Impaired consciousness, poor swallowing	Aspiration risk factors; consider in patients with recurrent infection
Nonrespiratory symptoms: falling, confusion, decreased functional status	May be the only symptoms related to pneumonia in the elderly
Respiratory rate	Rarely <20 if pneumonia, and mortality risk is increased if >30/min. Must be counted on admission for all patients.
Bronchial breath sounds, egophony, dullness, reduced breath sounds, crackles	Suggests pneumonia and should prompt a chest radiograph
Skin rash	*S. aureus, P. aeruginosa, Mycobacterium tuberculosis*, Endemic fungi, Aspergillus, Varicella- zoster, herpes simplex, *M. pneumoniae*
Elevated liver function tests	*S. pneumoniae*, *S. aureus*, *P. aeruginosa*, *M. tuberculosis*, *Legionella*, *H. influenzae*, *Coccidioides immitis*, Aspergillus, Herpes simplex, varicella -zoster, Q fever, *M. pneumoniae, C. psittaci*

capacity, or deterioration in a preexisting medical illness, such as congestive heart failure or dementia [3,4,5,7]. In one study, delirium or acute confusion were significantly more frequent in the elderly patients with pneumonia than in age-matched controls who did not have pneumonia [7]. In that study, there was no association between the etiologic pathogen and the symptoms of pneumonia, except for pleuritic chest pain, which was more common when *Streptocococcus pneumoniae* was the pathogen. Elderly patients are more commonly malnourished than other CAP patients (16% vs. 47% of controls), with kwashiorkor-like malnutrition being the predominant type of nutritional defect and one associated with delirium on initial presentation [7]. Several studies have documented a substantially higher mortality rate in the elderly than in other individuals with CAP and thus it is not surprising that in one study of 1812 patients of all ages, older patients tended to have a longer duration of symptoms, such as cough, sputum production, dyspnea, fatigue, anorexia, myalgia and abdominal pain, than did younger ones [3].

Physical Findings

Physical findings of pneumonia are not specific, but include tachycardia, tachypnea, crackles, rhonchi and signs of pulmonary consolidation (egophony, bronchial breath sounds, dullness to percussion). Patients may also have signs of pleural effusion. In some patients, the presence of extrapulmonary findings can help to diagnose metastatic infection (arthritis, endocarditis, meningitis), or add to the suspicion of an "atypical" pathogen such as *M. pneumoniae* or *C. pneumoniae*, the former of which can be accompanied by bullous myringitis, skin rash, pericarditis, hepatitis, hemolytic anemia, or meningoencephalitis. Measurement of respiratory rate is a key diagnostic and prognostic maneuver. For example, in elderly patients an elevation of respiratory rate can be the initial presenting sign of pneumonia, preceding other clinical findings by as much as 1–2 days. In a prospective study in a long term care setting, 19 of 21 patients who were diagnosed with lower respiratory tract infection had a respiratory rate above the normal range of 16–25, and in general the elevated rate preceded other clinical findings [8]. In another study, tachypnea was present in over 80% of all CAP patients, being present more often in the elderly than in younger patients with pneumonia [3]. Measurement of respiratory rate also is of prognostic significance, and the finding of a respiratory rate of more than 30 per minute is one of several factors associated with increased mortality [1].

Radiographic Features

Although most studies of CAP require the presence of a new radiographic infiltrate, not all patients will have this finding when first evaluated. Even when the radiograph is negative, if the patient has appropriate symptoms and focal physical findings, pneumonia may still be present. In one study, 47 patients with clinical signs and symptoms of CAP were evaluated with both a chest radiograph and a high-resolution CT scan of the chest and there were eight patients identified by CT scan as having pneumonia who had a negative chest radiograph. In many instances, there were more extensive abnormalities found on CT scan, with 16 patients shown to have bilateral infiltrates by this technique, compared to only 6 with this finding on chest radiograph [9]. Bronchopneumonia was the most common abnormality defined by either technique. The findings of this study confirm the need to repeat the chest film after 24–48 hours in certain symptomatic patients with an initially negative chest film. The reason for an initially negative chest film is not clear, but some studies have suggested that febrile and dehydrated patients can have a normal film when first admitted with pneumonia, but it is still uncertain if it is possible to "hydrate a pneumonia" after admission to the hospital [10]. In COPD patients, an exacerbation can be accompanied by the presence of an infiltrate (CAP), or without a radiographic abnormality (acute bronchitic exacerbation). One recent study has shown that if a radiographic abnormality is present, then the illness is more severe, and the complications greater, than if no infiltrate is present [11].

It is generally not possible to define the etiology of CAP on the basis of specific radiogaphic findings; however, there are certain patterns that have been associated with specific pathogens [10]. Focal consolidation can be seen with infections caused by pneumococcus, *Klebsiella*, aspiration (especially if in the lower lobes or other dependent segments), *S. aureus*, *L. pneumophila*, *H. influenzae*, *M. pneumoniae*, and *C. pneumoniae*. Interstitial infiltrates are present in patients with viral pneumonia as well as infection due to *M. pneumoniae*, *C. pneumoniae*, *C. psittaci*, and *P. carinii*. Lymphadenopathy with an interstitial pattern should raise concerns about anthrax, *Francisella tularensis* and *C. psittaci*; adenopathy can be seen with focal infiltrates in tuberculosis, fungal pneumonia, and bacterial pneumonia. Cavitation can be the result of an aspiration lung abscess, or infection with *S. aureus*, aerobic gram-negatives (including *P. aeruginosa*), tuberculosis, fungal infection, nocardia and actinomycosis.

Pleural effusion may be present, and it is necessary to sample the pleural fluid in order to distinguish empyema from a simple parapneumonic effusion. In some studies, the presence of bilateral pleural effusion was an independent predictor of short-term mortality in CAP [12]. Pneumococcal pneumonia is the infection most commonly complicated by effusion (36–57% of patients), but other pathogens causing effusion include *H. influenzae*, *M. pneumoniae*, *Legionella*, anthrax, tularemia and tuberculosis [13,14].

Typical vs. Atypical Pneumonia Syndromes

Using clinical patterns of pneumonia symptoms and findings to define the etiology of CAP is generally not helpful, and separating features into either "typical" or "atypical" pneumonia is of historic interest but cannot directly aid patient management. The typical pneumonia syndrome is characterized by sudden onset of high fever, shaking chills, pleuritic chest pain, lobar consolidation, a toxic-appearing patient, and the production of purulent sputum. Although this pattern has been attributed to pneumococcus and other bacterial pathogens, these organisms do not always lead to such classic symptoms. The atypical pneumonia syndrome, which is characterized by a subacute illness, nonproductive cough, headache, diarrhea, or other systemic complaints, is usually the result of infection with *Mycoplasma pneumoniae*, *C. pneumoniae*, *Legionella* sp., or viruses. However, patients with impaired immune responses (especially the elderly with chronic illness) may present in this fashion, even when bacterial pneumonia is present, and thus it is usually not possible to use the features on clinical presentation to predict the likely etiologic agent [1,15–18]. In fact, in one study the clinical features were no more than 42% accurate in differentiating pneumococcus, *Mycoplasma pneumoniae*, and other pathogens from one another [16].

ETIOLOGIC PATHOGENS

Diagnostic testing has limited value in patients with CAP, and can define an etiologic agent in only about half of all patients, raising the possibility that we do not know all the organisms that can cause CAP [1,17]. In the past three decades, a variety of new pathogens for this illness have been identified, including *Legionella pneumophila*, *Chlamydia pneumoniae*, and hantavirus. In addition, antibiotic-resistant variants of common pathogens such as *Streptococcus pneumoniae* and *H. influenzae* have become increasingly common. In an era where bioterrorism remains a threat, it is important to consider such organisms as *Bacillus anthracis*, *Yersinia pestis*, and *Francisella tularensis* in patients who present with a syndrome of CAP.

Streptococus pneumoniae

The most common pathogen for CAP in any patient population is *S. pneumoniae*, and this organism may even be responsible for many episodes of inpatient CAP that go undiagnosed by standard testing. In one study using transthoracic needle aspirates in patients with no organisms recovered by conventional diagnostic testing, half of the patients in whom the needle provided a diagnosis had pneumococcus identified as the pathogen [19]. Pneumococcal infection is more common in the elderly; those with asplenia, multiple myeloma, congestive heart failure, alcoholism; after influenza; and in patients with chronic lung disease. In patients with HIV infection, pneumococcal pneumonia with bacteremia is more common than in healthy populations of the same age. The classic radiographic pattern is a lobar consolidation, but bronchopneumonia can also occur, and in some series, this is the most common pattern [20]. Bacteremia is present in up to 20% of hospitalized patients with this infection, but the impact of this finding on mortality is uncertain [21]. Extrapulmonary complications include meningitis, empyema, arthritis, endocarditis, and brain abscess.

In the past decade, antibiotic resistance among pneumococci has become increasingly common, and penicillin resistance, along with resistance to other common antibiotics (macrolides, trimethoprim/sulfamethoxizole, selected cephalosporins), is present in over 40% of these organisms [1,22]. Because most penicillin resistance is of the "intermediate" type (penicillin minimum inhibitory concentration, or MIC, of 0.1 to 1.0 mg/L) and not of the high-level type (penicillin MIC of 2.0 or more), the clinical significance of these organisms is uncertain. Although not all resistance is likely to be relevant, experts believe that CAP with organisms having a penicillin minimum inhibitory concentration (MIC) of $\geq$ 4 mg/L can lead to an increased risk of death [1,14,21,23].

Although Pallares et al. were unable to show an impact of resistance (penicillin MIC $>$ 0.12 mg/L) on mortality, after adjusting for severity of illness in a population of 504 infected patients, Turrett and colleagues found that high-level resistance was a predictor of mortality in a population of 462 patients with pneumococcal bacteremia, of whom more than half were HIV positive [24,25]. In other studies, investigators did not find an increased risk of death from infection with resistant organisms but did find an enhanced likelihood of suppurative complications (empyema), and a more prolonged hospital length of stay [26,27]. While these studies involved relatively small number of patients, Feikin et al. studied the impact of pneumococcal resistance in 5837 patients with bacteremic CAP [23]. They found an increased mortality for patients with a penicillin MIC of at least 4 mg/L or greater, or with a cefotaxime MIC of 2.0 mg/L or more. However, this increased mortality was only present if patients who died in the first 4 days of therapy were excluded from analysis. One limitation of this study was a failure to correct for severity of illness or accuracy of therapy. More recently, Moroney et al. used both cohort study and matched-control methods and found that severity of illness, and not resistance or accuracy of therapy, was the most important predictor of mortality [28]. Interestingly, in the case-control part of the study, severity of illness was greater in patients without resistant organisms, implying a loss of virulence among organisms that become resistant, a finding echoed in another study that found absence of invasive illness to be a risk factor for pneumococcal resistance [29].

Atypical Pathogens

Although the term atypical should not be used to describe a specific clinical syndrome, the term can be used to refer to a group of pathogens that includes

M. pneumoniae, *C. pneumoniae*, and *Legionella*, all organisms that must be treated with a macrolide, tetracycline, or a quinolone. Infection with these pathogens is common in patients of all ages, not just young and healthy individuals, and these organisms have even been reported among the elderly in nursing homes [1,30,31]. In addition, they can occur as either primary pathogens or may be part of a mixed infection, along with traditional bacterial pathogens. When mixed infection is present, it may lead to a more complex course and a longer length of stay than if a single pathogen is present. There may be a particular synergy between *C. pneumoniae* and pneumococcus, with either sequential or mixed infection with *C. pneumoniae* leading to a more severe course for pneumococcus [32]. The frequency of atypical pathogens can be as high as 60% in some series, with as many as 40% of all CAP patients having mixed infection [33]. Although the exact frequency of infection with these organisms is uncertain, their importance has been suggested in studies of inpatients, which have shown a reduced mortality and length of stay when patients received empiric therapy that accounted for these organisms, compared to regimens that do not account for these organisms [34,35]. Although these organisms may be important, there may be both temporal and geographic variability in their occurrence. In one study, the benefit of providing empiric therapy directed at atypical pathogens was variable, being more important in some calendar years than in others [35].

The incidence of *Legionella* infection among admitted patients has varied from 1% to 15% or more and is also a reflection of geographic and seasonal variability in infection rates, as well as a reflection of the extent of diagnostic testing. This organism is a particular problem in patients with severe CAP, but its frequency is varable. In one report, atypical pathogens were present in almost 25% of all ICU CAP patients, but the responsible organism varied over time, with *Legionella* being common in one time period; but in the same hospital a decade later, it had been replaced by *Mycoplasma* and *Chlamydia* infection [36].

Although it is very difficult to use clinical features to predict the microbial etiology of CAP, there are descriptions of a classic *Legionella* syndrome, which is characterized by high fever, chills, headache, myalgias, and leukocytosis, along with preceding diarrhea, early onset of mental confusion, hyponatremia, relative bradycardia, and liver function abnormalities. This syndrome is usually not present, and the illness can be rapidly progressive, with the patient appearing to be quite toxic, and thus this diagnosis should always be considered in all patients admitted to the ICU with CAP.

Gram-Negative Bacteria

The most common gram-negative organism causing CAP is *H. influenzae*, a common pathogen in the elderly and in those who smoke cigarettes or who have chronic bronchitis [1]. *H. influenzae* can be either a typable (encapsulated) or nontypable organism, and can lead to bronchopneumonia and, rarely, empyema. Enteric gram-negatives are generally not common in CAP, unless the patients are elderly and have chronic cardiac or pulmonary disease or are alcoholics. In these patients, organisms such as *E. coli* and *Klebsiella pneumoniae* can be found. *Pseudomonas aeruginosa* is an uncommon cause of CAP but can be isolated from patients with CAP and bronchiectasis, and in those with severe forms of CAP, particularly in elderly patients older than 75 [1,37]. In one recent study, enteric gram-negative bacteria were present in 11% of 559 hospitalized CAP patients, with *P. aeruginosa* being the dominant pathogen. Pneumonia due to these organisms was associated with a 3.4-fold increased risk of mortality. Risk factors for gram-negative infection were probable aspiration, prior antibiotic therapy, prior hospitalization, and the presence of pulmonary comorbidity. The last two factors were also risk factors for infection with *P. aeruginosa* [38]. In very elderly (> age 75) patients admitted to the ICU with CAP, *P. aeruginosa* has also been identified, particularly in nursing home residents who have bronchiectasis and impaired functional status [37].

Other Organisms

CAP can also be caused by *S. aureus*, which can lead to severe illness and to cavitary lung infection. This organism can also seed the lung hematogenously from a vegetation in patients with right-sided endocarditis or from septic venous thrombophlebitis (from central venous catheter or jugular vein infection). The role of anaerobes in CAP in uncertain, but they may be

TABLE 2 Common Pathogens Causing Inpatient CAP

With Cardiopulmonary Disease and/or Modifying Factors
S. pneumoniae (including DRSP), *H. influenzae*, *M. pneumoniae*, *C. pneumoniae*, mixed infection (bacteria plus atypical pathogen), enteric gram-negatives, aspiration (anaerobes), viruses, *Legionella* sp., others (*M. tuberculosis*, endemic fungi, *Pneumocystic carinii*)
With No Cardiopulmonary Disease or Modifying Factors
All of the above, but DRSP and enteric gram-negatives are not likely
Severe CAP, with No Risks for *P. Aeruginosa*
S. pneumoniae (including DRSP), *Legionella* sp., *H. influenzae*, enteric gram-negative bacilli, *S. aureus*, *M. pneumoniae*, respiratory viruses, others (*C. pneumoniae*, *M. tuberculosis*, endemic fungi)
Severe CAP, with Risks for *P. Aeruginosa*
All of the pathogens above. plus *P. aeruginosa*

important in patients with aspiration risk factors (neurologic illness, impaired swallowing, esophageal disease), and may cause lung abscess in dependent lung segments. The need to treat these organisms when they are part of a mixed infection with aerobic organisms is uncertain [1,14]. The incidence of viral pneumonia is difficult to define, but during epidemic times, influenza should be considered; it can lead to a primary viral pneumonia or to secondary bacterial infection with pneumococcus, *S. aureus*, or *H. influenzae*. Finally, it important to always consider the diagnosis of tuberculosis in patients with CAP, and, in endemic areas, fungal infection with coccidiodomycosis and histoplasmosis, especially in HIV-infected persons.

TABLE 3 Clinical Associations with Specific Pathogens

Condition	Commonly Encountered Pathogens
Alcoholism	Streptococcus pneumoniae (including PRSP), anaerobes, gram-negative bacilli (possibly *K. pneumoniae*)
COPD/current or former smoker	*S. pneumoniae*, *H. influenzae*, *Moraxella catarrhalis*, *Legionella*. Role of atypicals uncertain
Residence in nursing home	*S. pneumoniae*, gram-negative bacilli, *H. influenzae*, *S. aureus* (including methicillin-resistant organisms), anaerobes, *C. pneumoniae*; consider *M. tuberculosis*. Modify considerations based on local epidemiology
Poor dental hygiene	Anaerobes
Bat exposure	*Histoplasma capsulatum*
Bird exposure	*Chlamydia psittaci*, *Cryptococcus neoformans*, *H. capsulatum*
Rabbit exposure	*Francisella tularensis*
Travel to SW USA	Coccidioidomycosis; hantavirus in selected areas
Exposure to farm animals or parturient cats	*Coxiella burnetii* (Q fever)
Post-influenza pneumonia	*S. pneumoniae*, *S. aureus*, *H. influenzae*
Structural disease of lung (bronchiectasis, cystic fibrosis, etc.)	*P. aeruginosa*, *P. cepacia* or *S. aureus*
Bioterrorism	*Bacillus anthracis*, *Yersinia pestis*, *Francisella tularensis*

Predicting Pathogens for Specific Patient Populations

Table 2 summarizes the common pathogens causing CAP in inpatients, both on the medical ward and in the ICU. The classification is based on the severity of illness and the presence of clinical risk factors for specific pathogens, referred to as "modifying factors." Patients with severe CAP may have a slightly different spectrum of organisms than other patients with this illness, being commonly infected with pneumococcus, atypical pathogens, enteric gram-negatives (including *P. aeruginosa*), *S. aureus*, and *H. influenzae*.

The modifying factors for DRSP are age greater than 65 years, β-lactam therapy within the past 3 months, alcoholism, immune suppressive illness (including therapy with corticosteroids), multiple medical comorbidities, and exposure to a child in a day-care [1,29,39]. The modifying factors for enteric gram-negatives include residence in a nursing home, underlying cardiopulmonary disease, multiple medical comorbidities, and recent antibiotic therapy. The risk factors for *P. aeruginosa* infection are structural lung disease (bronchiectasis), corticosteroid therapy (> 10 mg prednisone / day), broad-spectrum antibiotic therapy for more than 7 days in the past month, and malnutrition [1]. Table 3 shows that certain clinical conditions are associated with specific pathogens, and these associations should be considered in all patients when obtaining a history.

ASSESSMENT OF SEVERITY OF ILLNESS

Hospitalization Decision

Given the economic and social impact of pneumonia, the decision about site of initial care is one of the most important in disease management. Generally severity of illness should be determined in order to decide whether the patient should be hospitalized and whether ICU admission is needed. Although a number of prediction models have been developed to guide the admission decision, no rule is absolute and the decision to admit a patient should be based on social as well as medical considerations, and it remains an "art of medicine" determination. In general, the hospital should be used to observe patients who have multiple risk factors for a poor outcome, those who have decompensation of a chronic illness, or those who need therapies not easily administered at home (oxygen, intravenous fluids, cardiac monitoring) [1]. Risk factors for a poor outcome include respiratory rate greater than 30/minute, systolic blood pressure less than 90 mm Hg, diastolic BP less than 60 mm Hg, multilobar pneumonia, confusion, BUN greater than 19.6 mg/dl, PaO2 less than 60 mm Hg, PaCO2 greater than 50 mm Hg, respiratory or metabolic acidosis, or signs of systemic sepsis [1,40,41]. The British Thoracic Society (BTS) rule states that patients have a 9- to 21-fold increased risk of death if they have at least two of the following four criteria present: respiratory rate equal to or greater than 30/min, diastolic BP equal to or less than 60 mm Hg, BUN greater than 19.6 mg/dL, and confusion [41,42].

One approach to the admission decision was developed by the investigators in the Pneumonia Outcomes Research Team (PORT) study who developed a mortality prediction rule that classifies all patients into one of five groups (classes I through V), each with a different risk of death [40]. In the Infectious Disease Society of America (IDSA) guidelines for CAP, this mortality risk score, the Pneumonia Severity Index (PSI), has been used to guide the admission decision, recommending admission for patients in classes IV and V, with a predicted mortality risk of 8.2–9.3% and 27–31.1%, respectively, while outpatient care was recommended for patients in classes I and II, with a mortality risk of 0.1–0.4% and 0.6–0.7%, respectively [14]. Patients in class III had an intermediate risk of death, 0.9–2.8%, and the recommendation was that the admission decision be individualized for these patients. The scoring system is complex, and patients have points calculated based on such factors as age, sex, the presence of comorbid medical disease, certain physical findings, and certain laboratory data [40].

In prospective studies, the limitations of the PORT model have been identified, particularly the finding that as many as 30–40% of those who are admitted based on clinical judgment fall into the low-risk groups [43,44]. In one such study, 166 out of 826 patients presenting to the emergency department fell into classes I–III, and when the rule was used to guide the admission decision rule, 57% of the low-risk patients were discharged, compared to only 42% in a preceding period when clinical judgment was used [43]. However, in the period when the prediction rule was used, 9% of the discharged patients failed outpatient therapy, whereas no patients fell into this category during the period when clinical judgment was used to make this decision. In another study, 70% of low-risk patients were sent home when the admission decision rule was applied, compared to approximately 50% when clinical judgment was used [44]. Thus, in both studies, clinical judgment (probably appropriately) led to many patients being admitted, in spite of the model suggesting that they be discharged. One problem with the PORT model is that points are assigned on the basis of dichotomous variables, and thus if vital sign abnormalities are present but below the threshold for assigning points, severity of illness can be underestimated. The cut-off points in this model are heart rate greater than 125/min, respiratory rate greater than 30/min, systolic blood pressure less than 90 mm Hg, fever under 35° or over 40°C, PaO2 less than 60 mm Hg, BUN greater than 30 mg/dL, and glucose greater than 250 mg/dL [40].

Another limitation of the PORT model is that points are based on age and comorbid illness, and older patients will often have a high score, even if the illness is mild. Thus, in one recent study, when elderly individuals with CAP were admitted, most fell into risk classes III through V, and the risk of death increased along with the category [45]. However, it is uncertain how many older patients in higher risk classes can be safely managed out of the hospital. Recently, Lim et al. have shown that the BTS rule does not work as well in the elderly as in younger patients, reflecting the altered clinical presentations of pneumonia in this population. In one study, the rule had a 66% sensitivity and a 73% specificity for predicting mortality in a population that included 48% who were at least 75 years of age [46,47].

The BTS rule may be useful for avoiding the problem of overlooking a sick patient: in one study, the BTS critieria identified 19 of 20 patients, in a population of 255, who were destined to die, whereas clinical criteria identified only 12 of the 19 as being seriously ill [42]. However, the BTS rule may not be optimal in an elderly population, and in recent studies, it did not work as well as it did in other populations, although it had a higher sensitivity for predicting mortality than the Prognostic Scoring Index (PSI), derived from the PORT study [40,46]. It is clear that all rules can be problematic, and thus the admission decision remains a clinical judgment.

Need for ICU Care

There is no specific rule for who should be admitted to the ICU, but in general the ICU is used for approximately 10% of all admitted CAP patients, and this population has a mortality rate of at least 30%, compared to a mortality rate of 12% for all admitted patients [48]. There is some uncertainty about the benefit of ICU care for patients with CAP, but mortality rates are lower if patients are admitted early in the course of severe illness than if they are admitted only after the onset of respiratory failure [49].

The 1993 ATS guidelines used data from the literature to define 10 criteria for severe CAP, saying that the ICU admission was needed for anyone having one of these features present [50]. However, subsequent studies demonstrated that this definition was too inclusive, and 65% of all admitted CAP patients (not needing ICU care) met one of these criteria [51]. To better define the need for ICU care in CAP, Ewig et al. applied these 10 criteria to 64 patients who were admitted to the ICU and compared the findings to those in 331 patients admitted to the hospital but not the ICU [51]. With this approach, a better definition of severe CAP was derived, with a sensitivity of 78%, a specificity of 94%, a positive predictive value of 75%, and a negative predictive value of 95%. This definition required the presence of either two of three "minor criteria" present on admission, or one of two "major criteria" present on admission or later in the hospital course. The minor criteria were systolic blood pressure lower than 90 mm Hg, PaO2/FiO2 ratio less than 250, or multilobar infiltrates. The major criteria were need for mechanical ventilation or septic shock. In a subsequent study of 1339 patients, 170 were admitted to the ICU and no prediction rule was completely accurate for deciding need for ICU admission [52]. Overall the presence of one of two major criteria or two of three minor criteria was the most accurate rule, with a sensitivity of 71% and a specificity of 72% and a negative predictive value of 94%. A high score using the PORT model had a specificity of only 50% for defining need for ICU admission [52]. As discussed above, another way to identify patients with more severe illness is to apply the BTS rule in its original or modified version, but this approach had a sensitivity of 40% and a specificity of 78% when used to define need for ICU admission [52]. In the future, we will need to determine if there is a better way to prospectively define the need for ICU admission.

DIAGNOSTIC TESTING (Table 4)

Once the history and physical examination suggest the presence of pneumonia, the diagnosis should be confirmed by chest radiograph. Although some patients may have clinical findings of pneumonia (focal crackles, bronchial breath sounds), and a negative chest radiograph, the need for antibiotic therapy of CAP has been established in patients with a radiographic infiltrate. In some patients, findings of pneumonia may be present, but the chest radiograph is negative, and the correct diagnosis is bronchitis, an illness that may not require antibiotic therapy, unless patients have chronic underlying lung disease. However, in other populations, such as the elderly and chronically ill, the clinical diagnosis is difficult, and these patients can have pneumonia but present only with nonrespiratory findings; for these individuals, a chest radiograph is essential to define the presence of parenchymal lung infection. A chest radiograph not only confirms the presence of pneumonia but can be used to identify complicated illness and to grade severity of disease, by noting such findings as pleural effusion and multilobar illness [1].

Although defining a specific etiologic diagnosis of CAP allows for focused antibiotic therapy, most patients do not have a specific pathogen identified, and many who do, have this diagnosis made days or weeks later, as the results of cultures or serologic testing become available. In addition, recent studies have emphasized the mortality benefit of prompt administration of effective antibiotic therapy, with a goal of administering intravenous antibiotics within 8 hours of admission to the hospital, for those with moderate to severe illness [53]. Thus, therapy should never be delayed for the purpose of diagnostic testing, and the diagnostic workup should be streamlined, with all patients receiving empiric therapy based on algorithms as soon as possible. With such empiric regimens, as many as 90% of admitted patients will have a prompt response to therapy [54].

TABLE 4 Diagnostic Testing for CAP

Test	Comment
Chest radiograph	CT scan may show infiltrates that are absent on routine radiograph
CT scan	Not a routine test, but can be used in nonresponding patients to identify cavitation or loculated pleural fluid. Contrast study can demonstrate pulmonary embolus
Blood cultures	Pneumococcus is the usual organism (in 50–80% of positive samples). Can define antibiotic susceptibility pattern.
Sputum Gram stain	Patients are rarely able to give an adequate specimen. Can correlate with sputum culture to define predominant organism and can use to identify unsuspected pathogens
Sputum culture	Use if suspect drug-resistant or unusual pathogen, but positive result cannot separate colonization from infection
Oximetry or arterial blood gas	Both tests define severity of infection and the need for oxygen; a blood gas should be done if hypercarbia is suspected.
Serologic testing for *Legionella*, *C. pneumoniae*, *M. pneumoniae*, viruses	Usually requires acute and convalescent titers collected 4–6 weeks apart, and is impractical for guiding management
Legionella urinary antigen	Specific to serogroup 1, but the best diagnostic test for *Legionella* at the time of admission

Recommended testing for admitted patients includes a chest radiograph, assessment of oxygenation (pulse oximetry or blood gas, the latter if retention of carbon dioxide is suspected), routine admission blood work and two sets of blood cultures [1]. If the patient has a pleural effusion, this should be tapped and the fluid sent for culture and biochemical analysis. Although blood cultures are positive in only 10–20% of CAP patients, they can be used to define a specific diagnosis and to define the presence of drug- resistant pneumococci [21]. Sputum culture should be limited to patients suspected of having an infection with a drug-resistant or unusual pathogen.

The role of gram stain of sputum to guide initial antibiotic therapy is controversial, but this test can guide the interpretation of sputum culture results by defining the predominant organism present in the sample. The role of gram stain in focusing initial antibiotic therapy is uncertain because the accuracy of the test to predict the culture recovery of an organism such as pneumococcus depends on the criteria used. If the finding of any gram-positive diplococcus is used to define a positive test, then the test will be sensitive but not very specific. On the other hand, the finding of a predominance of gram-positive diplococci will be specific, but not sensitive, for predicting the culture recovery of pneumococcus [1,55]. In a recent study, the practical limitations of the test were demonstrated: out of 116 patients with CAP, only 42 could produce a sputum sample of which 23 were valid, and only 10 samples were diagnostic, with antibiotics directed to the diagnostic result in only one patient [56]. Even if gram stain findings were used to focus antibiotic therapy, this would not allow for empiric coverage of mixed infection with both bacteria and atypical pathogens. In the ATS guidelines, the recommendation is to use the gram stain to broaden initial empiric therapy, if the findings suggest an organism that is not covered in routine empiric therapy (such as *S. aureus* being suggested by the presence of clusters of gram-positive cocci, during a time of epidemic influenza) [1].

Routine serologic testing is not recommended. However, in patients with severe illness, the diagnosis of *Legionella* infection can be made by urinary antigen testing, which is the test that is most likely to be positive at the time of admission, but it is a test that is specific only for serogroup I infection [57]. Commercially available tests for pneumococcal urinary antigen have been developed, but their role in the clinical management of CAP has not been defined. Bronchoscopy is not indicated as a routine diagnostic test and should be restricted to immune-compromised patients, and to selected individuals with severe forms of CAP.

THERAPY OF CAP

General Principles

The goal of empiric therapy of patients with CAP is to target the likely etiologic pathogens by categorizing patients on the basis of place of therapy (inpatient, ICU), severity of illness, and the presence or absence of cardiopulmonary disease or specific "modifying" factors. By using these factors, a set of likely pathogens can be predicted for each patient (Table 2), and this information can be used to guide initial empiric therapy. If a specific pathogen is subsequently identified by diagnostic testing, then therapy can be focused.

In choosing empiric therapy of CAP, certain principles should be followed, as outlined in Table 5 [1,58]. For the non-ICU inpatient therapy can be an intravenous macrolide (azithromycin) alone, provided that the patient has no underlying cardiopulmonary disease and no risk factors for infection with DRSP, enteric gram-negatives, or anaerobes. Although very

TABLE 5 Principles in Antibiotic Therapy of CAP

Principle
Administer first dose of antibiotics within 8 hr of arrival in hospital
Treat all patients for the possibility of infection with "atypical pathogens" and pneumococcus
Monotherapy with a macolide can be given to inpatients with no risk factors for DRSP, gram-negatives or aspiration
For inpatients with risk factors for DRSP and/or gram-negatives, use either a β-lactam/macrolide combination or monotherapy with an anti-pneumococcal quinolone. Quinolone therapy should be used in penicillin-allergic patients.
For inpatients with clinical risks for DRSP intravenous β-lactam therapy should be with either cefotaxime, cefriaxone, ampicillin/sulbactam, or high-dose ampicillin
Limit anti-pseudomonal antibiotics to patients with pseudomonal risk factors
For severe CAP, use a β-lactam with either a macrolide or a quinolone, but no patient should get quinolone monotherapy
Limit the use of vancomycin to empiric therapy of patients with severe illness, especially with suspected meningitis

few patients of this type are admitted to the hospital, macrolide monotherapy has been documented to be effective in this population and may be more cost-effective than combination therapy [59,60]. The majority of admitted patients will have cardiopulmonary disease and/or modifying factors, and they can be treated with either a selected (see Table 5) intravenous β-lactam combined with a macrolide, or they can receive an intravenous antipneumococcal quinolone (gatifloxacin, levofloxacin, moxifloxacin) alone. From the available data, it appears that either regimen is therapeutically equivalent; and although not proven, it may be useful to use these two types of regimens interchangeably, striving for "antibiotic heterogeneity" in the hospital, so that one regimen is not used exclusively in all patients [1]. This type of approach has the theoretic advantage of minimizing selection pressure for antibiotic resistance.

Although oral quinolones may be as effective as intravenous quinolones for admitted patients with moderately severe illness, all admitted patients should receive initial therapy intravenously to be sure that the medication has been absorbed [1]. Once the patient shows a good clinical response (defined below), oral therapy can be started. Selected inpatients with mild to moderate disease can initially be treated with the combination of an intravenous β-lactam and an oral macrolide, switching to exclusively oral therapy once the patient shows a good clinical response.

In the ICU population, all individuals should be treated for DRSP and atypical pathogens, but only those with appropriate risk factors (above) should have coverage for *P. aeruginosa* [1]. The efficacy, dosing, and safety of quinolone monotherapy has not been established for ICU-admitted CAP patients, so the therapy for such patients, in the absence of pseudomonal risk factors, should be a selected intravenous β-lactam, combined with either an intravenous macrolide or an intravenous quinolone. For patients with pseudomonal risk factors, therapy can be with a two-drug regimen, using an anti-pseudomonal β-lactam (cefepime, imipenem, meropenem, piperacillin/tazobactam) plus ciprofloxacin (the only anti-pseudomonal quinolone); or alternatively with a three-drug regimen, using an anti-pseudomonal β-lactam plus an aminoglycoside plus either an intravenous non-pseudomonal quinolone or macrolide. In a study of patients admitted to the ICU with severe CAP, mortality was reduced whenever a macrolide was included, which was usually in combination with a β-lactam (either a cephalosporin or β-lactam/β-lactamase inhibitor) [61]. Similar outcome was seen with quinolone monotherapy, although few patients received this regimen, and thus it should not be used until more patients have been studied using this regimen [61]. The existing guideline recommendations for the therapy of CAP in inpatients on the medical ward, or in the ICU, are summarized in Table 6 [58].

The anti-pneumococcal quinolones have assumed great importance in the therapy of CAP because it is possible to cover pneumococcus (including DRSP), gram-negatives, and atypical pathogens with a single drug, given once daily. Quinolones penetrate well into respiratory secretions and are highly bioavailable, achieving the same serum levels with oral or intravenous therapy, thereby allowing a rapid switch from intravenous to oral antibiotic therapy. The possibility of quinolones promoting an early switch from intravenous to oral therapy was demonstrated in a study comparing moxifloxacin to a β-lactam/β-lactamase inhibitor, with or without a macrolide. In that study, therapy with the quinolone was associated with significantly more patients being afebrile at day 2 and switching to oral therapy by day 3 than those receiving the comparator regimen (50% vs. 18%) [62].

Although all of the anti-pneumococcal quinolones are available orally and intravenously, and all have been effective for the therapy of CAP, there are differences among the available agents in their intrinsic activity against pneumococcus [1,63,64]. Based on the minimum inhibitory concentration (MIC) against *S. pneumoniae*, these agents can be ranked, from most to least active, as moxifloxacin, gatifloxacin, and levofloxacin. Some data suggest a lower likelihood of both clinical failures and the induction of pneumoccal resistance to quinolones, if the more active agents are used in place of the less active agents [64,65]. In addition, there are now reports of failures in pneumococcal pneumonia with levofloxacin, and these have occurred in

TABLE 6 In-patient Therapy of CAP in Existing Guidelines

Non-ICU

IDSA 2000[a]:
- Selected β-lactam *plus* a macrolide
- *or* monotherapy with a respiratory fluoroquinolone
- No preference for either regimen

Canadian Consensus 2000[b]:
- Respiratory fluroquinolone
- *or* Second-, third-, or fourth-generation cephalosporin *plus* a macrolide
- Quinolone as first choice

CDC 2000[c]:
- Selected β-lactam *plus* a macrolide
- *or* Monotherapy with a respiratory fluoroquinolone
- Quinolone to be used only if β-lactam allergic, β-lactam failure, or documented high-level penicillin resistance.

ATS 2001[d]:
- *No cardiopulmonary disease or modifying factors*:
- IV azithromycin
- *Cardiopulmonary disease or modifying factors*:
- Selected β-lactam *plus* a macrolide or tetracycline
- *or* monotherapy with a fluoroquinolone
- *No* preference for either regimen

ICU

IDSA 2000[a]
- *No structural lung disease*:
- β-Lactam *plus either* a respiratory fluoroquinolone *or* a macrolide
- *Structural lung disease*:
- Anti-pseudomonal β-lactam *plus* a fluoroquinolone

Canadian Consensus 2000[b]:
- *No pseudomonal risks*:
- Cefotaxime, ceftriaxone, β-lactam/β-lactamase inhibitor *plus either* a respiratory fluoroquinolone *or* a macrolide
- *Pseudomonal risks*:
  1. Ciprofloxacin *plus either* an anti-pseudomonal β-lactam *or* aminoglycoside
  2. Anti-pseudomonal β-lactam *plus* aminoglycoside *plus* macrolide

CDC 2000[c]:
- β-Lactam *plus either* a macrolide *or* fluoroquinolone

ATS 2001[d]:
- *No pseudomonal risks*:
- β-Lactam *plus either* a macrolide *or* respiratory fluoroquinolone
- *Pseudomonal risks*:
  1. Anti-pseudomonal β-lactam *plus* ciprofloxacin
  2. Anti-pseudomonal β-lactam *plus* aminoglycoside *plus either* respiratory fluroquinolone *or* a macrolide

Note: Selected β-lactams are listed in Table 5. In the ATS guidelines, anti-pseudomonal agents (cefepime, piperacillin-tazobactam, imipenem, meropenem) are only to be used if pseudomonal risk factors are present (generally ICU patients), but the IDSA and Canadian guidelines permit some of these agents in non-ICU patients.

[a] Ref. 14.

[b] Ref. 21.

[c] Ref. 76.

[d] Ref 1.

patients who were infected with levofloxacin-resistant organisms, after a recent course of quionolone therapy or who acquired this resistance during therapy (after having an initially sensitive organism) [65,66]. Based on these data, and on the finding that recent therapy with a macrolide, β-lactam, or quinolone can predispose to resistance to other agents in the same class, a recent history of antibiotic therapy should guide initial therapy selection. If the patient has been on any antibiotic in the past 3 months, it may be preferable to choose an agent in a totally different therapeutic class for CAP therapy.

In addition to the general approach to therapy outlined above, there are several other therapeutic issues to consider in the management of CAP.

Timing of Initial Antibiotic Therapy

For inpatients with CAP, the use of timely and accurate therapy is essential to reduce mortality. In patients with severe CAP, improved survival has occurred if initial empiric therapy is accurate and if it leads to a rapid clinical response [67]. In one study, if initial therapy led to a clinical response within 72 hr, mortality of severe CAP was approximately 10%, compared to a mortality rate of 60% in patients who had initially ineffective therapy [67]. Another recent finding is the need to provide initial intravenous antibiotic therapy within 8 hr of the patient's arrival at the hospital [53]. In a large Medicare study of 14,069 patients, mortality at 30 days was significantly reduced for the 75% of patients who received their first dose of therapy within 8 hr of coming to the hospital [53]. Although this has become the target time frame for initial therapy, there was additional benefit for therapy given even sooner. To achieve the goal of early therapy, it may be necessary to assure that the first dose of antibiotics is administered in the emergency department. In one study of 700 patients with CAP, length of stay was significantly reduced in patients who received the first dose of antibiotic therapy in the emergency department rather than the medical floor. Patients treated in the emergency department received therapy at a mean of 3.5 hr, compared to a mean of 9.5 hr for those first treated on the medical floor [68].

The Role of Routine Therapy for Atypical Pathogens in All Hospitalized Patients

In most available North American guidelines, initial empiric therapy of CAP provides for all inpatients to be treated for the possibility of atypical pathogen infection, either as primary infection, or as part of a mixed infection [1,14,21]. A number of outcome studies of large populations, of primarily inpatients, have shown that when therapy includes a macrolide or a quinolone, outcomes (including mortality) are improved, compared to when a β-lactam is used by itself [34,35]. In one study of 13,000 Medicare patients, mortality at 30 days was reduced if a macrolide was added to a second- or third-generation cephalosporin, or a quinolone was used alone, compared to therapy with a third-generation cephalosporin by itself [34]. These findings support a potentially important role for atypical pathogens and may explain the findings of one recent study that mortality is increased for patients with bacteremic pneumococcal pneumonia when a single effective agent was used, compared to dual effective therapy [69]. In that study, it is of interest that monotherapy with a third-generation cephalosporin was associated with a higher mortality than if the same agent was used along with an agent that provided atypical pathogen coverage (i.e., a macrolide or quinolone), implying that coinfection with atypical pathogens may even be important in patients with bacteremic pneumococcal pneumonia.

The Role of DRSP in the Empiric Therapy of CAP

As discussed above, both the ATS and IDSA guidelines have identified risk factors for infection with DRSP, but the IDSA approach is to treat all inpatients for the possibility of DRSP, whereas the ATS approach is to use these risk factors to decide which inpatients should be targeted for DRSP and which do not need this therapy [1,14]. If an inpatient is at risk for infection with DRSP, therapy should be with any of the following intravenous agents: cefotaxime, ceftriaxone, ampicillin/sulbactam, high-dose ampicillin, or an anti-pneumococcal quinolone (considering the issues mentioned above). When a β-lactam is used, a macrolide should be added for the reasons previously discussed.

The rationale for using specific agents in patients with risk factors for DRSP is not only to minimize the risk of treatment failure, but also to rapidly and reliably eradicate pneumococcal organisms that have low levels of resistance, so that there is less selection pressure for emergence of organisms with high-level resistance. It is unlikely that targeting at-risk patients with highly active regimens will improve outcomes, because the clinically relevant level of pneumococcal resistance is a penicillin MIC value of at least 4 mg/L, a level of resistance that is relatively uncommon today [22,23]. The clinical relevance of cephalosporin resistance is also being studied. Recently, the breakpoints for defining cephalosporin-resistant pneumococci have been changed to an MIC of at least 4 mg/L for nonmeningeal infection. Pallares et al. found that when ceftriaxone or cefotaxime were used to treat organisms having MIC values up to 2 mg/L, the outcome was the same as if the organisms were not resistant. If penicillins were used for DRSP organisms, the mortality was higher than if the same therapy was used for sensitive organisms. However, cefotaxime and ceftriaxone were effective for penicillin-resistant organisms [70].

EVALUATION OF RESPONSE TO THERAPY

The majority of outpatients and inpatients will respond rapidly to the empiric therapy regimens suggested above, with clinical response usually occurring within 24 to 72 hours [1,71]. Clinical response for inpatients is defined as improvement in symptoms of cough, sputum production, and dyspnea, along with ability to take medications by mouth, declining white blood cell count, and an afebrile status for at least two occasions 8 hr apart. When a patient has met these criteria for clinical response, it is appropriate to switch to an oral therapy regimen and to discharge the patient, if he or she is otherwise medically and socially stable [1,71,72]. Observation in the hospital during oral therapy is generally not necessary, since patients usually do not have clinical deterioration after reaching signs of stability and after being able to switch to oral therapy [72]. If patients are discharged when not clinically stable, there is an increased risk of mortality and readmission [73]. In one study, instability was defined as any of the following within 24 hours of discharge: fever higher than 37.8°C, HR greater than 100/min, respiratory rate greater than 24/min, systolic BP less than 90 mm Hg, oxygen saturation less than 90%, inability to maintain oral intake, and abnormal mental status. Readmission or death was at least 3 times more likely for patients with at least two of these factors present, compared to none or one factor present, but only 2% of patients fell into this category [73].

Radiographic improvement lags behind clinical improvement, and in a responding patient, a repeat chest radiograph is not necessary until 2 to 4 weeks after starting therapy. In general, 50% of patients with pneumococcal pneumonia have radiographic clearing at 5 weeks, with the majority clear in 2 to 3 months. With bacteremic disease, 50% have clear chest radiographs at 9 weeks, and most are clear by 18 weeks [74,75]. Radiographic resolution in community-acquired pneumonia is most influenced by the number of lobes involved and the age of the patient. Radiographic clearance of community-acquired pneumonia decreases by 20% per decade, after age 20, and patients with multilobar infiltrates take longer to clear than those with unilobar disease [74].

If the patient fails to respond to therapy in the expected time interval, then it is necessary to consider infection with a drug-resistant or unusual pathogen (tuberculosis, anthrax, *C. burnetii*, *Burkholderia pseudomallei*, *C. psittaci*, *Pasteurella multocida*, endemic fungi, or viruses); a pneumonic complication (lung abscess, endocarditis, empyema); or a noninfectious process that mimics pneumonia (bronchiolitis obliterans with organizing pneumonia, hypersensitivity pneumonitis, pulmonary vasculitis, bronchoalveolar cell carcinoma, lymphoma, pulmonary embolus) [1]. The evaluation of the non-responding patient should be individualized but may include CT scanning of the chest, pulmonary angiography, bronchoscopy, and occasionally open lung biopsy.

REFERENCES

1. Niederman MS, Mandell LA, Anzueto A, et al. Guidelines for the management of adults with community-acquired lower respiratory tract infections: diagnosis, assessment of severity, antimicrobial therapy and prevention. Am J Respir Crit Care Med 2001; 163:1730–1754.
2. Niederman MS, McCombs JI, Unger AN, Kumar A, Popovian R. The cost of treating community-acquired pneumonia. Clin Ther 1998; 20:820–837.
3. Metaly JP, Schulz R, Li Y-H, Singer DE, Marrie TJ, Coley CM, et al. Influence of age on symptoms at presentation in patients with community-acquired pneumonia. Arch Intern Med 1997; 157:1453–1459.
4. Marrie TJ, Blanchard W. A comparison of nursing home-acquired pneumonia patients with patients with community-acquired pneumonia and nursing home patients without pneumonia. J Am Geriatr Soc 1997; 45:50–55.
5. Starczewski AR, Allen SC, Vargas E, Lye M. Clinical prognostic indices of fatality in elderly patients admitted to hospital with acute pneumonia. Age Aging 1988; 17:181–186.
6. Fine MJ, Orloff JJ, Arisumi D, et al. Prognosis of patients hospitalized with community-acquired pneumonia. Am J Med 1990; 88:1N–8N.
7. Riquelme R, Torres A, El-Ebiary, et al. Community-acquired pneumonia in the elderly: clinical and nutritional aspects. Am J Crit Care Med 1997; 156:1908–1914.
8. McFadden JR, Price RC, Eastwood HD, Briggs RS. Raised respiratory rate in elderly patients: a valuable physical sign. Br Med J 1982; 284:626–627.
9. Syrjala H, Broas M, Suramo I, Ojala A, Lahde S. High resolution computed tomography for the diagnosis of community-acquired pneumonia. Clin Infect Dis 1998; 27:358–363.
10. Katz DS, Leung AN. Radiology of pneumonia. Clin Chest Med 1999; 20:549–562.
11. Lieberman D, Lieberman D, Gelfer Y, Varshavsky R, Dvoskin B, Leinonen M, Friedman MG. Pneumonic vs nonpneumonic acute exacerbations of COPD. Chest 2002; 122:1264–1270.
12. Hasley PB, Albaum MN, Li YH, et al. Do pulmonary radiographic findings at presentation predict mortality in patients with community-acquired pneumonia? Arch Intern Med 1996; 156:2206–2212.
13. Sahn SA. Management of complicated parapneumonic effusions. Am Rev Respir Dis 1993; 148:813–817.
14. Bartlett JG, Dowell SF, Mandell LA, File TM, Musher DM, Fine MJ. Practice guidelines for the management of community-acquired pneumonia in adults. Clin Infect Dis 2000; 31:347–382.
15. Woodhead MA, MacFarlane JT. Comparative clinical laboratory features on

Legionella with pneumococcal and Mycoplasma pneumonias. Br J Dis Chest 1987; 81:133–139.
16. Farr BM, Kaiser DL, Harrison BW, Connolly CK. Prediction of microbial aetiology at admission to hospital for pneumonia from presenting clinical features. Thorax 1989; 44:1031–1035.
17. Fang GD, Fine M, Orloff J, Arisumi D, Yu VL, Kapoor W, et al. New and emerging etiologies for community-acquired pneumonia with implication for therapy; a prospective multicenter study of 359 cases. Medicine (Baltimore) 1990; 69:307–316.
18. Macfarlane JT, Miller AC, Roderick Smith WH, Morris AH, Rose DH. Comparative radiographic features of community acquired Legionnaires' disease, pneumococcal pneumonia, mycoplasma pneumonia, and psittacosis. Thorax 1984; 39:28–33.
19. Ruiz-Gonzalez A, Falguera M, Nogues A, Rubio-Caballero M. Is Streptococcus pneumonia the leading cause of pneumonia of unknown etiology? A microbiologic study of lung aspirates in consecutive patients with community-acquired pneumonia. Am J Med 1999; 106:385–390.
20. Ort S, Ryan JL, Barden G, et al. Pneumococcal pneumonia in hospitalized patients: clinical and radiological presentations. JAMA 1983; 249:214–218.
21. Mandell LA, Marrie TJ, Grossman RF, Chow AW, Hyland RHthe Canadian CAP Working GroupCanadian Guidelines for the Initial Management of Community-acquired Pneumonia: an Evidence-Based Update by the Canadian Infectious Diseases Society and the Candian Thoracic Society. Clin Infect Dis 2000; 31:383–421.
22. Doern GV, Pfaller MA, Kugler K, Freeman J, Jones RN. Prevalence of antimicrobial resistance among respiratory tract isolates of Streptococcus pneumoniae in North America: 1997 results from the SENTRY antimicrobial surveillance program. Clin Infect Dis 1998; 27:764–770.
23. Feikin DR, Schuchat A, Kolczak M, et al. Mortality from invasive pneumococcal pneumonia in the era of antibiotic resistance, 1995–1997. Am J Public Health 2000; 90:223–229.
24. Pallares R, Linares J, Vadillo M, et al. Resistance to penicillin and cephalosporin and mortality from severe pneumococcal pneumonia in Barcelona, Spain. N Engl J Med 1995; 333:474–480.
25. Turett GS, Blum S, Fazal BA, Justman JE, Telzak EE. Penicillin resistance and other predictors of mortality in pneumococcal bacteremia in a population with high human immunodeficiency virus seroprevalence. Clin Infect Dis 1999; 29: 321–327.
26. Plouffe JF, Breiman RF, Facklam RR. Bacteremia with Streptococcus pneumoniae. Implications for therapy and prevention. Franklin County Pneumonia Study Group. JAMA 1996; 275:194–198.
27. Metlay JP, Hoffman J, Cetron MS, et al. Impact of penicillin susceptibility on medical outcomes for adult patients with bacteremic pneumococcal pneumonia. Clin Infect Dis 2000; 30:520–528.
28. Moroney JF, Fiore AE, Harrison LH, Patterson JE, Farley MM, Jorgensen

JH, Phelan M, Facklam RR, Cetron MS, Breiman RF, Kolczak M, Schuchat A. Clinical outcomes of bacteremic pneumococcal pneumonia in the era of antibiotic resistance. Clin Infect Dis 2001; 33:797–805.

29. Clavo-Sánchez AJ, Girón-González JA, López-Prieto D, et al. Multivariate analysis of risk factors for infection due to penicillin-resistant and multidrug-resistant Streptococcus pneumoniae: a multicenter study. Clin Infect Dis 1997; 24:1052–1059.
30. Marston BJ, Plouffe JF, File TM Jr, Hackman BA, Salstrom SJ, Lipman HB, Kolczak MS, Breiman RF. Incidence of community-acquired pneumonia requiring hospitalization. Results of a population-based active surveillance Study in Ohio. The Community-Based Pneumonia Incidence Study Group. Arch Int Med 1997; 157:1709–1718.
31. Troy CJ, Peeling RW, Ellis AG, et al. Chlamydia pneumoniae as a new source of infectious outbreaks in nursing homes. JAMA 1997; 277:1214–1218.
32. Kauppinen MT, Saikku P, Kujala P, Herva E, Syrjala H. Clinical picture of *Chlamydia pneumoniae* requiring hospital treatment: a comparison between chlamydial and pneumococcal pneumonia. Thorax 1996; 51:185–189.
33. Lieberman D, Schlaeffer F, Boldur I, Lieberman D, Horowitz S, Friedman MG, Leiononen M, Horovitz O, Manor E, Porath A. Multiple pathogens in adult patients admitted with community-acquired pneumonia: a one year prospective study of 346 consecutive patients. Thorax 1996; 51:179–184.
34. Gleason PP, Meehan TP, Fine JM, Galusha DH, Fine MJ. Associations between initial antimicrobial therapy and medical outcomes for hospitalized elderly patients with pneumonia. Arch Intern Med 1999; 159:2562–2572.
35. Houck PM, MacLehose RF, Niederman MS, Lowery JK. Empiric antibiotic therapy and mortality among Medicare pneumonia inpatients in 10 Western states: 1993, 1995, 1997. Chest 2001; 119:1420–1426.
36. Ruiz M, Ewig S, Torres A, Arancibia F, Marco F, Mensa J, Sanchez M, Martinez JA. Severe community-acquired pneumonia: risk factors and follow-up epidemiology. Am J Respir Crit Care Med 1999; 160:923–929.
37. El Solh AA, Sikka P, Ramadan F, Davies J. Etiology of severe pneumonia in the very elderly. Am J Respir Crit Care Med 2001; 163:645–651.
38. Arancibia F, Bauer TT, Ewig S, Mensa J, Gonzalez J, Niederman MS, Torres A. Community-acquired pneumonia due to gram-negative bacteria and pseudomonas aeruginosa: incidence, risk, and prognosis. Arch Intern Med 2002; 162:1849–1858.
39. Nava JM, Bella F, Garau J, et al. Predictive factors for invasive disease due to penicillin-resistant *Streptococcus pneumoniae*: a population-based study. Clin Infect Dis 1994; 19:884–890.
40. Fine MJ, Auble TE, Yealy DM, et al. A prediction rule to identify low-risk patients with community-acquired pneumonia. N Engl J Med 1997; 336:243–250.
41. Farr BM, Sloman AJ, Fisch MJ. Predicting death in patients hospitalized for community-acquired pneumonia. Ann Int Med 1991; 115:428–436.
42. Neill AM, Martin IR, Weir R, et al. Community-acquired pneumonia: aetiol-

ogy and usefulness of severity criteria on admission. Thorax 1996; 51:1010–1016.
43. Atlas SJ, Benzer TI, Borowsky LH, et al. Safely increasing the proportion of patients with community-acquired pneumonia treated as outpatients: an interventional trial. Arch Intern Med 1998; 158:1350–1356.
44. Marrie Tj, Lau CY, Wheeler SL, Wong CJ, Vandervoort MK, Feagan BG, et al. A controlled trial of a critical pathway for treatment of community-acquired pneumonia. JAMA 2000; 283:749–755.
45. Mody L, Sun R, Bradley S. Community-acquired pneumonia in older veterans: does the pneumonia prognosis index help? J Am Geriatr Soc 2002; 50: 434–438.
46. Lim WS, Lewis S, Macfarlane JT. Severity prediction rules in community acquired pneumonia: a validation study. Thorax 2000; 55:219–223.
47. Lim WS, Macfarlane JT. Defining prognostic factors in the elderly with community acquired pneumonia: a case controlled study of patients aged $\geq$ 75 years. Eur Respir J 2001; 17:200–205.
48. Fine MJ, Smith MA, Carson CA, et al. Prognosis and outcomes of patients with community-acquired pneumonia: a meta-analysis. JAMA 1996; 275:134–141.
49. Hook EW, Horton CA, Schaberg DR. Failure of intensive care unit support to influence mortality from pneumococcal bacteremia. JAMA 1983; 249:1055–1060.
50. Niederman MS, Bass JB, Campbell GD, Fein AM, Grossman RF, Mandell LA, Marrie TJ, Sarosi GA, Torres A, Yu VL. Guidelines for the initial management of adults with community-acquired pneumonia: diagnosis, assessment of severity, and initial antimicrobial therapy. Am Rev Respir Dis 1993; 148: 1418–1426.
51. Ewig S, Ruiz M, Mensa J, Marcos MA, Martinez JA, Arancibia F, Niederman MS, Torres A. Severe community-acquired pneumonia: assessment of severity criteria. Am J Respir Crit Care Med 1998; 158:1102–1108.
52. Angus DC, Marrie TJ, Obrosky DS, Clermont G, Dremsizov TT, Coley C, Fine MJ, Singer DE, Kapoor WN. Severe community-acquired pneumonia: use of intensive care services and evaluation of American and British Thoracic Society diagnostic criteria. Am J Respir Crit Care Med 2002; 166:717–723.
53. Meehan TP, Fine MJ, Krumholz HM, Scinto JD, Galusha DH, Mockalis JT, et al. Quality of care, process, and outcomes in elderly patients with pneumonia. JAMA 1997; 278:2080–2084.
54. Sanyal S, Smith PR, Saha AC, Gupta S, Berkowitz L, Homel P. Initial microbiologic studies did not affect outcome in adults hospitalized with community-acquired pneumonia. Am J Respir Crit Care Med 1999; 160:346–348.
55. Rein MF, Gwaltney JM Jr., O'Brien WM, et al. Accuracy of Gram's stain in identifying pneumococci in sputum. JAMA 1978; 239:2671–2673.
56. Ewig S, Schlochtermeier M, Goke N, Niederman MS. Applying sputum as a diagnostic tool in pneumonia: limited yield, minimal impact on treatment decisions. Chest 2002; 121:1486–1492.

57. Plouffe JF, File TM Jr, Breiman RF, et al. Reevaluation of the definition of Legionnaires' disease: use of the urinary antigen assay. Community Based Pneumonia Incidence Study Group. Clin Infect Dis 1995; 20:1286–1291.
58. Niederman MS. Guidelines for the management of community-acquired pneumonia. Current recommendations and antibiotic selection issues. Med Clin North Am 2001; 85:1493–1509.
59. Plouffe J, Schwartz DB, Kolokathis A, Sherman BW, Arnow PM, Gezon JA, Suh B, Anzuetto A, Greenberg RN, Niederman M, Paladino JA, Ramirez JA, Inverso J, Knirsch CA. Clinical efficacy of intravenous followed by oral azithromycin monotherapy in hospitalized patients with community-acquired pneumonia. Antimicrob Agents Chemother 2000; 44:1796–1802.
60. Paladino JA, Gudgel LD, Forrest A, Niederman MS. Cost-effectiveness of IV-to-oral switch therapy: azithromycin vs cefuroxime with or without erythromycin for the treatment of community-acquired pneumonia. Chest 2002; 122: 1271–1279.
61. Rello J, Catalan M, Diaz E, Bodi M, Alvarez B. Associations between empirical antimicrobial therapy at the hospital and mortality in patients with severe community-acquired pneumonia. Intensive Care Med 2002; 28:1030–1035.
62. Finch R, Schurmann D, Collins O, Kubin R, McGivern J, Bobbaers H, Izquierdo JL, Nikolaides P, Ogundare F, Raz R, Zuck P, Hoeffken G. Randomized controlled trial of sequential intravenous (i.v.) and oral moxifloxacin compared with sequential i.v. and oral co-amoxiclav with or without clarithromycin in patients with community-acquired pneumonia requiring initial parenteral treatment. Antimicrob Agents Chemother 2002; 46:1746–1754.
63. Niederman MS. Treatment of respitory infections with quinolones. In: Andriole V, ed. The Quinolones. 2d ed. San Diego, CA: McGraw-Hill, 1998:229–250.
64. Chen DK, McGeer A, DeAzavedo JC, Low DE, et al. Decreased susceptibility of Streptococcus pneumoniae to fluoroquinolones in Canada. N Engl J Med 1999; 341:233–239.
65. Davidson R, Cavalcanti R, Brunton JL, Bast DJ, de Azavedo JC, Kibsey P, Fleming C, Low DE. Resistance to levofloxacin and failure of treatment of pneumococcal pneumonia. N Engl J Med 2002; 346:747–750.
66. Ho PL, Tse WS, Tsang KW, Kwok TK, Ng TK, Cheng VC, Chan RM. Risk factors for acquisition of levofloxacin-resistant Streptococcus pneumoniae: a case-control study. Clin Infect Dis 2001; 32:701–707.
67. Leroy O, Santre C, Beuscart C. A 5-year study of severe community-acquired pneumonia with emphasis on prognosis in patients admitted to an ICU. Intensive Care Med 1995; 21:24–31.
68. Battleman DS, Callahan M, Thaler HT. Rapid antibiotic delivery and appropriate antibiotic selection reduce length of hospital stay of patients with community-acquired pneumonia: link between quality of care and resource utilization. Arch Intern Med 2002 Mar 25; 162(6):682–688.
69. Waterer GW, Somes GW, Wunderink RG. Monotherapy may be suboptimal for severe bacteremic pneumococcal pneumonia. Arch Intern Med 2001; 161: 1837–1842.

70. Pallares R, Capdevila O, Linares J, Grau I, Onaga H, Tubau F, Schulze MH, Hohl P, Gudiol F. The effect of cephalosporin resistance on mortality in adult patients with nonmeningeal systemic pneumococcal infections. Am J Med 2002; 113:120–126.
71. Ramirez JA, Vargas S, Ritter GW, Brier ME, Wright A, Smith S, et al. Early switch from intravenous to oral antibiotics and early hospital discharge: a prospective observational study of 200 consecutive patients with community-acquired pneumonia. Arch Intern Med 1999; 159:2449–2454.
72. Rhew DC, Hackner D, Henderson L, Ellrodt AG, Weingarten SR. The clinical benefit of in-hospital observation in "low risk" pneumonia patients after conversion from parenteral to oral antimicrobial therapy. Chest 1998; 113:142–146.
73. Halm EA, Fine MJ, Kapoor WN, Singer DE, Marrie TJ, Siu AL. Instability on hospital discharge and the risk of adverse outcomes in patients with pneumonia. Arch Intern Med 2002; 162:1278–1284.
74. Mittl RL, Schwab RJ, Duchin JS, et al. Radiographic resolution of community-acquired pneumonia. Am J Respir Crit Care Med 1994; 149:630–635.
75. Jay S, Johanson W, Pierce A. The radiologic resolution of streptococcal pneumoniae pneumonia. N Engl J Med 1975; 293:798–801.
76. Hefflefinger JD, Dowell SF, Jorgensen JH, et al. Management of community-acquired pneumonia in the era of pneumococcal resistance: a report from the drug-resistant Streptococcus pneumoniae Therapeutic Working Group. Arch Intern Med 2000; 160:1399–1408.

15

Anaerobic Pleuropulmonary Infection

Matthew E. Levison
Drexel University College of Medicine
Medical College of Pennsylvania Hospital
Philadelphia, Pennsylvania, U.S.A.

INTRODUCTION

Bacteria can be classified by the type of oxidation-reduction reactions used to generate energy needed for growth and multiplication. Anaerobic bacteria are grouped as facultative, microaerophilic, or obligate anaerobes, depending on their degree of oxygen tolerance. Facultative anaerobes tolerate the presence or absence of oxygen, and microaerophils tolerate only no or low concentrations of oxygen. Obligate anaerobes, however, cannot survive long even when exposed to very low concentrations of oxygen. Indeed, obligate anaerobes tolerate only an environment with an oxidizing capacity (as measured by the redox potential) lower than would occur following total removal of oxygen; these very low redox potentials result from the additional presence of reducing agents, such as devitalized tissue in vivo. Similarly, devitalized tissue (e.g., chopped meat or liver) or reducing agents (cysteine or thioglycollate) are used in culture systems to lower the redox potential sufficiently to permit growth of obligate anaerobes in vitro. Obligate anaerobes are the predominant constituents of the normal microflora of the gingival crevice. The crevicular microflora is a complex ecosystem composed of several hundred different bacterial species. Its bacterial density approximates that of solid packed bacteria, as are found in colonies growing on an agar plate (i.e., 10^{12} colony-forming units [CFU]/gram). The crevicular microflora is normally predominantly gram-positive and the predominant anaerobic bacterial species is *Actinomyces*; but in the presence of periodontitis, the gingival crevice deepens as the epidermal dentine junction recedes toward the tooth apex. The bacterial microflora in the abnormal periodontal pocket becomes predominantly gram-negative, and the predominant anaerobic bacterial species are *Porphyromonas*, *Prevotella*, *Bacteroides*, and *Fusobacterium* species [1]. Saliva that bathes these surfaces contains gingival crevice microorganisms in addition to organisms that colonize the nasopharynx, tongue, and buccal mucosa, such as viridans streptococci and known aerobic pulmonary pathogens, such as *Streptococcus pneumoniae* and *Hemophilus influenzae*.

PATHOGENESIS

Anaerobic pulmonary infection usually is acquired by aspiration of oropharyngeal contents that includes these salivary microorganisms. Aspiration occurs among normal people, especially during deep sleep, but in certain patients aspiration is thought to be of sufficient magnitude or the aspirated material may contain adjuvants, such as necrotic tissue, food or foreign bodies, or particularly virulent pathogens or synergistic combinations of microorganisms to overcome lung defenses. However, the virulence of the organism is usually less important in the pathogenesis of anaerobic infection than defects in host defenses—for example, a predisposition to aspirate (such as occurs after a loss of consciousness from epilepsy, diabetic coma, general anesthesia, head trauma, or intoxication because of alcoholism or other drug abuse or overdose, or with a neurologic disorder of swallowing or with esophageal diseases) and periodontal disease that would favor the presence of large numbers of potential anaerobic pathogens and possibly necrotic periodontal debris in aspirated oropharyngeal secretions. Anaerobic pulmonary infection is less common among edentulous individuals. Indeed, the development of primary anaerobic pulmonary infection in edentulous patients should prompt a search for a neoplastic process in the nasopharynx or lower respiratory tract that would result in endobronchial obstruction and provide a focus of anaerobic microbial proliferation in necrotic neoplastic tissue.

Anaerobic pulmonary infection developing as a consequence of bronchogenic spread to the lung of endogenous microorganisms in the oropharyngeal microflora is usually referred to as primary. Hematogenous anaerobic pulmonary infection is referred to as secondary, because in this instance the primary infection (bacteremia, endocarditis, or suppurative thrombophlebitis, be it jugular or pelvic) will usually be clinically evident. Unresolved anaerobic bacterial pneumonitis will undergo necrosis in 1 to 2 weeks and result in one or more discrete cavities. The necrotizing infection is referred to as a lung abscess if each cavity is 2 cm or more in diameter. If there are multiple, small cavities, each less than 2 cm in diameter, the process is usually referred to as necrotizing pneumonia. Both lung abscess and necrotizing pneumonia are thought to be different manifestations of the same pathogenetic processes. Extension of the anaerobic pulmonary infection to the pleural space may result in anaerobic empyema.

MICROBIOLOGY

When microorganisms are aspirated into the lower respiratory tract, there is a marked simplification of the flora, so that only about four or five microbial species are isolated from minimally contaminated lower respiratory secretions in these patients. The pathogenic obligate anaerobes are usually more oxygen-tolerant than most obligate anaerobic members of the microflora. Anaerobic species, such as *Prevotella melaninogenica*, *Fusobacterium nucleatum*, and *Peptostreptococcus species*, usually predominate [2]. Microaerophilic and facultative streptococci are also frequently present. In some patients, the obligate anaerobes may be mixed with facultative respiratory pathogens, such as *S. pneumoniae*, *Staphylococcus aureus*, *H. influenzae*, or *Klebsiella pneumoniae*. The obligate anaerobic species, unlike facultative microorganisms, typically produce a foul odor in clinical specimens, in part due to various volatile short chain fatty acids.

Bacteriologic studies in the early 1970s of lower respiratory tract secretions obtained by methods (such as transtracheal aspiration that minimize contamination with oropharyngeal microbial flora), established that polymicrobial anaerobic bacterial flora are the cause of the infection in about one-third of patients with community-acquired pneumonia, one-third of non-intubated patients with nosocomial pneumonia, and in most patients with putrid lung abscess [3–8]. In a more recent study that used fiberoptic bronchoscopy and protected specimen brush to obtain samples from the involved area of lung prior to antimicrobial therapy [9], pathogens were recovered in 96% of patients with pneumonia and obligate anaerobes in 46% of these patients. Ventilator-associated pneumonia (VAP) is also thought to result from aspiration of oropharyngeal material. Indeed, using rigorous anaerobic methods and protected specimen brush sampling within 24 hr after development of pneumonia, anaerobes have been found in 23% of patients with VAP [10]. However, other studies using fiberoptic bronchoscopy and protected specimen brush to obtain cultures have failed to recover anaerobes in aspiration pneumonia and VAP [11,12], perhaps because the patients in these studies received antibiotic therapy prior to bacteriologic sampling [12].

ACTINOMYCOSIS

Actinomyces species, which are part of the normal gingival, intestinal, and vaginal flora, can produce a clinically distinct endogenous craniofacial, thoracic, abdominal, or pelvic infection. Actinomycosis is often polymicrobial, and the copathogens include anaerobic cocci, *Prevotella*, and *Actinobacillus actinomycetemcomitans* (microaerophilic gram-negative bacillus), and *Hemophilus* species. *Actinomyces* is an obligate anaerobic, delicate, filamentous gram-positive bacillus that branches to form Y, V, or T configurations and is often beaded. The bacilli are non–acid-fast, unlike the obligate aerobe, *Nocardia*, which they otherwise resemble morphologically. Colonies may appear in cultures, pus, and tissue as hard white-yellow granules, the so-called sulfur granule, which is 1–2 mm in diameter and composed of a mass of tangled filaments cemented together by a matrix secreted by the organism.

Routes of infection for thoracic actinomycosis include aspiration of oral contents or contiguous spread from craniofacial or abdominal-pelvic foci. Thoracic actinomycosis is characterized pathologically by the presence of sulfur granules and chronic inflammation, necrosis, and fibrosis, which crosses adjacent tissue plains and may involve contiguous regions of lung, pleura, ribs, vertebrae, mediastinum, esophagus, pericardium, and subcutaneous tissue, eventually to drain via multiple cutaneous sinuses on the chest wall. Hematogenous dissemination from the primary location can also occur.

EMPYEMA

Empyema can occur by contiguous spread from the infected lung or by hematogenous dissemination. Obligate anaerobes account for 25–40% of cases in most studies of empyema; the highest reported frequency of 76% was from a series of patients with empyema from a large city hospital and two Veterans Affairs hospitals [13].

CLINICAL PRESENTATION

The clinical presentation of aspiration pneumonia is usually acute and similar to that of pneumococcal pneumonia. However, about three-quarters of patients with primary lung abscess have an indolent febrile, wasting illness with respiratory symptoms (cough, sputum production, pleuritic chest pain, blood-streaked sputum) of several weeks duration, similar to that of tuberculosis or lung cancer, except over 50% of patients with lung abscess will produce sputum that has a foul odor or complain of a foul odor to their breath (although in early infection the putrid odor is often absent). One-quarter of patients with lung abscess will present with a more acute illness similar to that of pneumococcal pneumonia. Actinomycosis presents clinically as a chronic wasting febrile illness with pleuritic chest pain and cough productive of purulent, and, at times, blood-tinged sputum.

DIAGNOSIS

The anaerobic etiology of aspiration pulmonary infection is frequently presumptive and its therapy is consequently empirical because of the difficulties in obtaining uncontaminated respiratory secretions from the lung, in recovering of obligate anaerobes from clinical specimens, and in determining of antimicrobial susceptibility of the anaerobic isolates [14]. Patients who present with typical features of lung abscess that include a predisposition for aspiration, periodontal disease, a sputum with foul odor, one or more thick-walled cavities in dependent bronchopulmonary segments (e.g., superior segment of the lower lobe or posterior segment of the upper lobe when aspirating in the supine position), with air-fluid levels, should need little further initial diagnostic work-up and be treated presumptively for a polymicobial anaerobic infection. Although of no value for detecting anaerobes, culture of expectorated sputum is useful for excluding the presence of other pulmonary pathogens. Febrile patients should also have blood cultures to identify possible hematogenous anaerobic pneumonia (e.g. Lemierre's syndrome; i.e., *Fusobacterium* bacteremia, septic pulmonary emboli, and suppurative jugular thrombophlebitis) or exclude aerobic or facultative organisms capable of causing lung abscess (e.g., *S. aureus*). Pleural fluid, if present, should also be obtained for stains and cultures.

Upper lobe cavities without air-fluid levels suggest tuberculosis and require exclusion of *M. tuberculosis* with three morning sputum collections for mycobacterial stains and cultures. Also, in patients who fail to respond to empirical therapy for putative anaerobic pneumonia, in patients suspected of pulmonary neoplasm, and in immunocompromised patients, more rigorous diagnostic testing is usually indicated; such testing includes bronchoscopy, protected brushing, and collection of bronchoalveolar lavage fluid for stains and cultures for routine bacteria, *Rhodococcus equi* (in patients with AIDS), legionella, nocardia and fungi, if expectorated sputum studies fail to disclose the presence of these organisms. Computed tomography (CT) of the chest may be important to define pathologic anatomy in patients with a pyopneumothorax. CT, bronchoscopy, and biopsy may also be necessary in some patients, especially those who do not respond to empirical therapy for lung abscess to exclude conditions such as cystic bronchiectasis, cavitating neoplasms, and Wegener's granulomatosis, which may also produce cavitation and be confused with lung abscess.

ANTIMICROBIAL TREATMENT

Older Antimicrobial Agents

Penicillin, either 500–750 mg every 6 hours orally or 10–20 million unit intravenously per day, or tetracycline had been the standard antimicrobial agents used in empirical regimens to treat putative anaerobic lung abscess [13]. However, many obligate anaerobic gram-negative respiratory pathogens are now found to be penicillin-resistant as a consequence of β-lactamase production [9] and are also tetracycline-resistant. Indeed, two studies comparing penicillin to clindamycin in the treatment of putrid lung abscess found shorter time to defervescence and time to loss of the putrid odor to the sputum and less frequent relapse with clindamycin [15,16]. Clindamycin can be used intravenously in doses of 600 mg every 8 hr initially in hospitalized patients unable to tolerate oral therapy, or orally in doses of 300 mg every 6 hr.

Other older agents that are active against both the oral anaerobes and microaerophilic streptococci include the carbapenems, (e.g., imipenem and meropenem), cefoxitin, and β-lactamase/β-lactam antibiotic combinations (e.g., amoxicillin/clavulanate, ampicillin/sulbactam, ticarcillin/clavulanate or piperacillin/tazobactam) [14,17,18]. These drugs, however, do not have the proven efficacy of clindamycin, although susceptibility of anaerobes to clindamycin is no longer as predictable as when this drug was first used [17]. Metronidazole, although it is reliably active against gram-negative anaerobes [17], has been found to be inadequate therapy for anaerobic pleuropulmonary infections when used alone [19], apparently because it is inactive against microaerophilic streptococci. Chloramphenicol is reliably active in vitro against anaerobes [14,17], and is effective in treatment of anaerobic infections, but this drug is rarely used any longer because it can cause fatal aplastic anemia and alternative drugs are available.

Actinomyces is susceptible to penicillin, ampicillin, cephalosporins, carbapenems, macrolides, tetracycline, and clindamycin. However, intravenous administration of high-dose penicillin G remains the treatment of choice (10–20 million units daily) for actinomycosis. The duration of intravenous therapy for actinomycosis is 4–6 weeks, especially when there is extensive tissue destruction, followed by oral administration of penicillin 2–4 g daily or amoxicillin for up to one year to prevent relapse [20]. Tetracycline is an alternate option in patients allergic to penicillin. Antibiotic coverage of all the isolated pathogens involved in actinomycosis is often not necessary;

however, if clindamycin is used alone and *Actinobacillus* is a copathogen, persistent infection can occur with this clindamycin–resistant organism.

New Antimicrobial Agents: the Newer Fluoroquinolones, Ketolides, Oxazolidinones, and Carbapenems

In addition to these older drugs, several new antimicrobial agents with in vitro activity against obligate anaerobes have been approved for treatment of respiratory tract infections because of demonstrated efficacy in clinical trials of community-acquired pneumonia. However, none of these drugs have been studied in series of patients with bacteriologically confirmed anaerobic pleuropulmonary infections, or with putative anaerobic infections, such as putrid lung abscess. These drugs have reliable activity against aerobic respiratory

TABLE 1 Antimicrobial Regimens to Treat Anaerobic Pleuropulmonary Infections[a]

	Intravenous	Oral
Clindamycin	600–900 mg q8h	300 mg q6h
Cefoxitin	2 g q8h	
Amoxicillin plus metronidazole		500 mg q8h or 875 mg q12h 500 mg q6h
Ampicillin/sulbactam[b]	2 g ampicillin/1g sulbactam q6h	
Amoxicillin/clavulanate[b]		875 mg amoxicillin/125 mg clavulanate q12h or 500 mg amoxicillin/125 mg clavulanate q8h
Piperacillin/tazobactam[b]	3 g piperacillin/0.375 g tazobactam q6h	
Ticarcillin/clavulanate[b]	3 g ticarcillin/1g clavulanate q6h	
Imipenem[b]	500 mg q6h	
Meropenem[b]	1 g q8h	
Gatifloxacin[b]	400 mg q24h	400 mg q24h
Moxifloxacin[b]	400 mg q24h	400 mg q24h
Linezolid[b]	600 mg q12h	600 mg q12h

[a] Duration of therapy is at least 4–6 weeks. Intravenous can be switched to oral therapy when the patient has been afebrile for 4–5 days.
[b] This antibiotic has not been approved by the FDA for treatment of pleuropulmonary infection caused by anaerobic bacteria.

pathogens, such as *S. pneumoniae*, *H. influenzae*, and *Moraxella catarrhalis*, which have emerged resistant to the older agents. Except for ertapenem, they are also active against pathogens that cause the so-called atypical pneumonia syndrome (*Chlamydia pneumoniae*, *Mycoplasma pneumoniae*, and *Legionella pneumophila*). The in vitro activity demonstrated against a variety of anaerobic bacteria suggests that these drugs may have clinical efficacy in anaerobic pleuropulmonary infections. However, the sources for isolates in these studies have not necessarily been lower respiratory tract secretions or pleural fluid; when the source is other than pleuropulmonary, the published data may not be predictive of efficacy for infection caused by anaerobic pleuropulmonary pathogens.

New Fluoroquinolones

The older fluoroquinolones, such as ciprofloxacin, ofloxacin, and norfloxacin, are inactive against anaerobes. Trovafloxacin, gatifloxacin, moxifloxacin, and gemifloxacin, and to a limited extent levofloxacin, are active against anaerobes [21–26]. Use of trovafloxacin is now limited by the rare occurrence of hepatotoxicity that has been fatal in some cases. Side effects with levofloxacin, gatifloxacin, and moxifloxacin have been minimal, although prolongation of the QTc interval in some patients with sparfloxacin, gatifloxacin, and moxifloxacin has resulted in the recommendation that their use be avoided in patients with known prolongation of the QTc interval, in patients with uncorrected hypokalemia, and in patients receiving class 1A or class III antiarrhythmic agents. FDA approval of gemifloxacin is still pending. Because of their broad spectrum of activity for respiratory pathogens and infrequency of significant side effects, these newer fluoroquinolones have been used commonly for empirical therapy of community-acquired pneumonia. Indeed, the latest Infectious Disease Society of America (IDSA) guidelines for the treatment of community-acquired pneumonia [27] recommended their use, either (1) alone for treatment of outpatients or (2) combined with a β-lactam, such as ceftriaxone, for the treatment of patients requiring ICU admission. Combination therapy was recommended because efficacy of the newer fluoroquinolones when used alone in severe pneumonia has not been documented. For suspected aspiration, the IDSA recommended a newer fluoroquinolone, with or without a β-lactam/β-lactamase inhibitor combination (such as ampicillin/sulbactam or piperacillin/tazobactam), metronidazole, or clindamycin. They specifically commented, though, that the newer fluoroquinolones might not require additional anaerobic coverage, because of their in vitro activity against anaerobes.

A CDC panel that was convened to consider treatment of community-acquired pneumonia in the face of emerging antimicrobial resistance was hesitant to recommend the newer fluoroquinolones for fear that their widespread use may lead to development of fluoroquinolone resistance among the respiratory pathogens (as well as other microorganisms that colonize the treated patients) [28]. The CDC panel did not specifically comment on treatment of anaerobic pulmonary infection.

Ketolides

The ketolides are a new family of antimicrobial agents that are structurally related to the macrolides. Their mechanism of action, similar to that of the macrolides, involves blocking protein synthesis by binding to the ribosomal RNA complex; but bacteria that either display MLSb type of resistance (i.e., cross-resistance to macrolides, clindamycin, and streptogramin B) as a result of decreased affinity to an altered ribosomal target or display efflux type of resistance (i.e., resistance to macrolides, but susceptibility to clindamycin) are still susceptible to the ketolides. Telithromycin, a ketolide whose approval by the FDA for therapy of respiratory tract infection is pending, has been shown to be active against streptococci and staphylococci resistant to the macrolides. This ketolide is also active against many anaerobes, with minimal inhibitory concentrations (MIC) of ≤ 0.5 μg/mL [29]. Telithromycin is well absorbed and, when given in doses of 800 mg every 24 hr orally, achieves peak and tough serum levels of about 2 μg/ml and 0.05 μg/ml, respectively, with a serum half-life of 10 hr. It is concentrated ≥ 100-fold within phagocytes and about five-fold in the epithelial lining fluid of the alveoli.

Oxazolidinones

Linezolid, a member of a new class of synthetic antimicrobial agents, the oxazolidinones, has been approved by the FDA for therapy of respiratory tract infection. Because of its unique mechanism of action, cross-resistance with other antimicrobial agents does not occur. Linezolid has been found to be active against *Fusobacterium spp.*, *Prevotella* spp., *Porphyromonas* spp., *Bacteroides* spp., and peptostreptococci at MIC of $\leq$μg/mL [30] in addition to facultative respiratory pathogens. Linezolid is given in doses of 600 mg I.V. or orally every 12 hr. Its peak and trough serum levels are 12 and 4 μg/mL, and its serum half-life is about 4 hr. Doses do not have to be changed for renal failure. Side effects have been minimal, although reversible thrombocytopenia has been reported in about 3% of treated patients when the duration of therapy is greater than 2 weeks.

Carbapenems

Ertapenem is a new member of the carbapenem family of β-lactam antibiotics. The antimicrobial spectrum of ertapenem is similar to that of imipenem and meropenem, except ertapenem is not active against enterococci, *P.*

aeruginosa, and *Acinetobacter*. Specifically, ertapenem is active against *S. pneumoniae* (except highly penicillin-resistant strains), *H. influenzae*, obligate anaerobes [31,32] and *S. aureus* (excluding MRSA). Ertapenem has FDA approval for treatment of community-acquired pneumonia. The approved dose is 1 g every 24 hr for a total duration of therapy of up to 14 days for I.V. administration or 7 days I.M. administration, with an option to switch to an appropriate oral agent after at least 3 days of clinical improvement on ertapenem for a total of 10–14 days of therapy. However, anaerobic lung infection will usually require a longer duration of antibiotic therapy. The dose of ertapenem should be reduced to 500 mg daily if the creatinine clearance is less than 30 mL/min.

Duration of Antibiotic Therapy

Patients with anaerobic pulmonary infection on effective therapy can be expected to defervesce, and in patients with putrid lung abscess the sputum will become odorless within a week. Chest radiographic findings may take at least several weeks to resolve. The duration of therapy is controversial. The recommended duration of therapy for aspiration pneumonia is 14 days and for anaerobic lung abscess it is usually at least 4 to 6 weeks to prevent relapse, or until the abscess completely resolves or there is a small, stable residual scar. However, many patients will cease to take medication on their own after several weeks and return at a later point in time for other reasons with a clear chest radiogram. Failure to adequately respond to therapy (persistent fever, worsening of the pulmonary radiographic findings, or development of empyema) should prompt more intensive investigation to exclude the presence of resistant pathogens, endobronchial obstruction, or a noninfectious etiology.

PREVENTION

Because the usual pathogenesis of anaerobic pleuropulmonary infection involves aspiration of oral anaerobes, prevention is mainly directed at reducing the risk for aspiration of mouth contents in aspiration-prone patients (i.e., patients with a depressed state of consciousness, gastroesophageal regurgitation, or defective swallowing). Aspiration may be diminished in aspiration-prone patients who require long-term feeding tubes by maintaining them in a semi-recumbent position, by careful monitoring of their gastric volumes, and by use of percutaneous endoscopic gastrostomy or enterostomy tubes rather than naso-enteral feeding tubes. Prudent use of naso-enteral tubes, treatment of seizures, avoiding oversedation, and correction of reversible causes of gastroesophageal reflux are other measures to diminish aspiration. Liquids should be thickened in patients having difficulty swallowing these types of materials. Endobronchial obstruction, which impedes clearance of aspirated material, should be alleviated by removal of foreign bodies and shrinkage of endobronchial neoplasms, if possible. In addition, treatment of periodontal disease can diminish the size of the bacterial inoculum and virulence of the oral flora in aspirated material.

ANCILLARY MANAGEMENT

Surgery is rarely indicated for putrid lung abscess, except for the rare complication of massive hemoptysis. Postural and bronchoscopic drainage and chest physiotherapy traditionally have been recommended to enhance antimicrobial therapy. However, caution should be exercised to avoid sudden massive emptying of pus-filled cavities into the airways and previously uninvolved bronchopulmonary segments. Surgery for actinomycosis may be indicated for resection of necrotic soft tissue and bone and excision of sinus tracts. Anaerobic empyema will require complete drainage, usually by insertion of a chest tube, although thoracotomy and rib resection may be necessary to break loculations to accomplish this.

CONCLUSION

Obligate anaerobes are the predominant constituents of normal oropharyngeal flora and produce pleuropulmonary infection in patients who are prone to aspirate. The diagnosis of anaerobic pulmonary infection is frequently presumptive and therapy consequently empirical. Clindamycin has been shown in clinical trials to be more efficacious than penicillin for treatment of anaerobic lung abscess. Use of alternate agents (such as imipenem or meropenem, cefoxitin, β-lactamase/β-lactam antibiotic combinations (e.g., amoxicillin/clavulanate, ampicillin/sulbactam, ticarcillin/clavulanate, or piperacillin/tazobactam), is guided by published studies of their in vitro activity against collected clinical isolates of obligate anaerobic bacteria. Several new drugs (e.g., ertapenem [a carbapenem], new fluoroquinolones, ketolides, and linezolid) that also have in vitro activity against obligate anaerobes have recently become available for the empirical treatment of pneumonia.

REFERENCES

1. Slots J. Sub gingival microflora and periodontitis. J Clin Periodont 1979; 6:351–382.
2. Marina M, Strong CA, Civen R, et al. Bacteriology of anaerobic pleuropulmonary infection. Preliminary Report. Clin Infect Dis 1993; 16(suppl 4):S256–S262.

3. Levison ME, Bran JL, Ries K. Treatment of anaerobic bacterial infections with clindamycin 2 phosphate. Antimicrob Agents Chemother 1974; 5:276–280.
4. Gonzalez-C CL, Calia FM. Bacteriologic flora of aspiration-induced pulmonary infections. Arch Intern Med 1975; 135:711–714.
5. Lorber B, Swenson RM. Bacteriology of aspiration pneumonia, a prospective study of community and hospital acquired cases. Ann Intern Med 1974; 81: 329.
6. Bartlett JG, O'Keefe P, Tally FP, Louie TJ, Gorbach SL. Bacteriology of hospital-acquired pneumonia. Arch Intern Med 1986; 146:868–871.
7. Bartlett JG, Gorbach SL, Finegold SM. The bacteriology of aspiration pneumonia. Am J Med 1974; 56:202–207.
8. Bartlett JG, Gorbach SL. Treatment of aspiration pneumonia and primary lung abscess: penicillin G vs clindamycin. JAMA 1975; 234:935–937.
9. Pollack HM, Hawkins EL, Bonner JR, et al. Diagnosis of bacterial pulmonary infections with quantitative protected catheter cultures obtained during bronchoscopy. J Clin Microbiol 1983; 17:255–259.
10. Dore P, Robert R, Grolier G, et al. Incidence of anaerobes in ventilator-associated pneumonia with use of a protected specimen brush. Am J Respir Crit Care Med 1996; 153:1292–1298.
11. Mier L, Dreyfuss D, Darchy B, et al. Is penicillin G adequate initial treatment for aspiration pneumonia? A prospective evaluation using a protected specimen brush and quantitative cultures. Intensive Care Med 1993; 19:279–284.
12. Marik PE, Careau P. The role of anaerobes in patients with ventilator-associated pneumonia and aspiration pneumonia, a prospective study. Chest 1999; 115:178–183.
13. Bartlett JG. Anaerobic bacterial infections of the lung and pleural space. Clin Infect Dis 1993; 16(suppl 4):S248–S255.
14. Jorgensen JH, Ferraro MJ. Antimicrobial susceptibility testing: special needs for fastidious organisms and difficult to detect resistance mechanisms. Clin Infect Dis 2000; 30:799–808.
15. Levison ME, Mangura CT, Lorber B, et al. Clindamycin compared with penicillin for the treatment of anaerobic lung abscess. Ann Intern Med 1983; 98:466–471.
16. Gudiol F, Manresa F, Pallares R, et al. Clindamycin vs. penicillin for anaerobic lung infections. High rate of penicillin failures associated with penicillin-resistant *Bacteroides melaninogenicus*. Arch Intern Med 1990; 150:2525–2529.
17. Kasten MJ. Clindamycin, metronidazole and chloramphenicol. Mayo Clin Proc 1999; 74:825–833.
18. Falagas ME, Siakavellas E. Bacteroides, Prevotella and Porphyromonas species: a review of antibiotic resistance and therapeutic options. Int J Antimicrob Agents 2000; 15:1–9.
19. Perlino CA. Metronidazole vs clindamycin treatment of anaerobic pulmonary infection: failure of metronidazole therapy. Arch Intern Med 1981; 141:1424–1427.
20. Smego RA, Foglia G. Actinomycosis. Clin Infect Dis 1998; 26:1255–1261.

21. Appelbaum PC. Quinolone activity against anaeobes. Drugs 1999; 58:60–64.
22. Schaumann R, Ackerman G, Pless B, et al. In vitro activities of gatifoxacin, two other quinolones, and five nonquinolone antimicrobials against obligately anaerobic bacteria. Antimicrob Agents Chemother 1999; 43:2783–2786.
23. Goldstein EJ. Review of the in vitro activity of gemifloxacin against gram-positive and gram-negative anaerobic pathogens. J Antimicrob Chemother 2000; 45:55–65.
24. Goldstein EJ, Citron DM, Vreni Merriam C, et al. Activities of gemifloxacin (SB 265805, LB 20304) compared to those of other oral antimicrobial agents against unusual anaerobes. Antimicrob Agents Chemother 1999; 43:2726–2730.
25. Goldstein EJ, Citron DM, Merriam CV, et al. Activity of gatifloxacin compared to five other quinolones versus aerobic and anaerobic isolates from skin and soft tissue samples of human and animal bite wound infections. Antimicrob Agents Chemother 1999; 43:1475–1479.
26. Ackerman G, Schaumann R, Pless B, et al. Comparative activity of moxifoxacin in vitro against obligately anaerobic bacteria. Eur J Clin Microbiol Infect Dis 2000; 19:228–232.
27. Bartlett JG, Dowell SF, Mandell LA, et al. Practice guidelines for the management of community-acquired pneumonia in adults. Clin Infect Dis 2000; 31:347.
28. Heffelfinger JD, Dowell SF, Jorgensen JH, et al. Management of community-acquired pneumonia in the era of pneumococcal resistance. A report from the drug-resistant Streptococcus pneumoniae therapeutic working group. Arch Intern Med 2000; 160:1400.
29. Goldstein EJ, Citron DM, Merriam CV, et al. Activities of telithromycin (HMR 3647, RU 66647) compared to those of erythromycin, azithromycin, clarithromycin, roxithromycin, and other antimicrobial agents against unusual anaerobes. Antimicrob Agents Chemother 1999; 43:2801–2805.
30. Goldstein EJ, Citron DM, Merriam CV. Linezolid activity compared to those of other selected macrolides and other agents against aerobic and anaerobic pathogens isolated from soft tissues bite infections in humans. Antimicrob Agents Chemother 1999; 43:1469–1474.
31. Goldstein EJ, Citron DM, Merriam CV, et al. Comparative activity of ertapenem and 11 other antimicrobial agents against aerobic and anaerobic pathogens isolated from skin and soft tissue animal and human bite wound infections. J Antimicrob Chemother 2001; 48:641–651.
32. Hoellman DB, Kelly LM, Credito K, et al. In vitro antianaerobic activity of ertapenem (MK-0826) compared to seven other compounds. Antimicrob Agents Chemother 2002; 46:220–224.

16

Treatment of the Common Cold and Viral Bronchitis

Harley A. Rotbart
University of Colorado Health Science Center
Denver, Colorado, U.S.A.

> Wealth, honour, freedom, beauty are all his A very king, in short, of kings he is; In wind and limb sound, vigourous, and bold Except when troubled by a wretched cold.
>
> —Horace

The ancient poet aptly dispels the notion that the syndrome we know as the "cold" is common or trivial—indeed, "wretched cold" is a more appropriate name for this scourge of mankind. The common cold is responsible for 25 million days of missed work, 23 million days of missed school, and 84 million physician visits each year in the United States alone [1]. The common cold is also the most frequent cause of inappropriate antibiotic use in the United States [2,3]. Similarly, acute bronchitis is diagnosed millions of times each year in this country and is responsible for almost 30% of all antibiotic prescriptions—this despite the fact that the vast majority of cases, as with the common cold, are viral in origin [4]. Hence, the appropriate diagnosis and treatment of these two viral syndromes has important health implications for infected individuals as well as for society as a whole.

ETIOLOGY AND EPIDEMIOLOGY

The common respiratory viruses are responsible for the vast majority of cases of the common cold and acute bronchitis. Among these pathogens, the picornaviruses—rhinoviruses (RVs) and enteroviruses (EVs)—account for between 50 and 80% of all cases of the common cold [5,6]; influenza, adenoviruses, and picornaviruses are the leading causes of acute bronchitis [4]. The comparative roles of a variety of pathogens in the common cold and acute bronchitis syndromes are shown in Table 1.

The seasonalities of the common cold and acute bronchitis parallel the seasonalities of the major pathogens involved. Incidence of the common cold peaks in the late summer and fall each year with a smaller peak in the spring—both coincident with the seasonal variations of RV and EV infections [1]. In contrast, the winter "flu season" is also the season for acute bronchitic episodes dominated by influenza and adenovirus infections.

PATHOGENESIS

The pathogenesis of the common cold is incompletely understood. In persons lacking specific immunity to the infecting serotype, most exposures result in infection. Symptoms may begin within 12 hr of infection [7]. Transmission appears to be via hand-nose or hand-eye contact following contamination of the hand with nasal secretions from an infected index case. The initial event in cold production is viral infection of the nasal epithelium; the number of productively infected cells appears to be small [8,9] and nasal biopsy studies show little mucosal damage [10]. Elaboration of host inflammatory cytokines in response to viral infection is central in the pathogenesis of symptoms and in inducing immune responses. Respiratory epithelial cytokine production likely

TABLE 1 Major Pathogens of the Common Cold and Acute Bronchitis

Common cold	Acute bronchitis
Picornaviruses	Influenza viruses
Rhinoviruses	Picornaviruses
Enteroviruses	Rhinoviruses
Coronaviruses	Enteroviruses
Adenoviruses	Adenoviruses
Respiratory syncytial virus	*Mycoplasma pneumoniae*
Influenza viruses	*Chlamydia pneumoniae*
Parainfluenza viruses	*Bordetella pertussis*

contributes to airway hyperreactivity and to an influx of neutrophils in both nasal mucosa and secretions [11]. Cold symptoms also appear to be due to neurologic reflexes triggered by the infection [12]. Human HRV has been assumed to be restricted to the upper respiratory tract, but limited evidence indicates that the virus sometimes replicates in the tracheobronchial tree and lung [13,14].

The issue of viral invasiveness of the lower airways also plagues our understanding of acute bronchitis. Influenza viruses are known for their ability to invade the lower respiratory tract, whereas other etiologic agents of bronchitis (such as picornaviruses and coronaviruses, as noted above) are typically not. Hence, inflammatory mediators may be more important in the pathogenesis of bronchitis due to the viruses that are more restricted in their distribution within the respiratory tract. Destruction of the epithelial lining cells of the airways is typical of influenza bronchitis, but mucociliary dysfunction is probably more important for the virulence of non-influenzal pathogens. A component of bronchospasm in the pathogenesis of bronchitis has been suspected based on the increased incidence of asthma in patients with histories of bronchitis and, conversely, patients with histories of asthma appear to have increased likelihood of developing bronchitis episodes. Confounding this interpretation are recent data suggesting the presence of rhinoviruses in the lower airways detected by sensitive PCR techniques [14]. What role direct infection by these viruses has in acute viral bronchitis remains to be determined.

CLINICAL MANIFESTATIONS

Cough is a common clinical hallmark of both the common cold and acute bronchitis. In the former, cough is one of many concurrent symptoms, usually shadowed by nasal complaints, whereas in patients with bronchitis, cough becomes the major problem.

The usual incubation period of viral colds is 1 to 3 days. Rhinorrhea, nasal stuffiness, and sneezing are the commonest symptoms; other typical manifestations include sore or scratchy throat, facial pressure, headache, cough, hoarseness, and less often, malaise, chills, or feverishness [15]. Sore throat tends to be the first symptom and runny nose the most bothersome [16]. Significant fever is very uncommon in adults and should suggest an alternative diagnosis. Infants and young children have fever more often and may show only mucous nasal discharge. Red, sometimes macerated nostrils, and glassy nasal mucosa are also typically present but examination is primarily useful for excluding other diagnoses. In adults, nasal symptoms usually peak on the second or third day and then gradually subside. Cough usually persists until the end of the first week but may be protracted in smokers. The median duration of viral colds is one week, but up to one-quarter last 2 weeks or longer [16].

In patients with acute bronchitis, cough is the predominant symptom, but early in the course of the illness other symptoms typically associated with the common cold may also be present. The infection appears to "settle" in the lower respiratory tract, where it may result in sputum production, chest pain, rhonchi, rales, wheezing, and so forth. The patient may present for medical attention only after 1–2 weeks of "fighting a cold." The cough may last upwards of a month. Fever is more commonly seen in patients with influenza and adenovirus-associated bronchitis, less often in rhinovirus and coronavirus bronchitis. By definition, alveolar involvement, changes of pulmonary consolidation, and cyanosis are not classified as signs of bronchitis but instead imply pulmonary disease.

The common cold becomes even more the "wretched cold" when associated with any one of a number of frequently encountered upper and lower respiratory tract complications in both children and adults. Viral respiratory tract infections are the most important predisposing factor to *acute otitis media* (*AOM*). Viruses have been detected by culture or antigen assay in 11–41% of middle ear fluids from children with AOM [17,18], with rhinoviruses in up to 8% of such fluids. By polymerase chain reaction, rhinovirus infection is detectable in 35% of children with AOM, including the presence of rhinoviral RNA in 24% of middle ear fluids [19]. In adults, middle ear pressure abnormalities commonly develop during colds [20,21]. Coinfection with viruses and bacteria has been reported to predispose to failure of antibiotic therapy in AOM [22].

Most cases of acute *sinusitis* thought to result from bacterial disease are secondary to a preceding viral upper respiratory tract infection. Sinus abnormalities are frequently detectable during uncomplicated colds [23]. Consequently, distinguishing a primary viral rhinosinusitis from a secondary bacterial sinusitis is clinically difficult. Rhinovirus is detectable by culture or PCR in 40% of sinus brushings from patients with acute community-acquired sinusitis [24].

Respiratory virus infections are major factors in the induction of *acute exacerbations of asthma* in adults [25] and in children [26]. In a 2-year study of adult asthmatics 19–46 years of age, peak expiratory flow rate deteriorations occurred during 27% of respiratory illness episodes, and colds were associated with 71% of documented exacerbations [25]. Rhinoviruses are the most commonly identified pathogens found in asthma exacerbations and hospitalizations for those older than 2 years [27].

Respiratory virus infections are also associated with *lower respiratory tract syndromes* in other patient populations. Chronic obstructive pulmonary disease (COPD) is the second most common chronic, noncommunicable disease in the world [28]. Exacerbations of COPD can be shown to be due to respiratory viruses in more than 25% of all cases, with picornaviruses the leading cause [29]. Hospitalizations due to COPD exacerbations are even more strongly linked to viral infections, with as many as 45% of all such events proved to be triggered by viral infections [29]. Similarly, in children with cystic fibrosis, picornaviruses have been detected in more than 25% of exacerbations, and colds were associated with deterioration in pulmonary function testing [30]. Among adults 60–90 years of age residing in the community, rhinovirus infection was associated with lower respiratory tract symptoms in 65%; 40% consulted their doctor, and 76% of these received antibiotics [31]. The impact of rhinoviruses in elderly people, as measured by those indices, approaches that of influenza [31]. Up to 40% of exacerbations in patients with chronic bronchitis may be associated with RV infections [32]. In infants younger than 12 months, rhinovirus infections have been associated with hospitalization for lower respiratory tract illness, particularly bronchiolitis [33], and deterioration in those with bronchopulmonary dysplasia [34].

DIAGNOSIS

No rapid antigen detection or practical serologic tests exist for rhinovirus infections because of the multiplicity of serotypes. Viral culture takes 3–7 days and is of limited clinical use. PCR detection of RV RNA has been frequently positive in RV culture–negative samples [35] but currently is only a research tool. Diagnosis of influenza virus infection is possible using traditional culture techniques as well as a variety of rapid antigen assays that are commercially available. Similarly, respiratory syncytial virus infection is diagnosable by both culture and antigen assays. The other major viral pathogens of the common cold and of acute bronchitis are more difficult to diagnose and, as such, specific viral diagnostic tests are rarely performed for either of these clinical syndromes.

MANAGEMENT

Cold treatments are associated with subjectivity and strong placebo effects, so adequate blinding of studies is essential. It is difficult to draw positive or negative conclusions from many of these studies because of small sample sizes, limited micobiological support, and differing outcome measures. Recent examples of interventions shown to be of no real value include intranasal hyperthermia [36], zinc gluconate lozenges [37], and oral Echinacea [38].

Antivirals

A major hurdle to effective antiviral therapy for the cold and bronchitis syndromes is the unclear importance of ongoing viral replication in symptom pathogenesis after illness onset. Clinical trials of antiviral therapies for the cold and bronchitis have been limited to compounds with efficacy against the picornaviruses.

There are several steps in the replication cycle of the picornaviruses that are potential targets in antiviral therapy. Cell susceptibility, viral attachment, viral uncoating, viral RNA replication, and viral protein synthesis have all been studied as potential strategic targets of anti-picornaviral compounds (Table 2). The following sections briefly review these targets, the mechanisms of action of anti-picornavirus compounds directed at these targets, and the clinical trials performed to date.

Interferon

Interferons are potent, selective mediators of cellular changes that induce a number of antiviral, antiproliferative, and immunological effects, all of which collectively affect host cell susceptibility to picornavirus infection [39–47]. The cellular antiviral effects of interferons are mediated through specific receptor-signal transduction pathways. In conjunction with double-stranded RNA, interferons induce the expression of proteins, some of which mediate an antiviral activity. The best-described pathways are (1) 2′,5′-adenylate synthetase; (2) double-stranded RNA-dependent protein kinase; and (3) the Mx proteins. Through transfection/expression systems, an isoform of the 2′,5′adenylate synthetase system has been linked to the inhibition of replication of picornaviruses [48]. Clinically, children with acute EV meningitis have significant elevations in endogenous interferon levels in the CSF [49,50], which may be important in recovery from the infection. Although alfa interferon itself is a very potent inhibitor of picornavirus infection, additive

TABLE 2 Therapeutic Strategies and Candidate Compounds for Treatment of Picornaviral Infections

Target	Compound class
Cell susceptibility	Interferons
Viral attachment and binding to host cells	Antibodies, soluble ICAM
Viral uncoating/capsid function	Capsid-function inhibitors
Viral replication	Enviroxime-like compounds
Viral protein synthesis	3C protease inhibitors

or synergistic protective effects are seen when used in conjunction with capsid-inhibiting compounds [43], nucleoside analogues [46], or gamma interferon [51]. Interferons may also work in conjunction with humoral antibodies and macrophages to eliminate picornavirus infections [40].

Intranasal interferon has been shown to be effective as prophylaxis for RV colds in several studies [52–56]. Additional studies demonstrated significant efficacy against naturally acquired RV infections and against contact spread of RVs within family groups after experimental induction of a natural cold [52,57]. Side effects of interferon included nasal irritation and stuffiness, and mucosal ulceration [52,55]. Administered therapeutically 1 day after experimental RV infection, intranasal interferon had no effect on development of infection or symptoms, but did result in moderate reductions of virus shedding and cold symptoms [58]. Additional studies with low-dose intranasal interferon also demonstrated a lack of efficacy in post-exposure prophylaxis of RV infections in families [59].

Capsid-Inhibiting Compounds

Capsid-inhibiting compounds block viral uncoating and/or viral attachment to host cell receptors. The resolved three-dimensional structure of the EVs reveals a "canyon" formed by the junctions of VP1 and VP3. Beneath the canyon lies a "pore" that leads to a hydrophobic pocket into which a variety of diverse hydrophobic compounds can bind (Table 2). Although the compounds integrate into a virus capsid via a number of noncovalent, hydrophobic-type interactions, the affinity is high with constants ranging from 2.0×10^{-8} to 2.9×10^{-7} M [60]. Enhanced potency of the capsid-binding compounds appears to correlate with increased number of molecules of compound per pocket [60,61], proximity of compound to the opening of the pocket [61], increased hydrophobic energy resulting from filling a greater proportion of the pocket by the compound [60–62] and absence of bulky amino acid substitutions (mutations) within the pocket structure [63–65].

Several potential mechanisms of action of picornavirus inhibition by compounds that affect the function of the virus capsid have been hypothesized. Filling the hydrophobic pocket results in increased stability of the virus, making the virus more resistant to uncoating. The increased stability of the virus-compound complex is evidenced by the resistance to thermal inactivation [66]. This property can be used as a rapid screen in order to identify molecules with binding avidity; the majority of, but not all, compounds with potent antiviral activity also result in thermal stability. It is also possible that a degree of capsid flexibility may be required for uncoating, and activity of these compounds within the hydrophobic pocket may reduce this necessary flexibility, inducing a more rigid structure. Alternatively, changes in the conformation of the canyon floor as a result of drug activity within the underlying pocket may affect the attachment of the virus to the host cell receptor [44]. It has been shown, however, that such perturbations in the canyon floor do not absolutely correlate with antiviral potency [61,62]. The capsid-inhibiting compounds vary in their spectrum of activity, perhaps as a result of factors such as pocket fit discussed above. Certain compounds demonstrate both anti-EV and anti-RV activity [67 68]; others are more selective to one picornavirus genus or the other [69].

Trials of the “R” series of capsid-binding compounds have been limited to intranasal administration to patients with RV colds [70–72]. Pirodavir (R77975) and R61837 were efficacious in experimentally induced RV colds when these drugs were administered intranasally before or after infection, but prior to onset of symptoms [71,72]; pirodavir required 6 times daily dosing, with efficacy loss at 3 daily doses [72]. Another series of capsid-binding compounds, the phenoxyl imidazoles, are broad-spectrum inhibitors of the EVs and demonstrate therapeutic oral efficacy in animal models [69]. This series has limited potency against the RVs, and further development of candidate drugs has been discontinued.

The “WIN” series of compounds has been clinically evaluated in both RV and EV infections. The first compound of this group to advance to clinical trials was disoxaril (WIN 51711; Fig. 1). Disoxaril was moderately active against RVs in vitro and very active against EVs both in vitro and in vivo [67,73,74]. The appearance of asymptomatic crystalluria in healthy volunteers prevented further clinical study. Shortening of the aliphatic chain from $n = 7$ to $n = 5$ and adding chloro- groups to the phenyl ring (Fig. 1) resulted in WIN 54954, which had broad, potent anti-RV and anti-EV activity in vitro and in vivo [75], including oral therapeutic efficacy in mice. Clinical efficacy was assessed in two RV (rhinovirus 23 and rhinovirus 39) challenge trials [76] and one EV challenge trial (coxsackievirus A21) [77]. Despite administering the compound prior to infection and achieving serum concentrations above the in vitro minimal inhibitory concentrations, both RV trials failed to show efficacy of WIN 54954 [76]; very low concentrations of the drug were found in nasal wash samples, the site of the experimental infection. In contrast, WIN 54954 significantly reduced the number and severity of colds induced by coxsackievirus A21, and also significantly reduced nasal mucous discharge, respiratory and systemic symptoms, and viral titer [77]. The overall symptomatic attack rate was reduced from 15/23 patients in the placebo group to 3/27 in the WIN 54954–treated groups ($P = 0.0001$). This study represents the first demonstration of oral efficacy of an anti-EV agent; the differences in results compared with those in the RV studies using the same compound are enigmatic because the MIC for one of the RV serotypes was identical to that of the coxsackievirus A21 strain used. The fact that EV infections are systemic, usually with a viremic phase, may explain the enhanced EV efficacy of an orally active compound that achieves good blood levels over the effect seen in RV infections, which are limited to the upper airway where drug distribution may have been insufficient. WIN 54954 was not further developed for clinical use because of adverse reactions of flushing and rash, possibly related to concomitant alcohol ingestion by study volunteers.

Pleconaril (3-13,5-dimethyl-4- [[3-methyl-5-isoxazoly)propyl]phenyl]-5-(trifluoromethyl)-1,2,4-oxadiazole) is the first of a new generation of metabolically stable capsid function-inhibitors; this compound has been more extensively evaluated in clinical trials than any other anti-picomaviral agent. Pleconaril has demonstrated broad-spectrum and potent anti-EV and anti-RV activity and is highly orally bioavailable [78–81]. In a mouse model of multi-organ system infection following intracranial inoculation of EVs, pleconaril, a capsid-inhibitor compound, has been shown to reduce viral titers in all affected organs and to prevent death of the animals [78]. High levels of pleconaril are achieved in the central nervous system and in the nasal epithelium (M. McKinlay, personal communication). Pharmacokinetic studies of pleconaril have been undertaken in adults, children, and neonates [79–81]. In adults, the pharmacokinetics of pleconaril are best characterized as a one-compartment open model with first-order absorption [81], indicative of a compound that is readily absorbed into and distributed throughout the water compartment. Concentrations of pleconaril 12 hr after a single oral dose remain 2.5-fold greater than required to inhibit 95% of EVs in vitro. Neonates and older children have similar PK profiles [79,80]. Oral bioavailability, in animals and humans, approaches 70%.

In a challenge study of coxsackievirus A21 respiratory infection, 33 volunteers were randomized to receive either 400 mg of pleconaril or matching placebo, orally, 14 hr before inoculation with virus [82]. Beginning after inoculation, subjects received 200 mg capsules twice daily for 6 days. Pleconaril had a significant beneficial effect on symptom scores, global assessment, fever, and nasal mucus production, with 41% of placebo-treated subjects experiencing moderate colds versus none in the pleconaril-treated group. Peak viral titers, which occurred on the peak day of symptoms, were reduced by greater than 99% in the pleconaril group compared to the placebo group [82].

In a double-blind, placebo-controlled study of 1024 adults with viral respiratory infection during the fall rhinovirus season, patients receiving pleconaril recovered from all cold symptoms and returned to overall wellness (measured via a global assessment score) 3.5 days sooner than patients receiving placebo [83]. Individual symptoms (including nasal congestion, rhinorrhea, and pharyngitis) each resolved 1–2 days sooner in the pleconaril-treated patients.

In two follow-up double-blind, randomized, placebo-controlled studies of rhinoviral respiratory infection in adults involving more than 2000 patients in 200 centers across the United States and Canada, benefit of pleconaril was again demonstrated [84]. Pooled data from the two studies showed statistically significant differences in the median number of days to illness alleviation (approximately 1 day reduction with reduction in severity of symptoms seen within the first 24 hr), as well as statistically significant reductions in total symptom scores, days of cold medication use, nights of sleep disturbance, and nasal tissue use [84].

In all short-course (5 days) clinical studies of respiratory infections to date [82–84], a very favorable safety profile has been observed with pleconaril. There have been no differences in serious adverse events between treatment and placebo groups; a slight increase in the incidence of nausea has been seen in pleconaril-treated patients in certain studies and with certain dosing regimens [85]. Although safety data were favorable for pleconaril in these studies using 5-day therapy, longer treatment in other studies resulted in induction of the cyp 3A enzyme, raising the possibility of undesirable drug-drug interactions (M. McKinlay, personal communication). At this time, strategies to explore this safety concern are being investigated before further development of pleconaril is undertaken.

Enviroxime-Related Compounds

Enviroxime [2-amino-l-(isopropyisulfonyl)-6-bcnzimidazole phenyl ketone oxime is a prototype compound for a series of molecules with broad anti-EV and anti-RV activity [86–88]. The mechanism of action of these compounds has been suggested to be the inhibition of RNA replication via targeting the 3A protein coding region of the viruses [89]. The drugs apparently prevent formation of the RNA replicative intermediate, a complex dependent on both viral proteins 3A and 3AB [89], and, hence, the formation of new plus-strand RNA molecules. Vinyl acetylene benzimidazoles derivatives of enviroxime provide improved bioavailability of the compounds; fluoridation of these latter structures further enhances blood levels in animal models [90,91]. This class of compounds can be added to tissue culture systems several hours after viral inoculation without loss of antiviral activity, again reflecting their action at a later stage of the viral life cycle (i.e., RNA replication).

Enviroxime resulted in modest clinical and virologic benefit in some studies [92,93] and no benefit in others [94,95]. Problems with poor pharmacokinetics and undesirable toxicology and side effects resulted in discontinuance of that program. Newer derivatives of enviroxime promise better bioavailability and tolerance but have not been clinically evaluated.

Soluble ICAM

The majority of rhinoviruses bind to the intracellular adhesion molecule (ICAM) receptor on cell surfaces. A strategy to bind infecting virus with an intranasally applied soluble form of ICAM, named tremacamra, resulted in modest clinical benefits in a volunteer study with challenge infection. Statistically significant reductions in total symptom score, proportion of clinical colds, and nasal mucus weight were achieved [96]. Further development of this compound has not been undertaken as of this time.

3-C Protease Inhibitors

A series of compounds are under development that target the 3C protease of picornaviruses, resulting in inhibition of viral protein synthesis via blocking viral specific protein processing [97]. Published results are limited to those with tripeptide aldehydes derived from the sequence of a natural 3C cleavage site, Leu-Phe-Gln. Anti-enzyme activity is potent (K_I = 6 nM) with high therapeutic indices in vitro. Like the RNA inhibitors discussed above, time of addition with the protease inhibitors is several hours without loss of antiviral activity. These compounds appear to have both anti-RV activity and anti-EV activity and appear to have an antiviral effect even if initiated (in the animal model) several hours after infection. Clinical trials in RV upper respiratory infections for the lead compound, AG7088, have been discontinued as of this time in an attempt to improve characteristics of the formulation.

Ancillary Management

Symptomatic Therapies

Antihistamines have been frequently used for the treatment of common colds but their usefulness has been the subject of controversy [98]. Only first-generation antihistamines (e.g. chlorpheniramine, clemastine), which have anticholinergic and sedating effects, are useful in treating cold-associated rhinorrhea and sneezing [99,100]. Selective, nonsedating first-generation antihistamines (e.g., terfenadine, loratadine) are ineffective [101]. The anticholinergic nasal spray ipratropium bromide has been shown to reduce rhinorrhea by 30% in natural colds [102]. Corticosteroids do not provide clinically meaningful benefit in RV colds and may serve to increase viral replication [103]. Inhaled steroids, although used by many practitioners in treating bronchitis, have also not been proven to be beneficial [4]. Nonsteroidal anti-inflammatory agents variably benefit cold symptoms but certain ones (e.g., ibuprofen, naproxen) relieve discomfort and systemic symptoms [104]. These latter compounds do suppress cough. Both naproxen and ibuprofen have been shown in clinical trials to be active cough suppressants [4,105]. Expectorants have not been adequately studied in colds or viral bronchitis.

Antibiotics

Despite the frequent use of antibiotics during colds, no convincing evidence of benefit exists for their use. A recent meta-analysis [106] found that antibiotic treatment in over 1500 children did not affect the symptoms of common cold. A subset of about 20% of cold sufferers are colonized with pathogenic respiratory bacteria (*S. pneumoniae, H. influenzae, M. catarrhalis*) and may experience modest symptom benefit and lower rates of subsequent antibiotic use if treated with amoxicillin-clavulanate [107]. Noncolonized patients do not benefit, and gastrointestinal (GI) intolerance develops five-fold more often in amoxicillin-clavulanate recipients [107]. Determination of carriers of pathogenic bacteria is not practical in the office setting and of doubtful clinical value. Antibiotics should be withheld unless secondary bacterial infections are strongly suspected.

Alternative Therapies

A wide variety of alternative therapies have been tried over the past many years in attempts to alleviate the symptoms of the cold and bronchitis. Zinc lozenges have been subjected to numerous randomized clinical trials [37,108–110]. Although certain studies have shown modest effects in treating colds, the collective data from all studies show little benefit [37,108–110]. Even in those individual studies with positive results, undesirable side effects such as burning, tingling, bad taste, and nausea limit the utility of this treatment [109]. A zinc nasal gel has been studied in a single randomized clinical trial with highly positive results reported [111]. Study design flaws, including no standardized duration of therapy or monitoring of concomitant treatments, require confirmation of beneficial results with additional studies before this intervention can be recommended. Limited randomized clinical trials with echinacea have found no benefit [38]. Finally, high-dose vitamin C has been studied more than 20 times in randomized, controlled clinical trials for prevention and/or treatment of the common cold. When analyzed collectively, there is no apparent reduction in the incidence of colds when vitamin C is used prophylactically. However, the combined variables of duration and severity of the cold are improved by treatment with onset of cold symptoms. Among all studies, this reduction was of the order of magnitude of 23%, but in the largest and best controlled of the studies, it appears that duration and/or severity are reduced by up to 10% with vitamin C treatment [112].

Prevention

The only agent consistently shown to have prophylactic activity against RV infections is intranasal interferon [113]. Nonpharmacologic interventions effective in preventing these viral infections include the usual recommendations for careful handwashing and good hygiene.

REFERENCES

1. Rotbart HA, Hayden FG. Picornaviruses: a primer for the practitioner. Archives of Family Practice 2000; 9:913–920.
2. Gonzales R, Steiner JF, Sande MA. Antibiotic prescribing for adults with colds, upper respiratory tract infections, and bronchitis by ambulatory care physicians. JAMA 1998; 278:901–904.
3. Nyquist A-C, Gonzales R, Steiner JF, Sande MA. Antibiotic prescribing for children with colds, upper respiratory tract infections, and bronchitis. JAMA 1998; 279:875–877.
4. Gwaltney JM. Acute Bronchitis. In: Mandell GL, Bennett JE, Dolin R, eds. Principles and Practice of Infectious Diseases. 2000:703–710.
5. Makela MJ, Puhakka T, Ruuskanen O, et al. Viruses and bacteria in the etiology of the common cold. J Clin Microbiol 1998; 36:539–542.
6. Arruda E, Pitkaranta A, Witek TJ, et al. Frequency and natural history of rhinovirus infections in adults during autumn. J Clin Microbiol 1997; 35:2864–2868.
7. Harris JM, Gwaltney JM Jr. Incubation periods of experimental rhinovirus infection and illness. Clin Infect Dis 1996; 23:1287–1290.
8. Bardin PG, Johnston SL, Sanderson G, et al. Detection of rhinovirus infection of the nasal mucosa by oligonucleotide in situ hybridization. Am J Respir Cell Mol Biol 1994; 10:207–213.
9. Arruda E, Boyle TR, Winther B, Pevear DC, Gwaltney JM, Hayden FG. Localization of human rhinovirus replication in the upper respiratory tract by in situ hybridization. J Infect Dis 1995; 171:1329–1333.
10. Winther B. Effects on the nasal mucosa of upper respiratory viruses (common cold). Danish Med Bull 1994; 41:193–204.
11. Turner RB, Weingand K, Yeh CH, et al. Association between interleukin-8 (IL-8) and symptom severity in rhinovirus colds. Proceedings of the 36th Interscience Conference on Antimicrobial Agents and Chemotherapy. New Orleans, LA, 1996.
12. Igarashi Y, Skoner DP, Doyle WJ. Analysis of nasal secretions during experimental rhinovirus upper respiratory infections. J Allergy Clin Immunol 1993; 92:722–731.
13. Jacoby DB. Viral respiratory infection: a mechanism for the induction of airway inflammation and airway hyperreactivity. In: Shelhamer JH, moderator. Airway inflammation. Ann Intern Med 1995; 123:292–294.

14. Gern JE. Rhinovirus respiratory infections and asthma. Am J Med 2002; 112:19S–27S.
15. Gwaltney JM Jr, Rueckert RR. Rhinovirus, Chapter 43. In: Richman DD, Whitley RJ, Hayden FG, eds. Clinical Virology. New York, NY: Churchill Livingstone, 1997:1025–1047.
16. Arruda E, Pitkaranta A, Witek TJ, et al. Frequency and natural history of rhinovirus infections in adults during autumn. J Clin Microbiol 1997; 35: 2864–2868.
17. Heikkinen T, Thint M, Chonmaitree T. Prevalence of various respiratory viruses in the middle ear during acute otitis media. N Engl J Med 1999; 340: 260–264.
18. Arola M, Ruuskanen O, Ziegler T, et al. Clinical role of respiratory virus infection in acute otitis media. Pediatrics 1990; 86:848–855.
19. Pitkaranta A, Virolainen A, Jero J. Detection of rhinovirus respiratory syncytial virus and coronavirus infections in acute otitis media by reverse transcriptase polymerase chain reaction. Pediatrics 1998; 102:291–295.
20. Buchman CA, Doyle WJ, Skoner D, Fireman P, Gwaltney JM. Otologic manifestations of experimental rhinovirus infection. Laryngoscope 1994; 104:1295–1299.
21. Elkhatieb A, Hipskind G, Woerner D, Hayden FG. Middle ear abnormalities during natural rhinovirus colds in adults. J Infect Dis 1993; 168:618–621.
22. Patel JA, Reisner B, Vizirinia N, Owen M, Chonmaitree T, Howie V. Bacteriological failure of amoxicillin-clavulanate in treatment of acute otitis media caused by nontypeabale Haemophilus influenzae. J Pediatr 1995; 126: 799–806.
23. Gwaltney JM Jr, Phillips CD, Miller RD, Riker DK. Computed tomographic study of the common cold. N Engl J Med 1994; 330:25–30.
24. Pitkaranta A, Arruda E, Malmberg H, Hayden FG. Detection of rhinovirus in sinus brushings of patients with acute community-acquired sinusitis by reverse transcription-PCR. J Clin Microbiol 1997; 35:1791–1793.
25. Nicholson KG, Kent J, Ireland DC. Respiratory viruses and exacerbations of asthma in adults. BMJ 1993; 307:982–986.
26. Johnston SL, Pattemore PK, Sanderson G, Smith S, Lampe F, Josephs L. Community study of role of viral infections in exacerbations of asthma in 9-11 year old children. BMJ 1995; 310:1225–1229.
27. Johnston SL, Pattermore PK, Sanderson G, et al. The relationship between upper respiratory infections and hospital admissions for asthma: a time-trend analysis. Am J Respir Crit Care Med 1996; 154:654–660.
28. Murray CJ, Lopez AD. Evidence-based health policy—lessons from the global burden of disease study. Science 1996; 274:740–743.
29. Greenberg SB, et al. Respiratory viral infections in adults with and without chronic obstructive pulmonary disease. Am J Respir Crit Care Med 2000; 162: 167–173.
30. Collinson J, Nicholson KG, Gancio E, et al. Effects of upper respiratory tract infections in patients with cystic fibrosis. Thorax 1996; 51:1115–1122.

31. Nicholson KG, Kent J, Hammersley V, Gancio E. Risk factors for lower respiratory complications of rhinovirus infections in elderly people living in the community: prospective cohort study. BMJ 1996; 313:1119–1123.
32. Gwaltney JM Jr. Rhinoviruses. In: Evans, ed. Viral Infection of Humans. 1989:593.
33. Schmidt HJ, Fink RJ. Rhinovirus as a lower respiratory pathogen in infants. Pediatr Infect Dis J 1991; 10:700–702.
34. Chidekel AS, Bazzy AR, Rosen CL. Rhinovirus infection associated with severe lower respiratory tract illness and worsening lung disease in infants with bronchopulmonary dysplasia. Pediatr Pulm 1994; 18:261–263.
35. Gilbert LL, Dakharna A, Bone BM, Thomas EE, Hegele RG. Diagnosis of viral respiratory tract infections in children by using reverse transcription-PCR panel. J Clin Microbiol 1996; 34:140–143.
36. Hendley JO, Abbott RD, Beasley PB, Gwaltney JM Jr. Effect of inhalation of hot humidified air on experimental rhinovirus infection. JAMA 1994; 271: 1112–1113.
37. Mossad SB, Macknin ML, Medendorp SV, Mason P. Zinc gluconate lozenges for treating the common cold. A randomized, double-blind, placebo-controlled study. Ann Intern Med 1996; 125:81–88.
38. Grimm W, Muller H-H. A randomized controlled trial of the effect of fluid extract of Echinacea purpurea on the incidence and severity of colds and respiratory infections. Am J Med 1999; 106:138–143.
39. Capobianchi MR, Matteucci D, Glovannetti A, Soldaini E, Bendineiii M, Stanton JG, Dianzani F. Role of interferon in lethality and lymphoid atrophy induced by coxsackievirus S3 infection mice. Virol Immunol 1991; 5:103–110.
40. Geniteau-Legendre M, Forestier F, Quero AM, German A. Role of interferon, antibodies and macrophages in the protective effect of Corynebacterium parvum on encephalomyocarditis virus-induced disease in mice. Antiviral Res 1987; 7:161–167.
41. Kandolf R, Canu A, Hofschneider PH. Coxsackie B3 virus can replicate in cultured human foetal heart cells and is inhibited by interferon. J Mol Cell Cardiol 1985; 17:167–181.
42. Kishimoto C, Crumpacker CS, Abelmann WH. Prevention of murine Coxsackie B3 viral myocarditis and associated lymphoid organ atrophy with recombinant human leucocyte interferon alpha A/D. Cardiovasc Res 1988; 22: 732–738.
43. Langford MP, Barber JC, Sklar VE, Clark SW III. Patriarca PA, Onarato IM, Yin-Murphy M, Stanton GJ. Virus-specdic, early appearing neutralizing activity and interferon production in patients with acute hemorrhagic conjunctivitis. Curr Eye Res 1985; 4:233–239.
44. Langford MP, Kadi RM, Ganley JP, Yin-Murphy M. Inhibition of epidemic isolates of Coxsackie virus type A24 by recombinant and natural interferon alpha and interferon beta. Intervirology 1988; 29:320–327.
45. Lopez-Guerrero JA, Pimentel-Muinos FX, Fresno M, Alonso MA. Role of

soluble cytokines on the restricted replication of poliovirus in the monocylic U937 cell line. Virus Res 1990; 16:225–230.
46. Okada I, Matsumori A, Matoba Y, Tominaga M, Yamada T, Kowai C. Combination treatment with ribavirin and interferon for coxsackievirus B3 replication. J Lab Clin Med 1992; 120:569–573.
47. Sasaki O, Karaki T, Imanishi J. Protective effect of interferon on infections with hand, foot and mouth disease virus in newborn mice. J Infect Dis 1986; 153:498–502.
48. Chebath J, Benech P. Constituitive expression of (2′-5′) oligo A synthetase confers resistance to picornavirus infection. Nature 1987; 330:587–588.
49. Chonmaitree T, Baron S. Bacteria and viruses induce production of interferon in the cerebrospinal fluid of children with acute meningitis: a study of 57 cases and review. Rev Infect Dis 1991; 13:1061–1065.
50. Ichimura H, Shimase K, Tamura I, Kaneto E, Kurimura O, Aramftsu Y, Kurimura T. Neutralizing antibody and interferon-alpha in cerebrospinal fluids and sera of acute aseptic meningitis. J Med Virol 1985; 15:231–237.
51. Fleischmann WR Jr, Fleischmann CM, Fiers W. Potentialtion of interferon action by mixtures of recombinant DNA-derived human interferons. Antiviral Res 1984; 4:357–360.
52. Hayden F, Albrecht JK, Kaiser DL, Gwaltney JM. Prevention of natural colds by contact prophylaxis with intranasal alpha 2-interferon. N Engl J Med 1986; 314:71–75.
53. Hayden F, Gwaltney JM. Intranasal interferon alpha2 for prevention of rhinovirus infection and illness. J Infect Dis 1983; 148:543–550.
54. Merigan T, Reed S, Hall T, Tyrrell D. Inhibition of respiratory virus infection by locally applied interferon. Lancet 1973; 1:536–567.
55. Samo TC, Greenberg SB, Couch RB, Quarles J, Johnson PE, Hook S, Harmon MW. Efficacy and tolerance of intranasal applied recombinant leukocyte A interferon in normal volunteers. J Infect Dis 1983; 148:535–542.
56. Greenberg SB, Harmon MW, Couch RB, Johnson PE, Wilson SZ, Dacso CC, Bloom K, Quarles J. Prophylactic effect of low doses of human leukocyte interferon against infection with rhinovirus. J Infect Dis 1982; 145:542–546.
57. Douglas RM, Moore BW, Miles HB, Davies LM, Graham N, Ryan P, Worswick D, Albricht J. Prophylactic efficacy of intranasal alpha A2-interteron against rhinovirus infections in the family setting. N Engl J Med 1986; 314: 65–70.
58. Hayden F, Gwaltney JM. Intranasal interferon-α2 treatment of experimental rhinovirus colds. J Infect Dis 1984; 150:174–180.
59. Monto AS, Schwartz SA, Albrecht JK. Ineffectiveness of postexposure prophylaxis of rhinovirus infection with low-dose intranasal alpha 2b interferon in families. Antimicrob Agents Chemother 1989; 33:387–390.
60. Fox MP, McKinlay MA, Diana GD, Dutko FJ. Binding affinities of structurally related human rhinovirus capsid-binding compounds are related to their activities against human rhinovirus type 14. Antimicrob Agents Chemother 1991; 35:1040–1047.

61. Zhang A, Nanni RG, Arnold GF, Oren DA, Li T, Jacobo-Molkina A, William RL, Kamer G, Rubenstein DA, Li Y, Rozhon E, Cox S, Bumotempo P, O'Connell J, Schwartz J, Miller G, Nash C, Bauer B, Versace R, Ganguly A, Girijavallabhan V, Arnold E. Structure of a complex of human rhinovirus 14 with a water soluble antiviral compound SCH 38057. J Mol Biol 1991; 230:857–867.
62. Zhang A, Nanni RG, Oren DA, Rozhon EJ, Arnold E. Three-dimensional structure-activity relationships for antiviral agents that interact with picornavirus capsids. Semin Virol 1992; 3:453–471.
63. Heinz BA, Rueckert RR, Shepard DA, Dutko FJ, McKinlay MA, Fancher M, Rossmann MG, Badger J, Smith TJ. Genetic and molecular analysis of spontaneous mutants of human rhinovirus 14 that are resistant to an antiviral compound. J Virol 1989; 63:2476–2485.
64. Heinz BA. Escape mutant analysis of a drug-binding site can be used to map functions in the rhinovirus capsid. In: Laver WG, Air GA, eds. Use of X-Ray Crystallography in the Design of Antiviral Agents. San Diego, Calif.: Academic Press, Inc., 1990: 173–186.
65. Pevear DC, Fancher MJ, Felock PJ, Rossmann MG, Miller MS, Diana GD, Treasurywala AM, McKinlay MA, Dutko FJ. Conformational change in the floor of the human rhinovirus canyon blocks adsorption to HeLa Cell receptors. J Virol 1989; 63:2002–2007.
66. Rombaut B, Vrijsen R, Boeye A. Comparison of arildone and 3-methylquercetin as stabilizers of poliovirus. Antiviral Res Suppl 1985; 1:67–73.
67. Otto MJ, Fox MP, Fancher MJ, Huhrt MF, Diana GD, McKinlay MA. In vitro activity of WIN 5171 1, a new broad-spectrum antipicornavirus drug. Antimicrob Agents Chemother 1985; 27:883–886.
68. Pevear D. Antiviral therapy for picornavirus infections: pleconaril. Abstracts of the 15th Annual Clinical Virology Symposium, Clearwater, Fl., 1999.
69. Cox S, Bunotempo P, Wright-Minogue J, DeMartino, Skelton A, Ferrari E, Schwartz J, Rozhon E, Linn C, Girijavallabhan V, O'Connell JF. Antipicornavirus activity of SCH 47802 and analogues: in vitro and in vivo studies. Antiviral Res 1996; 32:71–79.
70. Al-Nakib W, Higgins PG, Barrow GI, Tyrrell DAJ, Andries K, Bussche GV, Taylor N, Janssen PAJ. Suppression of colds in human volunteers challenged with rhinovirus by a new synthetic drug (R61837). Antimicrob Agents Chemother 1989; 33:522–525.
71. Barrow GI, Higgins PG, Tyrrell DAJ, Andries K. An appraisal of the efficacy of the antiviral R 61837 in rhinovirus infections in human volunteers. Antiviral Chem Chemother 1990; 5:278–283.
72. Hayden FG, Andries A, Janssen PAJ. Safety and efficacy of Intranasal pirodavir (R77975) in experimental rhinovirus infection. Antimicrob Agents Chemother 1992; 36:727–732.
73. McKinlay MA, Frank JA, Steinberg BA. Use of WIN 51711 to prevent echovirus type 9- induced paralysis in suckling mice. J Infect Dis 1986; 154:676–681.

74. McKinlay MA, Steinberg BA. Oral efficacy of WIN 51711 in mice infected with human poliovirus. Antimicrob Agents Chemother 1986; 29:30–32.
75. Woods MG, Diana GD, Rogge MC, Otto MJ, Dutko FJ, McKinlay MA. In vitro and in vivo activities of WIN 54954, a new broad-spectrum antipicornavirus drug. Antimicrob Agents Chemother 1989; 33:2069–2074.
76. Turner RB, Dutko FJ, Goldstein NH, Lockwood G, Hayden FG. Efficacy of oral WIN 54954 for prophylaxis of experimental rhinovirus infection. Antimicrob Agents Chemother 1993; 37:297–300.
77. Schiff GM, Sherwood JR, Young EC, Mason LJ. Prophylactic efficacy of WIN 54954 in prevention of experimental human coxsackievirus A21 infection and illness. Antiviral Res 1992; 17(suppl):92.
78. Pevear DC, Tull TM, Seipel ME, Groarke JM. Activity of pleconaril against enteroviruses. Antimicrob Agents Chemother 1999; 43:2109–2115.
79. Kearns GL, Bradley JS, Jacobs RF, et al. Pleconaril pharmocokinetics in neonates. Abstracts of the 36th annual Infectious Diseases Society of America meeting, Denver, CO, 1998. Abstract 750.
80. Kearns GL, Abdel-Rahman SM, James LP, et al. Single-dose pharmacokinetics of a pleconaril oral solution in children and adolescents. Antimicrob Agents Chemother 1999; 43:634–638.
81. Abdel-Rahman SM, Kearns GL. Single oral dose escalation pharmacokinetics of pleconaril capsules in adults. J Clin Pharmacol 1999; 39:613–618.
82. Schiff GM, McKinlay MA, Sherwood JR. Oral efficacy of VP63843 in coxsackievirus A21 infected volunteers. Abstracts of the 36th Interscience Conference on Antimicrobial Agents and Chemotherapy, New Orleans, LA, 1996. Abstract H-43.
83. Hayden FG, Hassmann HA, Coats T, et al. Pleconaril treatment shortens duration of picornavirus respiratory illness in adults. Abstracts of the 39th Interscience Conference on Antimicrobial Agents and Chemotherapy, San Francisco, CA, 1999. Abstract.
84. Hayden FG, Kim K, Hudson S. Pleconaril treatment reduces duration and severity of viral respiratory infection (common cold) due to picornaviruses. Abstracts of the 41st Interscience Conference on Antimicrobial Agents and Chemotherapy, Chicago, IL, 2001. Abstract.
85. Rotbart HA, Liu S. Pleconaril safety—cumulative study data for a novel antiviral compound. Abstracts of the 39th Annual Meeting of the Infectious Diseases Society of America, San Francisco, CA, 2001. Abstract.
86. DeLong DC, Nelson JD, Wu E, Warren B, Wikel J, Templeton RJ, Dinner A. Virus inhibition studies with AR -36 III. Relative activity of syn and anti isomers, abstr. 34 In Program and abstracts of the 18th Interscience Conference on Antimicrobial Agents and Chemotherapy. American Society for Microbiology, Washington, DC, 1978a.
87. DeLong DC, Nelson JD, Wu CYE, Warren B, Wikel J, Chamberlin J, Montgomery D, Paget CJ. Virus inhibition studies with AR-336. 1. Tissue culture activity, abstr. S-128, p. 234. In Abstracts of the 78th Annual Meeting of the American Society for Microbiology 1978. American Society for Microbiology, Washington, DC, 1978b.

88. Wikel JH, Paget CJ, DeLong DC, Nelson JD, Wu CYE, Paschal JW, Dinner A, Templeton RJ, Chaney MO, Jones ND, Chamberlin JW. Synthesis of syn and anti isomers of 6-[(hydroxyimino)phenAmethA[-l-[(l-methyieth@l)sulfonyi]-i H-benzimidazol-2-amine. Inhibitors of rhinovirus multiplication. J Mod Chem 1980; 23:368–372.
89. Heinz BA, Vance LM. The antiviral compound enviroxime targets the 3A coding region of rhinovirus and poliovirus. J Virol 1995; 69:4189–4197.
90. Tebbe MJ, Spitzer WA, Tang J. Oral bioavailability screening of the antirhinoviral vinyl acetylene benzimidazoles. Abstracts of the 10th International Conference on Antiviral Research, Atlanta, GA, 1997:A89.
91. Tebbe MJ, Spitzer WA, Victor S, et al. Antirhinoviral vinyl acetylene benzimidazoles. Abstracts of the 10th International Conference on Antiviral Research, Atlanta, GA, 1997:A75.
92. Philipotts RJ, Wallace J, Tyrrell DAJ, Tagart VB. Therapeutic activity of onviroxime against rhinovirus infection in volunteers. Antimicrob Agents Chemother 1983; 23:671–675.
93. Philipotts RJ, DeLong DC, Wallace J, Jones RW, Reed SE, Tyrrell DAJ. The activity of enviroxime against rhinovirus infection in man. Lancet 1981; 2:1342–1344.
94. Hayden FG, Gwaltney JM Jr. Prophyiactic activity of intranasal enviroxime against experimentally induced rhinovirus type 39 infection. Antimicrob Agents Chemother 1982; 21:892–897.
95. Miller FD, Monto AS, DeLong DC, Exelby A, Bryan ER, Srivastava S. Controlled trail of enviroxime against natural rhinovirus infections in a community. Antimicrob Agents Chemother 1985; 27:102–106.
96. Turner R, Wecker Mt, Pohl G, et al. Efficacy of tremacamra, a soluble intercellular adhesion molecule 1, for experimental rhinovirus infection; a randomized clinical trial. JAMA 1999; 281:1797–1804.
97. Patick AK, Ford C, Binford S, et al. Evaluation of the antiviral activity and cytotoxicfty of peptide inhibitors of human rhinovirus 3C protease, a novel target for antiviral intervention. Abstracts of the 10th International Conference on Antiviral Research, Atlanta, GA, 1997:A75.
98. Luks D, Anderson MR. Antihistamines and the common cold. A review and critique of the literature. J Gen Intern Med 1996; 11:240–244.
99. Gwaltney JM Jr, Park J, Paul RA, Edelman DA, O'Connor RR, Turner RB. Randomized controlled trial of clemastine fumarate for treatment of experimental rhinovirus colds. Clin Infect Dis 1996; 22:656–662.
100. Turner RB, Sperber SJ, Sorrentino JV, et al. Effectiveness of clemastine fumarate for treatment of rhinorrhea and sneezing associated with the common cold. Clin Infect Dis. In press.
101. Berkowitz RB, Tinkelman DG. Evaluation of oral terfenadine for treatment of the common cold. Am Rev Respir Dis 1987; 136:556–560.
102. Hayden FG, Diamond L, Wood PB, Korts DC, Wecker MT. Effectiveness and safety of intranasal ipratropium bromide in common colds. A randomized, double-blind, placebo-controlled trial. Ann Intern Med 1996; 125:89–97.
103. Gustafson LM, Proud D, Hendley O, Hayden FG, Gwaltney JM. Oral pred-

nisone therapy in experimental rhinovirus infections. J Allergy Clin Immunol 1996; 97:1009–1114.
104. Sperber SJ, Hendley JO, Hayden FG, Riker DK, Sorrentino JV, Gwaltney JM Jr. Effects of naproxen on experimental rhinovirus colds. A randomized, double-blind, controlled trial. Ann Intern Med 1992; 117:37–41.
105. Gwaltney J. clinical and mechanistic perspectives on acute self-limited cough. Symposium Report from the World Congress of Pharmacy and Pharmaceutical Sciences. Int Pharm J 1997; 11:5–7.
106. Gadomski AM. Potential interventions for preventing pneumonia among young children: lack of effect of antibiotic treatment for upper respiratory infections. Pediatr Infect Dis J 1993; 12:115–120.
107. Kaiser L, Lew D, Hirschel B, et al. Effects of antibiotic treatment of the subset of common-cold patients who have bacteria in nasopharyngeal secretions. Lancet 1996; 347:1507–1510.
108. Jackson JL, Lesho E, Peterson C. Zinc and the common cold: a meta-analysis revisited. J Nutr 2000; 130(suppl 5S):1512S–1515S.
109. Marshall S. Zinc gluconate and the common cold. Review of randomized controlled trials. Can Fam Physician 1998; 44:1037–1042.
110. Macknin ML, Piedmonte M, Calendine C, Janosky J, Wald E. Zinc gluconate lozenges for treating the common cold in children: a randomized controlled trial. JAMA 1998; 279:1962–1967.
111. Hirt M, Nobel S, Barron E. Zinc nasal gel for the treatment of common cold symptoms; a double-blind, placebo-controlled trial. ENT Journal 2000; 79: 778–782.
112. Hemila H. Does Vitamin C alleviate the symptoms of the common cold—a review of current evidence. Scand J Infect Dis 1994; 26:1–6.
113. Arruda E, Hayden FG. Clinical studies of antiviral agents for picornaviral infections. In: Jeffries DJ, DeCierrq E, eds. Antiviral Chemotherapy. John Wiley & Sons Ltd, 1995.

17

Treatment of Influenza-Related Respiratory Tract Infections

Ann L. N. Chapman
Royal Hallamshire Hospital
Sheffield, England

Martin J. Wood[†]
Heartlands Hospital
Birmingham, England

INTRODUCTION

Influenza is one of the most widespread infectious diseases throughout the world, infecting many millions of people annually. It is of major importance for two reasons: first, its potential to cause massive-scale pandemics with significant mortality and major economic sequelae; and second, its preponderance in causing severe viral and secondary bacterial pneumonia, particularly in the elderly, the chronically infirm, and the immunosuppressed. Although vaccination is effective in preventing many cases of influenza in healthy and high-risk individuals, cases still occur due to incomplete coverage, poor vaccine-induced immunity in some groups, and variant viral strains

[†] Deceased.

not covered by the vaccine. Antiviral treatment for acute influenza has been available since the 1960s, but it is only in the past few years, with the development of the neuraminidase inhibitors, that specific treatment has been considered on a wide scale. In this chapter, we review the current state of knowledge and recommendations for the use of antiviral drugs for acute influenza, in particular for the respiratory complications.

VIROLOGICAL AND CLINICAL ASPECTS

The Virus

Influenza viruses are members of the orthomyxoviridae family. They are 100 nm diameter, spherical or rod-shaped, enveloped, single-stranded RNA (antisense) viruses, with three major subtypes: A, B, and C. Types A and B cause most clinically relevant disease. The virus encodes a number of proteins, including the neuraminidase and hemagglutinin glycoproteins embedded in the envelope; the matrix M1 protein, which forms a layer surrounding the viral nucleocapsid; nucleoproteins that associate closely with viral RNA; and several proteins involved in RNA transcription and processing. Influenza A also contains a further envelope protein, M2, which is not found in influenza B and C subtypes [1].

In addition to the A, B, and C subtypes, influenza viruses are classified further on the basis of the type of hemagglutinin (H) and neuraminidase (N) glycoproteins present. To date, there are 15 and 9 of these, respectively, and these two proteins are important targets for both antibody and cell-mediated immunity. Hemagglutinin is a highly variable glycopeptide that is involved in viral attachment and fusion with cells in the respiratory tract by binding to sialic acid–containing receptors on the cell surface. The neuraminidase is an enzyme that aids the release of newly formed virus from the surface of infected cells. It does this by cleaving terminal sialic acid residues from glycoproteins in the cell membrane. Because the hemagglutinin molecule itself contains sialic acid residues, the neuraminidase enzyme also cleaves these, preventing viral clumping and aiding dissemination. Furthermore, neuraminidase also inhibits virus binding to mucoprotein-rich respiratory secretions, allowing the virus to penetrate through the secretions to the surface of neighboring cells and to be transmitted to other individuals.

Emerging viral strains are classified not only on the basis of their core proteins (into A, B, and C subtypes) but also according to their geographic and species origin, year of isolation, and which hemagglutinin and neuraminidase types they possess. Currently there are two major strains of influenza A circulating: H1N1 and H3N2. The outbreak of avian-associated influenza in

1997 in Hong Kong was associated with an H5N1 strain, which did not disseminate widely [2].

Pandemics occur as a result of a process known as antigenic shift, in which a new viral strain emerges with a completely different hemagglutinin or neuraminidase type to circulating viruses [3]. This may arise due to recombination of avian and human viruses in an "intermediate" host—for example, a pig—resulting in a recombinant virus radically different from the prevailing strains, to which there is little or no human herd immunity. However, in the recent Hong Kong outbreak, it is thought that a viral strain found in domestic birds was able to transfer directly to humans without an intermediate species; this pattern of transmission may lead to explosive outbreaks and pandemics with little warning and is of major concern for the future. Both influenza A and B have the potential to cause epidemics and pandemics, although B viruses tend to be more genetically stable and result in less severe outbreaks due to higher levels of herd immunity.

In addition to this dramatic antigenic shift, a more gradual process of antigenic drift occurs constantly and results in the emergence of new viral strains every few years that resemble their "parent" strains to a varying extent—the degree of homology influences the level of herd immunity and thus clinical impact. Careful surveillance of such viral changes allows an approximate prediction to be made regarding which viral strains are likely to predominate during the coming year, enabling vaccination for at-risk groups [4].

Epidemiology

During most winters, an outbreak of influenza infection, lasting a few weeks, spreads rapidly throughout the population. The outbreaks vary in intensity but in an average year influenza is estimated to be responsible for from 18 to 20 million respiratory illnesses in the United States: 13.8 to 16.0 million of these are in individuals younger than 20 years and 4.1 to 4.5 million in persons 20 years of age or older [5]. In addition, complications of acute influenza are common, with 150,000 hospitalizations and 10–40,000 deaths yearly in the United States [6,7]. Most morbidity is seen in the largest proportion of the population (i.e., schoolchildren and healthy adults). The highest rates of morbidity and mortality, however, occur in persons over 65 years of age. In the United States alone, influenza virus infection results annually in 25 million visits to physicians and millions of days of work lost and costs the nation an estimated 12 billion [8,9].

As mentioned above, influenza viruses have the potential to cause massive pandemics, affecting up to 50% of the community with major associated morbidity and mortality [10,11] as a result of a genetic shift. There were three major pandemics in the twentieth century: the 1918 "Spanish flu" killed an estimated 20 million people worldwide and the pandemics of 1957 and 1968 each led to more than 100,000 deaths in the United States alone [12]. The recent outbreak of an H5N1 avian influenza virus A in Hong Kong [2] should serve as a warning that a further pandemic (probably in the near future) is inevitable and must be planned for [13,14].

Viral Pathogenesis

Influenza virus is predominantly spread via inhalation of small particle aerosols (<10 μm diameter) produced by sneezing, coughing, or even talking. It is highly transmissible, with an attack rate of up to 50% in epidemics, and stable for prolonged periods at a range of temperatures and humidities. The virus replicates only in the epithelial cells of the upper and lower respiratory tract. Cell death occurs as a result of necrosis and also, it is thought, apoptosis, with release of virions and infection of neighboring epithelial cells. Thus infection tends to spread along epithelial surfaces rather than occurring at discrete sites. Histologically, the respiratory epithelium shows edema, hyperemia, and superficial ulceration. As the infection spreads distally, the histological changes become more severe, with necrotizing tracheobronchitis, ulceration, and sloughing of the mucosa, and a hemorrhagic pneumonia with hyaline membrane formation. Secondary bacterial pneumonia may occur, with a neutrophilic infiltrate.

Clinical Features

Influenza is an acute respiratory tract infection affecting all ages. In its typical form, occurring in adolescents and young adults, it generally presents after a short incubation period of 1 to 3 days, with abrupt onset of fever (usually above 38°C) and chills, headache, dry cough, myalgia, and prostration. The patient may have sore throat, sneezing, and nasal discharge, but local symptoms tend to be less marked than systemic ones. Children seem more prone to having gastrointestinal symptoms, such as vomiting and abdominal pain, in addition. A typical case is associated with 5 to 6 days of limited activity, 3 to 4 days of bed rest, and about 3 days of lost school or work [15]. Convalescence occurs over the ensuing 1 to 2 weeks, although some individuals may experience prolonged cough and wheeze due to increased bronchial reactivity. Influenza A and B subtypes tend to produce similar illnesses, whereas type C results in a milder infection with fewer systemic symptoms and complications. Many infections with any of the viral strains are asymptomatic.

In the very young and very old this typical picture may not be seen. In the elderly, there may be fever and confusion without symptoms or signs localizing infection to the respiratory tract and presenting a diagnostic challenge. Some patients may present with deterioration in their chronic pulmonary disease or congestive cardiac failure. Infants may also develop fever, vomiting, and convulsions without localizing features, or may show clinical evidence of respiratory tract involvement with laryngotracheobronchitis or pneumonia. Although most infections occur in school-age children and young adults, it is the very young and very old who are most at risk of developing severe influenza and its complications [16–18]. These are more likely in the presence of chronic ill health: in young children, predisposing conditions include congenital heart disease, cystic fibrosis, asthma, sickle cell disease and neoplasm; in the older age group, chronic cardiovascular, respiratory and renal disease, diabetes mellitus, and immunosuppression increase the risk of complications and death.

Influenza pneumonia occurs uncommonly and mainly in the context of major influenza A epidemics. In the 1918–1919 pandemic, primary viral pneumonia was a major cause of death in young adults, particularly pregnant women. Subsequent work has shown that pregnancy is an independent risk factor for severe or complicated infection, the risk increasing as pregnancy progresses [19]. The illness starts with a typical pattern but progresses rapidly to fever, cough, dyspnea and hypoxia. The chest radiograph may show an interstitial pattern of shadowing, and examination of sputum yields no bacteria (initially) on microscopy or culture, but a positive viral culture. Influenza pneumonia has a high mortality and survivors may develop residual diffuse pulmonary fibrosis.

The more frequent respiratory complications of influenza, particularly in the elderly and in patients with a predisposing factor, are secondary bacterial pneumonia and bronchitis [20]. Such patients may have a typical pattern of infection, initially appearing to improve over a period of 1 to 2 weeks, but then become more unwell, with fever and productive cough. Secondary bacterial pneumonias are the major cause of death in nonpandemic influenza and are thought to occur because of local changes in the respiratory mucosa: impaired mucociliary clearance of secretions, increased amounts of extravascated tissue fluid providing a rich growth medium for bacteria, and altered adherence of bacteria to the respiratory epithelium. Local pro-inflammatory cytokines such as interleukins 6 and 8 and tumor necrosis factor–α may also play a role [21]. *Streptococcus pneumoniae* and *Haemophilus influenzae* are the main associated pathogens; the widespread introduction of pneumococcal vaccination for individuals with chronic ill health or immunosuppression may paradoxically reduce influenza mortality. *Staphylococcus aureus* pneumonia is less common but carries a high mortality.

In children, otitis media is a common complication [22]. Less common complications of influenza include encephalopathy and encephalitis, Reye's syndrome, Guillain-Barré syndrome, and myocarditis.

ANTIVIRAL AGENTS

There are four licensed anti-influenza agents available in the United States and Europe.

Adamantanes

Amantadine and rimantadine are drugs known as adamantanes that were recognized in the 1960s as having activity at concentrations below 1μg/mL against influenza A but not influenza B viruses [23]. During the initial stages of replication of influenza A viruses, the M1 protein needs to be dissociated from the ribonucleoprotein complexes before the latter can enter the cell nucleus and commence replication. This requires an acid milieu, and the M2 protein, which spans the viral membrane, acts as an ion channel through which hydrogen ions reach the center of the viral particle and facilitate the M1 protein/ribonucleoprotein dissociation [24]. Amantadine and rimantadine act by binding to the M2 ion channel and blocking its function, thus indirectly preventing the initiation of viral replication [25].

Amantadine was approved for chemoprophylaxis of influenza A in 1966 and in 1976 for treatment of influenza A virus infections in persons older than 1 year. Rimantadine was approved in the United States in 1993 for treatment and chemoprophylaxis of influenza A in adults but only for prophylaxis among children (Table 1). Both agents are almost completely absorbed after oral dosing, amantadine about twice as rapidly than rimantadine, and both are excreted in urine. The half-life of amantadine is about 15 hr in younger adults but twice as long in elderly individuals. Rimantadine has a half-life that is about 30 hr in all age groups [26]. Both amantadine and rimantadine are effective in reducing the intensity and duration of symptoms of influenza A if started within 2 days of onset of symptoms [27,28]. They appear to have similar efficacy, in general reducing the duration of illness by one day [29]. By preventing viral replication, they also reduce the amount of free virus in respiratory secretions and may therefore be of benefit in reducing transmission in an epidemic situation.

Amantadine and rimantadine are administered orally once or twice daily. The daily dose of either drug is 200 mg (100 mg in the elderly or those with renal impairment and 5 mg/kg body weight, to a maximum of 150 mg, in children from 1 to 9 years of age). The most prominent side effects of aman-

TABLE 1 Antiviral Agents for Influenza

Drug	Route	Age range approved for treatment/prophylaxis	Dose—adults[a]	Dose—children[a]	Side effects
Amantadine	Oral (tablets or syrup)	Treatment ≥ 1 year	100 mg twice daily[b]	<40 kg 5 mg/kg (to max 150 mg daily) >40 kg 100 mg twice daily (treatment and prophylaxis)	Confusion, anxiety, impaired concentration, seizures, nightmares, hallucinations; nausea and vomiting
		Prophylaxis ≥ 1 year	100 mg twice daily[b]		
Rimantadine	Oral (tablets or syrup)	Treatment ≥ 18 years	100 mg twice daily[b]	N/A	Nausea and vomiting, diarrhea
		Prophylaxis ≥ 1 year	100 mg twice daily[b]	As amantadine	
Zanamivir	Inhalation	Treatment ≥ 7 years	10 mg twice daily	N/A	Bronchospasm (uncommon)
		Prophylaxis not approved	N/A	N/A	
Oseltamivir	Oral (capsules or powder for oral suspension)	Treatment ≥ 1 year	75 mg twice daily[c]	See package insert	Nausea and vomiting
		Prophylaxis ≥ 13 years	75 mg once daily	N/A	

[a] Duration of treatment usually 5 days; prophylaxis for 7 days or until end of outbreak.
N/A not approved.
[b] Reduce dose to 100 mg daily in elderly patients and patients with renal impairment.
[c] Reduce dose for patients with serum creatinine clearance of <30 mL/min.

tadine are neuropsychological, since this agent promotes release of catecholamines [30]. Symptoms include anxiety, impaired concentration, depression, and insomnia; these occur in 10–20% of patients, probably more commonly in the elderly [31,32]. Side effects are related to the serum concentration and where levels are high—for example, in individuals with renal impairment—include hallucinations or seizures. Even with normal therapeutic serum levels, amantadine may induce fits in those with a predisposition, and thus the drug is contraindicated in patients with epilepsy. Rimantadine does not induce catecholamine release in the same way, and side effects are much less common and usually gastrointestinal in nature [33]. Rimantadine is the drug of choice when available because of its improved side-effect profile.

The main concern with these agents is the rapid development of resistance during a course of therapy. This occurs in between one-quarter and one-third of individuals taking either of these agents. The molecular basis of resistance is a point mutation at residue 26, 27, 30, 31, or 34 in the gene encoding the M2 protein, and development of resistance to one agent confers resistance to the other in this group [34]. The resistant strains can be transmitted to other persons and illnesses caused by resistant strains are indistinguishable from those caused by amantadine-susceptible strains[35–37]. Resistant virus may become the predominant viral type in an outbreak or epidemic, and may limit use of this group of antiviral agents for treatment or prevention of new infections [38]. However, although resistance emerges rapidly during treatment, natural resistance is uncommon and long-term resistance is unlikely because of the emergence of new drug-sensitive strains every few years by antigenic drift [39].

Neuraminidase Inhibitors

The neuraminidase enzyme is essential for the replication of influenza A and B viruses (see above). Studies have now shown that although most of the protein varies between strains, the amino acid residues that line the active site and interact with the sialic acid substrate are highly conserved in all strains that have been studied [40,41]. This finding suggested that competitive inhibitors that mimicked sialic acid might inhibit neuraminidase and hence have activity against a wide range of strains of influenza A and B [42]. To date, two such agents have been developed: zanamivir and oseltamivir. Both are analogues of N-acetylneuraminic acid, the cell-surface receptor for influenza viruses and potently inhibit influenza virus neuraminidase activity at low nanomolar concentrations [43].

Resistance to the neuraminidase inhibitors may develop either as a result of mutations altering the binding of the drug to the neuraminidase enzyme or due to a reduction in the affinity of the hemagglutinin-receptor binding so that there is less need for neuraminidase activity to enable virus to be released from infected cells [44]. Resistant strains appear only after several days of treatment; their emergence does not alter the time course of the illness. Studies in animals have suggested that resistant strains are less virulent [44].

Zanamivir

The first analogue of N-acetylneuraminic acid to be developed in 1969 was 2-deoxy-3,3-dihydro-*N*-acetyl neuraminic acid (also known as Neu5Acen), but this was found to be insufficiently specific for viral neuraminidase. Once the crystal structure of the viral enzyme was determined [40], then the affinity of compounds for the active site could be enhanced and this led to 4-guanido Neu5Acen (GG167 or zanamivir) [45,46].

Zanamivir is licensed for the treatment of influenza A and B infections in adults and adolescents of 12 years and older (Table 1). It has low oral bioavailability and needs to be administered by inhalation through the mouth or nose. In volunteers, scintigraphic studies have demonstrated that nearly 80% of a dose of zanamivir inhaled through the mouth is deposited in the oropharynx, and that only 15% or so reaches the tracheobronchial and pulmonary sites of viral replication [47]. About 10–20% of the inhaled dose is absorbed and then excreted unchanged in the urine [48].

The clinical efficacy of zanamivir given by intranasal administration was initially demonstrated in experimental influenza A (H1N1) infection of volunteers [49]. When given before experimental infection, zanamivir dosages of 3.6–16 mg, given two to six times daily, prevented 82% of labora-tory-proven infection and 95% of febrile illnesses, compared with placebo ($P < 0.001$). Early treatment of experimental infection reduced peak viral titers, duration of viral shedding, and the duration of illness compared with placebo [49].

Clinical studies of zanamivir have shown that inhaled zanamivir (10 mg twice daily for 5 days), given with or without concomitant intranasal zanamivir within 48 hours of natural influenza A or B infection, significantly shortens the duration of symptoms compared with placebo, on average by 1 to 1½ days [50,51]. Complications and antibiotic use for secondary bacterial infections were also reduced in previously healthy individuals [52] and this effect is also likely to occur in high-risk patients [51], although the number of such patients studied to date has been too small to give conclusive information.

No significant differences in side effects between placebo and zanamivir were reported in these trials. However, zanamivir can cause bronchospasm and airflow reduction and hence may need to be used with caution in patients with chronic respiratory disease: in one study of 11 patients with mild to moderate asthma, however, there was no reduction in pulmonary function or airway hyperreactivity to methacholine [53]. Despite this, the manufacturers recommend that patients on maintenance bronchodilator therapy use their brochodilator before taking zanamivir.

Zanamivir in a dose of 10 mg once daily was 30% effective in the prevention of infection and 67% effective in prevention of illness when given before exposure during a community epidemic [54]. In a family study, when zanamivir was given to family members 5 years of age or older who had been exposed to an index case, new cases were prevented in 79% of persons [55].

Resistance mutations were not detected in the trials of zanamivir but mutations in both the hemagglutinin and neuraminidase genes occurred in an immunocompromised patient treated with zanamivir for 2 weeks for an influenza B infection [56].

Oseltamivir

Incorporation of a carbocyclic structure into the neuraminidase inhibitor molecule improved the stability and activity of the compounds and led to the development of Ro640802 (oseltamivir carboxylate) [57]. Oseltamivir carboxylate is another potent and specific influenza neuraminidase inhibitor [43]. It is licensed for treatment of influenza A and B infections in individuals of 1 year and older, and for prophylaxis of patients of 13 years and older (Table 1). Although oseltamivir carboxylate is more lipophilic than zanamivir, its oral bioavailability is similarly low [58] and so an ethyl ester prodrug was developed. This compound, after oral administration as a capsule or liquid and gastrointestinal absorption, undergoes rapid enzymatic conversion on passage through the liver, resulting in an estimated 75% of the dose entering the systemic circulation [58]. After administration of oral oseltamivir, the area under the plasma concentration versus time curve (AUC) increases proportionately with dose over the range 20 mg to 1 g. Peak plasma concentrations are achieved between 2.5 hr and 6 hr after administration and the terminal plasma elimination half-life is between 6.8 hr and 9.3 hr. Oseltamivir is systemically distributed and maintains therapeutic concentrations in lung tissue at 24 hr post-dose: the elimination half-life in bronchoalveolar lavage fluid is fourfold longer than in plasma [59]. There is little penetration into the central nervous system. The pharmacokinetics (both absorption and elimination) of oseltamivir are similar in young and in healthy elderly volunteers. Reductions in the dose are recommended for individuals with a creatinine clearance of less than 30 mL/min.

As for zanamivir, the antiviral activity, clinical efficacy, and tolerability of oseltamivir have been evaluated in double-blind, placebo-controlled studies of experimental influenza A (H1N1) infection. In one such study, oseltamivir was assessed for both treatment and prevention of experimentally induced influenza [60]. In the treatment study, various dosages (20, 100, or 200 mg twice daily or 200 mg once daily for 5 days) of oral oseltamivir were initiated 28 hr after experimental infection. All dosages significantly reduced the titre and duration of virus shedding in nasal washes and significantly reduced the severity and duration of clinical symptoms. In naturally acquired infection, oseltamivir reduced duration of illness by 1 to 1½ days [61,62], with a suggestion that secondary complications such as bronchitis and sinusitis were also reduced [61].

Oseltamivir is associated with nausea and vomiting in about 10% of those treated but the incidence of gastrointestinal side effects is reduced (without altering the pharmacokinetics) by taking the drug with food.

Oseltamivir, in a dose of 75 mg once daily, was 50% effective in the prevention of influenza and 84% effective in the prevention of illness when given as prophylaxis during a community epidemic [63]. In the family setting, the same dose of oseltamivir prevented influenza in 89% of families when it was given to exposed family members 12 years of age or older [64].

Mutations in the neuraminidase gene resulting in resistance to oseltamivir were detected in about 1.5% (higher in children) of individuals treated with oseltamivir [26].

USE OF ANTIVIRAL AGENTS FOR TREATMENT OF INFLUENZA

When to Use

The pathogenesis of influenza, with virus replication present for 24–48 hr before symptom onset and reaching a peak within 48 hr, suggests that antiviral treatment would work best if taken early after the onset of symptoms. Studies of antiviral treatment of influenza to date have excluded patients presenting with symptoms for more than 48 hours because of this theoretical consideration, and at present zanamivir and oseltamivir are approved for the treatment of influenza only in patients who have been symptomatic for less than 48 hr. Some studies have shown added benefit for patients starting treatment within a shorter time; for example, Hayden and colleagues demonstrated that patients who received treatment with zanamivir within 30 hr of symptom onset recovered 2 days more quickly than patients receiving placebo [50]. Thus, antiviral therapy where recommended should be instituted as soon as possible. The exception to this is the patient with immunocompromise: such patients have increased and prolonged viral replication and it would seem appropriate to give antiviral therapy after a longer symptomatic period. There is no evidence that treatment courses of greater than 5 days are of any added benefit, and since the risk of drug resistance increases with time, treatment should not exceed this duration, except in the setting of immunocompromise where longer treatment courses have been used.

Choice of Antiviral Agent

Of the four agents currently available for the treatment of influenza, the neuraminidase inhibitors have the advantages of activity against both A and B influenza viruses, good tolerability, and favorable resistance profile. They are, however, more expensive than the adamantanes and there may be a role for amantadine or rimantadine in specific settings; for example, in an influenza A outbreak in a residential care facility, or where resistance to the neuramindase inhibitors is present. Rimantadine is preferred to amantadine because of the high incidence of neuropsychological side effects with amantadine but is currently not licensed in the United Kingdom. Oseltamivir is likely to be easier to administer than zanamivir in an elderly or pediatric population. There have, however, been no direct comparisons of these agents as regards efficacy and tolerability; such a study will be important for formulation of guidelines concerning influenza treatment.

Patient Groups

In previously fit individuals, influenza causes significant morbidity at an individual level, as well as significant economic impact in terms of lost productivity. Treatment with antiviral agents generally reduces the period of illness by one day and expedites return to usual activities. Several studies have attempted to analyze the cost-effectiveness of antiviral treatment in previously healthy individuals, offsetting the personal and economic impact of illness due to influenza against the cost of drugs and health-care services required for their administration [65–69]. Their conclusions have been conflicting, and antiviral agents for influenza in previously healthy adults are currently not recommended except in circumstances where there would be exceptional benefit from an earlier return to usual activities [26].

In the high risk patient, however, influenza is more likely to be severe and complicated and preliminary evidence suggests that early antiviral therapy has a significant impact on duration of illness and complication rate [51]. Assuming this to be the case, cost-benefit analysis of the use of antiviral treatment in high-risk patients demonstrates a benefit, particularly if treatment reduces the rate of hospitalization [70,71]. Antiviral treatment for high-risk patients with illness due to influenza is recommended both in the United States and Britain, although again no recommendations can be made regarding choice of agent because of the lack of comparative studies [72,73]. Treatment should be given regardless of prior vaccination status.

To date there is little experience of the use of antiviral drugs for influenza in patients with impaired immunity. Patients immunocompromised following bone marrow or solid organ transplantation, or because of chemotherapy or steroid use, are at increased risk of severe infection and it is not yet clear whether such patients should receive a prolonged course of antiviral therapy, with the associated risk of resistance [74]. Zanamivir was effective and well tolerated in one small observational study of seven children with influenza virus infection following stem cell transplantation; patients were treated with zanamivir until virus could no longer be isolated from nasopharyngeal secretions, the median duration being 15 days (range 5–44) [75]. HIV-infected individuals may be at risk of more severe influenza if significantly immunosuppressed, and antiviral treatment for influenza is probably indicated for those with a CD4 count of less than 200 cells/μL [76]. No interactions with antiretroviral medications have been described.

Method of Diagnosis

None of the anti-influenza drugs have any useful efficacy against other respiratory viruses, and their use should be based on proof or strong possibility of influenza. Viral culture or serological diagnosis, although of use for surveillance and epidemiological study, are not sufficiently rapid for the diagnosis of individual cases of influenza prior to antiviral therapy, and in recent years attention has focused on newer rapid diagnostic assays. Antigen detection tests using immunofluorescence or enzyme-linked immunoassay generally have limited sensitivity (approximately 70%) but high specificity (90%) and may be of use for the exclusion of influenza [77]. Several diagnostic kits are available that may be used outside the laboratory at the point of care [78]. Detection of viral nucleic acid by reverse-transcriptase polymerase chain reaction is more sensitive (around 90%) but may be less accessible for routine use [79,80]. Such tests are costly, and there has been debate regarding their cost-effectiveness compared to diagnosis on clinical grounds alone. Most treatment studies have shown that a clinical diagnosis is 60–70% accurate in an epidemic setting [50,51,61,62]; this increases to 79% if patients have high fever and cough [81,82]. The conclusion from these decision analyses is that in nonepidemic stages of the influenza cycle, cost-benefit analysis favors rapid testing to confirm influenza prior to antiviral therapy; in an epidemic, where the probability of a patient presenting with influenza-like symptoms having influenza exceeds 35–40%, empirical treatment on clinical grounds alone is the preferred option [83,84]. The success of this approach depends on accurate surveillance to determine influenza activity at a given time, and a cascade of information to primary care and hospital physicians when influenza is circulating [85].

PREVENTION OF INFLUENZA

Use of Antiviral Agents for Prophylaxis

All of the currently available antiviral drugs for influenza have been shown to be effective as prophylaxis if taken prior to or shortly after exposure. Prophylaxis has been shown to have additional benefit to vaccination, in part because of poor immune response to the vaccine, particularly in the elderly or immunosuppressed, or because of poor antigenic match between infecting and vaccine strains. Thus prophylaxis should be given where indicated regardless of vaccination history. Daily amantadine or rimantadine reduce infection rates by 50–80% during influenza A outbreaks, although again there is concern about the emergence and transmission of resistant virus [35,86]. Rimantadine is preferable to amantadine because of its side-effect profile. As described earlier, both zanamivir (at a dose of 10 mg daily by inhalation) and oseltamivir (75 mg daily or twice daily orally) have been shown to be protective against natural and experimental influenza infection [54,55,63,64], although zanamivir is currently not licensed for prophylactic use.

Prior to the influenza season, prophylaxis should be considered for individuals at high risk for severe and complicated influenza who have not been vaccinated or who have been vaccinated too recently for a protective immune response to develop. In an outbreak, residents and staff of residential care homes (whether vaccinated or not), and indeed household contacts of confirmed cases, benefit from prophylaxis [55,87]. In an outbreak situation, prophylaxis should be given for 14 days, or until 7 days have elapsed since the onset of the last confirmed case of influenza [88]. Other measures to reduce spread of infection include restricting visitors, instructing staff of hospitals or residential care homes to stay away if unwell, and respiratory isolation of ill patients [89].

Vaccination

In preventive terms, annual vaccination of high-risk individuals is the single most important and cost-effective intervention in the prevention of influenza [90–92]. Vaccination of staff caring for high-risk patients in hospitals or residential homes has also been shown to reduce mortality in their patients [93,94]. Current influenza vaccines are inactivated trivalent vaccines containing two influenza A subtypes (H1N1 and H3N2) and one influenza B subtype. Vaccine efficacy is high in healthy school-age children and adults, but reduced in infants, the elderly, and immunosuppressed persons [95–99]. To provide continuing protection, annual vaccination is necessary and vaccine is prepared each year using viral strains similar to those predicted to be circulating the forthcoming winter. Vaccination is generally well tolerated, with occasional local inflammation at the injection site, and rarely short-lived febrile symptoms [100,101]. An association with Guillain-Barré syndrome has been reported, but the risk is extremely low [102]. Egg hypersensitivity is the only absolute contraindication (since the vaccine virus is grown in eggs prior to inactivation), but the vaccine is not recommended in pregnancy.

Young children and elderly and immunosuppressed individuals respond relatively poorly to the inactivated vaccine, and in recent years, there has been interest in the development of a live attenuated vaccine for influenza. This would have the advantages of high antigenic load at the site of influenza infection—that is, the nasopharynx—and the possibility of a broader, more physiological immune response, including local IgA production as well as systemic antibody responses to a wider range of antigens [103,104]. Several studies have examined the protective efficacy of live vaccines and in general found comparable or improved efficacy compared to inactivated vaccines, including in children and high-risk patients [105–108]. One randomized placebo-controlled, double-blind study in nursing home residents compared live attenuated vaccine plus inactivated vaccine with inactivated vaccine alone, and found significantly lower rates of infection in those individuals who received both vaccines [109]. Future developments in influenza vaccines are likely to include the production of vaccine viruses using cell culture systems rather than eggs, the use of subunit or nucleic acid vaccines, and the development of adjuvants and delivery systems that may allow longer-lived immunity.

Influenza vaccine is currently recommended for all individuals at risk for severe and complicated influenza—that is, those individuals for whom antiviral treatment is recommended [110]. Despite this, uptake is generally poor. There are economic and social arguments for extending vaccination coverage to include healthy adults and school-age children [92].

CONCLUSIONS

The influenza virus is likely to coexist with the human race for the foreseeable future, and although we have made great advances in our understanding of viral pathogenesis and epidemiology, there is much work still to be done. The recent development of the neuraminidase inhibitors is an exciting advance, and novel diagnostic methods may also help in diagnosis of individual cases and study of the virus at a population level. However, there remain many unresolved issues. First, while the evidence to date suggests that all groups of patients benefit from antiviral therapy if administered early in their illness, the cost-effectiveness of such treatment has not been established in all groups. More research is required, particularly in patients at high risk for severe and complicated influenza, as well as other groups such as pregnant women, infants, and the immunosuppressed. A direct comparison between agents is required in order to formulate evidence-based guidelines recommending particular agents, and the possible benefits of multiple drug regimens explored. The issue of diagnostic testing as opposed to a clinical diagnosis needs to be clarified. As our experience with these antiviral agents grows, it will be important to be vigilant for development of resistance both locally and globally.

When considering treatment of influenza virus infections, it is important to consider the wider picture. Treatment of established influenza infection is a small part of this picture in terms of the control of influenza both locally and globally, the mainstay of prevention being annual vaccination using viral strains predicted to be circulating in the coming year. In cost-benefit terms, vaccination has a much greater (and additional) impact than antiviral treatment of ill patients, and it is important that vaccination remains the priority in any control strategy for influenza. Similarly, the use of antiviral agents for prophylaxis is an important element in control of infection in close contacts of cases, whether in a household or hospital.

In conclusion, the recent development of new agents and assays for influenza infection offers the potential for improved control over influenza in individuals and populations. It is to be hoped that our expanding knowledge of this infection will eventually allow us to control or influence the pandemics that have caused so much mortality and morbidity over past centuries.

REFERENCES

1. Lamb RA, Krug RM. Orthomyxoviridae: the viruses and their replication. In: Fields BM, Knipe DM, Howley PM, eds. Fields Virology. Vol. 1. 3rd ed. Philadelphia: Lippincott-Raven, 1996;1353–1395.
2. Yuen KY, Chan PKS, Peiris M, Tsang DN, Que TL, Shortridge KF, Cheung PT, To WK, Ho ET, Sung R, Cheng AF. Clinical features and rapid viral diagnosis of human disease associated with avian influenza H5N1 virus. Lancet 351:467–471.
3. Kendal AP. Epidemiologic implications of changes in the influenza virus genome. Am J Med 1987; 82(suppl 6A):4–14.
4. Meicklejohn G, Eickhoff TC, Graves P. Antigenic drift and efficacy of influenza virus vaccines. J Infect Dis 1978; 138:618–624.
5. Sullivan KM, Monto AS, Longini IM Jr. Estimates of the US health impact of influenza. Am J Public Health 1993; 83:1712–1716.
6. Schoenbaum SC. Economic impact of influenza. The individual's perspective. Am J Med 1987; 82:26–30.
7. Lui KJ, Kendal AP. Impact of influenza epidemics on mortality in the

United States from October 1972 to May 1985. Am J Public Health 1987; 77:712–716.

8. Nichol KL, Lind A, Margolis KL, Murdoch M, McFadden R, Hauge M, Magnan S, Drake M. The effectiveness of vaccination against influenza in healthy, working adults. N Engl J Med 1995; 333:889–893.
9. Nichol KL, Margolis KL, Lind A, Murdoch M, McFadden R, Hauge M, Magnan S, Drake M. Side effects associated with influenza vaccination in healthy working adults: a randomized, placebo-controlled trial. Arch Intern Med 1996; 156:1546–1550.
10. Monto AS. Influenza: Quantifying morbidity and mortality. Am J Med 1987; 82(suppl 6A):20–25.
11. Barker WH, Mullooly JP. Impact of epidemic type A influenza in a defined adult population. Am J Epidemiol 1980; 112:798–811.
12. Glezen WP. Emerging infections: pandemic influenza. Epidemiol Rev 1996; 18:64–76.
13. Hatta M, Kawaoka Y. The continued pandemic threat posed by avian influenza viruses in Hong Kong. Trends Microbiol 2002; 10:340–344.
14. Senior K. Are we ready for the next flu pandemic? Lancet Infect Dis 2001; 1:295.
15. Kavet J. A perspective on the significance of pandemic influenza. Am J Public Health 1977; 67:1063–1070.
16. Cate TR. Clinical manifestations and consequences of influenza. Am J Med 1987; 82(suppl 6A):15–19.
17. Munoz FM. The impact of influenza in children. Semin Pediatr Infect Dis 2002; 13:72–78.
18. Griffin MR, Coffey CS, Neuzil KM, Mitchel EF Jr, Wright PF, Edwards KM. Winter viruses: influenza and respiratory syncytial virus-related morbidity in chronic lung disease. Arch Intern Med 2002; 162:1229–1236.
19. Neuzil KM, Reed GW, Mitchel EF, Simonson L, Griffin MR. Impact of influenza on acute cardiopulmonary hospitalizations in pregnant women. Am J Epidemiol 1998; 148:1094–1102.
20. Sethi S. Bacterial pneumonia. Managing a deadly complication of influenza in older adults with comorbid disease. Geriatrics 2002; 57:56–61.
21. Hayden FG, Fritz RS, Lobo M, Alvord G, Strober W, Strauss SE. Local and systemic cytokine responses during experimental human influenza A virus infection. J Clin Invest 1998; 101:643–649.
22. Neuzil KM, Zhu Y, Griffin MR, Edwards KM, Thompson JM, Tollefson SJ, Wright PF. Burden of interpandemic influenza in children younger than 5 years: a 25-year prospective study. J Infect Dis 2002; 185:147–152.
23. Oxford JS, Galbraith A. Antiviral activity of amantadine: a review of laboratory and clinical data. Pharmacol Ther 1980; 11:181–262.
24. Bui M, Whittaker G, Helenius A. Effect of M1 protein and low pH on nuclear transport of influenza virus ribonucleoproteins. J Virol 1996; 70:8391–8401.
25. Hay AJ. The action of adamantanamines against influenza A viruses: inhibition of the M2 ion channel protein. Semin Virol 1992; 3:21–30.

26. Couch RB. Prevention and treatment of influenza. N Engl J Med 2000; 343: 1778–1787.
27. Wingfield WL, Pollack D, Grunert RR. Therapeutic efficacy of amantadine HCI and rimantadine HCI in naturally occurring influenza A2 respiratory illness in man. N Engl J Med 1969; 281:579–584.
28. Smorodintsev AA, Zlydnikov DM, Kiseleva AM, Romanov JA, Kazantsev AP, Rumovsky VI. Evaluation of amantadine in artificially induced A2 and B influenza. JAMA 1970; 213:1448–1454.
29. Van Voris LP, Betts RF, Hayden FG, Christmas WA, Douglas RG. Successful treatment of naturally occurring influenza A/USSR/77 H1N1. JAMA 1981; 245:1128–1131.
30. Vernier VG, Harmon JB, Stump Jm, Lynes TE, Marvel JP, Smith DH. The toxicologic and pharmacologic properties of amantadine hydrochloride. Toxicol Appl Pharmacol 1969; 15:642–665.
31. Dolin R, Reichman RC, Madore HP, Maynard R, Linton PN, Webbe Jones J. A controlled trial of amantadine and rimantadine in the prophylaxis of influenza A infection. N Engl J Med 1982; 307:580–584.
32. Bryson YJ, Monahan C, Pollack M, Shields WD. A prospective double-blind study of side-effects associated with the administration of amantadine for influenza A virus prophylaxis. J Infect Dis 1980; 141:543–547.
33. Hayden FG, Gwaltney JM Jr, Van de Castle RL, Adams KF, Giordani B. Comparative toxicity of amantadine hydrochloride and rimantadine hydrochloride in healthy adults. Antimicrob Agents Chemother 1981; 19:226–233.
34. Belshe RB, Smith MH, Hall CB, Betts R, Hay AJ. Genetic basis of resistance to rimantadine emerging during treatment of influenza virus infection. J Virol 1988; 62:1508–1512.
35. Hayden FG, Belshe RB, Clover RD, Hay AJ, Oakes MG, Soo W. Emergence and apparent transmission of rimantadine-resistant influenza A virus in families. N Engl J Med 1989; 321:1696–1702.
36. Hayden FG, Hay AJ. Emergence and transmission of influenza A viruses resistant to amantadine and rimantadine. Curr Top Microbiol Immunol 1992; 176:119–130.
37. Belshe RB, Burk B, Newman F, Cerruti RL, Sim IS. Resistance of influenza A virus to amantadine and rimantadine: results of one decade of surveillance. J Infect Dis 1989; 159:430–435.
38. Degelau J, Somani SK, Cooper SL, Guay DR, Crossley KB. Amantadine-resistant influenza A in a nursing facility. Arch Intern Med 1992; 152:390–392.
39. Ziegler T, Hamphill ML, Ziegler ML, Perez-Oronoz G, Klimov AI, Hampson AW, Regnery HL, Cox NJ. Low incidence of rimantidine resistance in field isolates of influenza A viruses. J Infect Dis 1999; 180:935–939.
40. Colman PM, Varghese JN, Laver WG. Structure of the catalytic and antigenic sites in influenza virus neuraminidase. Nature 1983; 303:41–44.
41. Colman PM, Hoyne PA, Lawrence MC. Sequence and structure alignment of paramyxovirus hemagglutinin-neuraminidase with influenza virus neuraminidase. J Virol 1993; 67:2972–2980.

42. Von Itzstein M, Wu W-Y, Kok GB, Peggs MS, Dyason JC, Jin B, Van Phan T, Smythe ML, White HF, Oliver SW, et al. Rational design of potent sialidase-based inhibitors of influenza virus replication. Nature 1993; 363:418–423.
43. Mendel DB, Tai CY, Escarpe PA, Li W, Sidwell RW, Huffman JH, Sweet C, Jakeman KJ, Merson J, Lacy SA, Lew W, Williams MA, Zhong L, Chen MS, Bischofberger N, Kim CU. Oral administration of a prodrug of the influenza virus neuramindase inhibitor GS 4071 protects mice and ferrets against influenza infection. Antimicrob Agents Chemother 1998; 42:640–646.
44. McKimm-Breschkin JL. Resistance of influenza viruses to neuraminidase inhibitors—review. Antiviral Res 2000; 47:1–17.
45. Woods JM, Bethell RC, Coates JA, Healy N, Hiscox SA, Pearson BA, Ryan DM, Ticehurst J, Tilling J, Walcott SM, et al. 4-Guanidino-2,4-dideoxy-2,3-dehydro-N-acetylneuraminic acid is a highly effective inhibitor both of the sialidase (neuraminidase) and of growth of a wide range of influenza A and B viruses in vitro. Antimicrob Agents Chemother 1993; 37:1473–1479.
46. Thomas GP, Forsyth M, Penn CR, McCauley JW. Inhibition of the growth of influenza viruses in vitro by 4-guanidino-2,4-dideoxy-N-acetylneuraminic acid. Antiviral Res 1994; 24:351–356.
47. Cass LM, Brown J, Pickford M, Fayinka S, Newman SP, Johansson CJ, Bye A. Pharmacoscintigraphic evaluation of lung deposition of inhaled zanamivir in healthy volunteers. Clin Pharmacokinet 1999; 36(suppl 1):21–31.
48. Cass LM, Efthymiopoulos C, Bye A. Pharmacokinetics of zanamivir after intravenous, oral, inhaled or intranasal administration to healthy volunteers. Clin Pharmacokinet 1999; 36(suppl 1):1–11.
49. Hayden FG, Treanor JJ, Betts RF, Lobo M, Esinhart JD, Hussey EK. Safety and efficacy of the neuraminidase inhibitor GG167 in experimental human influenza. JAMA 1996; 275:295–299.
50. Hayden FG, Osterhaus ADME, Treanor JJ, Fleming DM, Aoki FY, Nicholson KG, Bohnen AM, et al. Efficacy and safety of the neuraminidase inhibitor zanamivir in the treatment of influenzavirus infections. N Engl J Med 1997; 337:874–880.
51. The MIST (Management of Influenza in the Southern Hemisphere Trialists) Study Group. Randomised trial of efficacy and safety of inhaled zanamivir in treatment of influenza A and B virus infections. Lancet 1998; 352:1877–1881.
52. Kaiser L, Keene ON, Hammond JMJ, Elliott M, Hayden FG. Impact of zanamivir on antibiotic use for respiratory events following acute influenza in adolescents and adults. Arch Intern Med 2000; 160:3234–3240.
53. Cass LM, Gunawardena KA, Macmahon MM, Bye A. Pulmonary function and airway responsiveness in mild to moderate asthmatics given repeated inhaled doses of zanamivir. Respir Med 2000 Feb; 94:166–173.
54. Monto AS, Robinson DP, Herlocher ML, Hinson JM Jr, Elliott MJ, Crisp A. Zanamivir in the prevention of influenza among healthy adults: a randomized controlled trial. JAMA 1999; 282:31–35.
55. Hayden FG, Gubareva LV, Monto AS, Klein TC, Elliott MJ, Hammond JM,

Sharp SJ, Ossi MJ. Inhaled zanamivir for the prevention of influenza in families. Zanamivir Family Study Group. N Engl J Med 2000; 343:1282–1289.
56. Gubareva LV, Matrosovich MN, Brenner MK, Bethell RC, Webster RG. Evidence for zanamivir resistance in an immunocompromised child infected with influenza B virus. J Infect Dis 1998; 178:1257–1262.
57. Lew W, Chen X, Kim CU. Discovery and development of GS4104 (oseltamivir): an orally active influenza neuraminidase inhibitor. Curr Med Chem 2000; 7:663–672.
58. Li W, Escarpe PA, Eisenberg EJ, Cundy KC, Sweet C, Jakeman KJ, Merson J, Lew W, Williams M, Zhang L, Kim CU, Bischofberger N, Chen MS, Mendel DB. Identification of GS 4104 as an orally bioavailable prodrug of the influenza virus neuraminidase inhibitor GS 4071. Antimicrob Agents Chemother 1998; 42:647–653.
59. Eisenberg EJ, Bidgood A, Cundy KC. Penetration of GS4071, a novel influenza neuraminidase inhibitor, into rat bronchoalveolar lining fluid following oral administration of the prodrug GS4104. Antimicrob Agents Chemother 1997; 41:1949–1952.
60. Hayden FG, Treanor JJ, Fritz RS, Lobo M, Betts RF, Miller M, Kinnersley N, Mills RG, Ward P, Straus SE. Use of the oral neuraminidase inhibitor oseltamivir in experimental human influenza: randomized controlled trials for prevention and treatment. JAMA 1999; 282:1240–1246.
61. Treanor JJ, Hayden FG, Vrooman PS, Barbarash R, Bettis R, Riff D, Singh S, Kinnersley N, Ward P, Mills RG. Efficacy and safety of the oral neuraminidase inhibitor oseltamivir in treating acute influenza: a randomized controlled trial. JAMA 2000; 283:1016–1024.
62. Nicholson KG, Aoki FY, Osterhaus AD, Trottier S, Carewicz O, Mercier CH, Rode A, Kinnersley N, Ward P. Efficacy and safety of oseltamivir in treatment of acute influenza: a randomised controlled trial. Lancet 2000; 355:1845–1850.
63. Hayden FG, Atmar RL, Schilling M, Johnson C, Poretz D, Paar D, Huson L, Ward P, Mills RG. Use of the selective oral neuraminidase inhibitor oseltamivir to prevent influenza. N Engl J Med 1999; 341:1336–1343.
64. Munoz FM, Galasso GJ, Gwaltney JM Jr, Hayden FG, Murphy B, Webster R, Wright P, Couch RB. Current research on influenza and other respiratory viruses: II international symposium. Antiviral Res 2000; 46:91–124.
65. Lee PY, Matchar DB, Clements DA, Huber J, Hamilton JD, Peterson ED. Economic analysis of influenza vaccination and antiviral treatment for healthy working adults. Ann Intern Med 2002; 137:225–231.
66. Muennig PA, Khan K. Cost-effectiveness of vaccination versus treatment of influenza in healthy adolescents and adults. Clin Infect Dis 2001; 33:1879–1885.
67. Pitts SR. Evidence-based emergency medicine/systemic review abstract. Use of the neuraminidase inhibitor class of antiviral drugs for the treatment of healthy adults with an acute influenza like illness. Ann Emerg Med 2002; 39:552–554.
68. Demicheli V, Jefferson T, Rivetti D, Deeks J. Prevention and early treatment of influenza in healthy adults. Vaccine 2000; 18:957–1030.

69. Smith KJ, Roberts MS. Cost-effectiveness of newer treatment strategies for influenza. Am J Med 2002; 113:300–307.
70. Mauskopf JA, Cates SC, Griffin AD, Neighbors DM, Lamb SC, Rutherford C. Cost effectiveness of zanamivir for the treatment of influenza in a high risk population in Australia. Pharmacoeconomics 2000; 17:611–620.
71. Griffin AD, Perry AS, Fleming DM. Cost-effectiveness analysis of inhaled zanamivir in the treatment of influenza A and B in high-risk patients. Pharmacoeconomics 2001; 19:293–301.
72. Roach JO. NICE recommends flu drug for 'at risk' patients. BMJ 2000; 321:1305.
73. Bridges CB, Fukuda K, Uyeki TM, Cox NJ, Singleton JA. Prevention and control of influenza. Recommendations of the Advisory Committee on Immunization Practices (ACIP). MMWR Morb Mortal Wkly Rep 2002; 51(RR03): 1–31.
74. Ison MG, Hayden FG. Viral infections in immunocompromised patients: what's new with respiratory viruses. Curr Opin Infect Dis 2002; 15:355–367.
75. Johny AA, Clark A, Price N, Carrington D, Oakhill A, Marks DI. The use of zanamivir to treat influenza A and B infection after allogeneic stem cell transplantation. Bone Marrow Transplant 2002; 29:113–115.
76. Couch RB. Influenza, influenza virus vaccine, and human immunodeficiency virus infection. Clin Infect Dis 1999; 28:548–551.
77. Noyola DE, Clark B, O'Donnell FT, Atmar RL, Greer J, Demmler GJ. Comparison of a new neuraminidase detection assay with an enzyme immunoassay, immunofluorescence, and culture for rapid detection of influenza A and B viruses in nasal wash specimens. J Clin Microbiol 2000; 38:1161–1165.
78. Poehling KA, Griffin MR, Dittus RS, Tang YW, Holland K, Li H, Edwards KM. Bedside diagnosis of influenzavirus infections in hospitalized children. Pediatrics 2002; 110:83–88.
79. Demmler GJ. Laboratory diagnosis of influenza: recent advances. Semin Pediatr Infect Dis 2002; 13:85–89.
80. Ellis JS, Zambon MC. Molecular diagnosis of influenza. Rev Med Virol 2002; 12:375–389.
81. Monto AS, Gravenstein S, Elliott M, Colopy M, Schweinke J. Clinical signs and symptoms predicting influenza infection. Arch Intern Med 2000; 160:3243–4347.
82. Boivin G, Hardy I, Tellier G, Maziade J. Predicting influenza infections during epidemics with use of a clinical case definition. Clin Infect Dis 2000; 31:1166–1169.
83. Blitz SG, Cram P, Chernew ME, Monto AS, Fendrick AM. Diagnostic testing or empirical neuraminidase inhibitor therapy for patients with influenza-like illness: what a difference a day makes. Am J Manag Care 2002; 8:221–227.
84. Sintchenko V, Gilbert GL, Coiera E, Dwyer D. Treat or test first? Decision analysis of empirical antiviral treatment of influenza virus infection versus treatment based on rapid test results. J Clin Virol 2002; 25:15–21.

85. Brammer TL, Murray EL, Fukuda K, Hall HE, Klimov A, Cox NJ. Surveillance for influenza-United States, 1997–98, 1998–99, and 1999–00 seasons. MMWR Surveill Summ 2002; 51:1–10.
86. Mast EE, Harmon MW, Gravenstein S, Wu SP, Arden NH, Circo R, Tyszka G, Kendal AP, Davis JP. Emergence and possible transmission of amantadine-resistant viruses during nursing home outbreaks of influenza A (H3N2). Am J Epidemiol 1991; 13:988–997.
87. Arden NH. Control of influenza in the long-term-care facility: a review of established approaches and newer options. Infect Control Hosp Epidemiol 2000; 21:59–64.
88. Drinka PJ, Gravenstein S, Schilling M, Krause P, Miller BA, Shult P. Duration of antiviral prophylaxis during nursing home outbreaks of influenza A: a comparison of 2 protocols. Arch Intern Med 1998; 158:2155–2159.
89. Bradley SF. Prevention of influenza in long-term-care facilities. Infect Control Hosp Epidemiol 1999; 20:629–637.
90. Nichol KL, Lind A, Margolis KL, Murdoch M, McFadden R, Hauge M, Magnan S, Drake M. The effectiveness of vaccination against influenza in healthy, working adults. N Engl J Med 1995; 333:889–893.
91. Nichol KL, Margolis KL, Wuorenma J, Von Sternberg T. The efficacy and cost effectiveness of vaccination against influenza among elderly persons living in the community. N Engl J Med 1994; 331:778–784.
92. Nichol KL, Wuorenma J, Von Sternberg T. Benefits of influenza vaccination for low-, intermediate-, and high-risk senior citizens. Arch Intern Med 1998; 158:1769–1776.
93. Potter J, Stott DJ, Roberts MA, Elder AG, O'Donnell B, Knight PV, Carman WF. Influenza vaccination of health care workers in long-term-care hospitals reduces the mortality of elderly people patients. J Infect Dis 1997; 175: 1–6.
94. Carman WF, Elder AG, Wallace LA, McAulay K, Walker A, Murray GD, Stott DJ. Effects of influenza vaccination of health-care workers on mortality of elderly people in long-term care: a randomised controlled trial. Lancet 2000; 355:93–97.
95. La Montagne Jr, Noble GR, Quinnan GV, Curlin GT, Blackwelder WC, Smith JI, Ennis FA, Bozeman FM. Summary of clinical trials of inactivated influenza vaccine–1978. Rev Infect Dis 1983; 5:723–736.
96. Keitel WA, Cate TR, Couch RB, Huggins LL, Hess KR. Efficacy of repeated annual immunization with inactivated influenza virus vaccines over a five year period. Vaccine 1997; 15:1114–1122.
97. Gross PA, Hermogenes AW, Sacks HS, Lau J, Levandowski RA. The efficacy of influenza vaccine in elderly persons: a meta-analysis and review of the literature. Ann Intern Med 1995; 123:518–527.
98. Piedra PA, Glezen WP. Influenza in children: epidemiology, immunity and vaccines. Semin Pediatr Infect Dis 1991; 2:140–146.
99. Kroon FP, van Dissel JT, de Jong JC, van Furth R. Antibody response to influenza, tetanus and pneumococcal vaccines in HIV-seropositive individuals in relation to number of CD4+ lymphocytes. AIDS 1994; 8:469–476.

100. Margolis KL, Nichol KL, Poland GA, Pluhar RE. Frequency of adverse reactions to influenza vaccine in the elderly: a randomized placebo-controlled trial. JAMA 1990; 264:1139–1141.
101. Govaert TME, Dinant GJ, Aretz K. Adverse effects to influenza vaccine in elderly people: randomised double-blind placebo controlled trial. BMJ 1993; 307:988–993.
102. Lasky T, Terracciano GJ, Magder L. The Guillain-Barre syndrome and the 1992–93 and 1993–94 influenza vaccines. N Engl J Med 1998; 339:1797–1802.
103. Betts RF, Treanor JJ. Approaches to improved influenza vaccination. Vaccine 2000; 18:1690–1695.
104. Belshe RB, Gruber WL, Mendelson PM, Mehta HB, Mahmood K, Reisinger K, Treanor J, Zangwill K, Hayden FG, Bernstein DI, Kotloff K, King J, Piedra PA, Block SL, Yan L, Wolff M. Correlates of immune protection induced by live attenuated cold adapted trivalent intranasal influenza virus vaccine. J Infect Dis 2000; 181:1133–1137.
105. Edwards KM, Dupont WD, Westrich MK, Plummer WD Jr, Palmer PS, Wright PF. A randomised controlled trial of cold-adapted and inactivated vaccines for the prevention of influenza A disease. J Infect Dis 1994; 169:68–76.
106. Treanor J, Dumyati G, O'Brien D, Riley MA, Riley G, Erb S, Betts R. Evaluation of cold adapted, reassortant influenza B virus vaccines in elderly and chronically ill patients. J Infect Dis 1994; 169:402–407.
107. Gruber WC, Belshe RB, King JC, Treanor JJ, Piedra PA, Wright PF, Reed GW, Anderson E, Newman F. Evaluation of live attenuated influenza vaccine in children of 6-18 months: safety, immunogenicity and efficacy. J Infect Dis 1996; 173:1313–1319.
108. Belshe RB, Mendelman PM, Treanor J, King J, Gruber WC, Piedra P, Bernstein DI, Hayden FG, Kotloff K, Zangwill K, Iacuzio D, Wolff M. The efficacy of live attenuated cold adapted trivalent intranasal influenza virus vaccine in children. N Engl J Med 1998; 338:1405–1412.
109. Treanor JJ, Mattison HR, Dumyati G, Yinnon A, Erb S, O'Brien D, Dolin R, Betts RF. Protective efficacy of combined live intranasal and inactivated influenza A virus vaccines in the elderly. Ann Intern Med 1992; 117:625–633.
110. Nicholson KG, Snacken R, Palache AM. Influenza immunisation policies in Europe and the United States. Vaccine 1995; 13:365–369.

18

Severe Acute Respiratory Syndrome

Thomas M. File, Jr.
Northeastern Ohio Universities College of Medicine, Rootstown
and Summa Health System
Akron, Ohio, U.S.A.

INTRODUCTION

From late February through mid-March 2003, public health officials from several countries worldwide had identified a newly described atypical respiratory illness, which was termed severe acute respiratory syndrome (SARS). This was first recognized in Guandong Province in southeast China in late 2002 and subsequently spread globally during March and April 2003. This newly described infectious disease appears to be highly contagious by close contact and has been associated with significant morbidity and mortality. Within a matter of weeks after the World Health Organization (WHO) issued its global health alert on March 15, 2003, an unprecedented amount of information has become known about this disease. This has in part been due to a coordinated effort of several international organizations, but most notably the World Health Organization (WHO) and the Centers for Disease Control and Prevention (CDC).

SARS—DEFINITION

As determined by a consensus of worldwide public health officials in March 2003, surveillance case definitions for SARS included both "suspect" and "probable" cases [1,2].

A suspect case includes a respiratory illness of unknown etiology with onset since February 1, 2003, and with the following criteria: (1) measured temperature higher than 100.4°F (>38.0°C); (2) one or more clinical findings of respiratory illness (e.g., cough, shortness of breath, difficulty breathing, hypoxic, or radiographic findings of either pneumonia or acute respiratory distress syndrome); (3) travel within 10 days of onset of symptoms to an area with suspected or documented community transmission of SARS (excluding areas with secondary cases limited to health care workers or direct household contacts or close contact within 10 days of onset of symptoms with either a person with a respiratory illness and travel to a SARS area or a person under investigation or suspected of having SARS).

A probable case is defined as a suspect case with either radiographic evidence of pneumonia or respiratory distress syndrome or autopsy findings consistent with respiratory distress syndrome without an identifiable cause.

On April 29, 2003, the CDC's interim surveillance case definition for SARS had been updated to include laboratory criteria for evidence of infection with the SARS-associated coronavirus (see etiology), (Table 1) [2]. Although at the time of this writing no instances of SARS-associated coronavirus had been detected in persons who were asymptomatic, there remained the possibility of subclinical infection; and in such cases, laboratory detection might be able to identify patients with mild respiratory illness or those who are asymptomatic (Fig. 1).

EPIDEMIOLOGY

As of the end of April 2003, over 5500 cases of suspect or probable SARS had been identified in approximately 26 countries [3]. The syndrome was observed primarily in adults ages 25 through 70, and children have been relatively spared. There appears to be no significant underlying predisposing condition to the development of SARS; however, the elderly and patients with underlying conditions are at greater risk of dying. Earlier in the evaluation of this syndrome most of the descriptions were of patients who required hospitalization. However, as more cases have been identified, particularly in the Western countries, it has become apparent that many patients have not required hospitalization.

SARS appears to be transmitted by close contact, most probably via direct contact with respiratory secretions [4,5]. The majority of early cases

TABLE 1 Updated U.S. Surveillance Case Definition for Severe Acute Respiratory Syndrome (SARS)—April 29, 2003

- Clinical criteria
  - Asymptomatic or mild respiratory illness
  - Moderate respiratory illness
    - Temperature of >100.4°F (>38°C), and
    - One or more clinical findings of respiratory illness (such as cough, shortness of breath)
  - Severe respiratory illness
    - Same as for moderate, plus
    - Radiographic evidence of pneumonia, or
    - Respiratory distress syndrome, or
    - Autopsy findings consistent with pneumonia or respiratory distress syndrome without an identifiable cause
- Epidemiological criteria
  - Travel within 10 days of onset of symptoms to an area with current or recently documented or suspected community transmission of SARS (China, Hong Kong, Singapore, Taiwan, Toronto, Hanoi)
  - Close contact within 10 days of onset of symptoms with a person known or suspected to have SARS infection. Close contact is defined as having cared for or lived with a person known to have SARS or having a high likelihood of direct contact with respiratory secretions and/or body fluids of a patient known to have SARS. Examples include kissing or embracing, sharing eating or drinking utensils, close conversation (<3 feet), physical examination, and any other direct contact between persons. Close contact does not include activities such as walking by a person or sitting across a waiting room or office for a brief period of time.
- Laboratory criteria
  - Confirmed
    - Detection of antibody to SARS-CoV in specimens obtained during acute illness or > 21 days after illness onset, or
    - Detection of SARS-CoV RNA by RT-PCR confirmed by a second PCR assay, by using a second specimen
    - Isolation of SARS-CoV
  - Negative
    - Absence of antibody to SARS-CoV in convalescent serum obtained > 21 days after symptom onset
  - Undetermined: laboratory testing either not performed or incomplete
- Case classification[a]
  - Probable case: meets the clinical criteria for severe respiratory illness of unknown etiology with onset since February 2003, and epidemiological criteria; laboratory criteria confirmed, negative, or undetermined
  - Suspect case: meets the clinical criteria for moderate respiratory illness of unknown etiology with onset since February 2003, and epidemiologic criteria; laboratory criteria as for probable case

[a] Asymptomatic SARS CoV infection or clinical manifestations other than respiratory illness might be identified as more is learned about SARS-CoV infection.
Source: Ref. 2.

Patient Sticker or Addressograph

SEVERE ACUTE RESPIRATORY SYNDROME (SARS)
EMERGENCY DEPARTMENT SURVEILLANCE PROJECT
(4/8/03)

EMERGENCY DEPARTMENT TRIAGE:
Complete this form for every patient with FEVER.

- **Apply patient stamp (addressograph) to upper right corner of form**
- **Visit Date: ____________________________**
- **Circle YES or NO as applicable**

1	Does the patient have fever (>38 degrees Celsius, >100.4 degrees Fahrenheit)?	YES ☐ Go to 2a	NO ☐ STOP
2a	Does the patient have respiratory complaints (cough, shortness of breath, difficulty breathing, or current pneumonia/ARDS)?	YES ☐ Go to 2b	NO ☐ Go to 2b
2b	Is the patient's pulse oximetry reading <94% while on room air?	YES ☐ Go to 3	NO ☐ Go to 3
3	Travel to Ontario, Canada; People's Republic of China (both mainland China and Hong Kong); Hanoi, Vietnam; Taiwan; and/or Singapore within the 10 days preceding symptom onset? <u>OR</u> Close contact with a person meeting criteria 1, 2 and 3 within the 10 days preceding symptom onset? (Close contact – cared for, lived with or direct contact with respiratory secretions or body fluids)	YES ☐ Go to 4	NO ☐ STOP
4	If the answer to questions 1 **AND** (2a **or** 2b), **AND** 3 are **<u>ALL</u>** yes, follow the instructions below:		

IF THE ANSWERS TO QUESTIONS 1, 2 (either part), and 3 are yes:

- **Place patient in negative pressure room with strict respiratory precautions, including use of N-95 masks.**
- **Notify charge nurse and charge physician immediately.**
- **Notify RN from Infection Control (pager #).**

IMPORTANT:

Please keep forms together by date of triage each day (midnight to midnight), so that each day's frequency of YES responses, can be easily counted.

Please maintain a file of these forms in the ED until you are advised by your local public health authority they are no longer needed.

Produced by the SARS-SP task force in cooperation with EMSystem

FIGURE 1 Checklist for evaluation of patient with possible SARS.

have been reported among health care workers and family members of affected persons. However, evidence of community spread of the disease is emerging, suggesting that other modes of transmission, such as airborne or direct contact, may also have a role. Clusters of cases in community settings such as hotels and apartment buildings demonstrate that transmission can be efficient. Many household contacts have become ill. Early epidemiological evidence indicates that the transmission of SARS is facilitated by face-to-face contact, and this still appears to be the most common mode of spread. However, airborne transmission may have a role in some settings, and it could account for extensive spread within buildings and other confined areas that has been observed in some places in Asia.

ETIOLOGY

Several different laboratories have identified a novel coronavirus in Vero E6 cell cultures inoculated with respiratory secretions and lung tissue of infected patients [6,7]. Other techniques, including electron microscopy, RT-PCR, and serovonversion, have also pointed to this as the causative agent. The sequence of the viral genome has been determined: it indicates no close relationship with any of the known human or animal coronaviruses. Although there is speculation the virus originated in animals, at the time of this report, the source of the virus is undetermined.

Of the 50 patients with clinical SARS described by Peiris et al. 45 had serological or PCR evidence of SARS-associated coronavirus infection; and of the five cases which were unconfirmed, four had serological testing prior to 14 days of onset of illness (possibly prior to the time of seroconversion—see Diagnosis, below) [8].

CLINICAL MANIFESTATIONS

The initial descriptions of the clinical manifestations of SARS have come from reports of patients who have required hospitalization [9–11]. In such patients the disease is often reported as a biphasic illness: an initial acute febrile phase followed by a lower respiratory illness phase. At the time of this writing, the mortality of probable SARS cases is 217/3816 (5.6%). It is possible, as more data become available from sero-epidemiological studies, that a milder form of the infection (including subclinical infection) will emerge.

The illness generally begins with a prodrome of fever, often associated with chills, rigors, and myalgia. Headache and severe malaise may accompany this phase. Rash and gastrointestinal symptoms have been absent in most cases, although in one outbreak within an apartment complex in Hong Kong, diarrhea was found in 66% of cases. After a typical period of 3–7 days, a lower respiratory phase may begin with the onset of nonproductive cough and progressive pneumonia. In the initial reports of cases, 10–20% of patients required intensive care unit management and mechanical ventilation. The presenting symptoms of patients admitted to the hospital for SARS from three published series is presented in Table 2 [8,10,12]. Most patients were admitted to the hospital several days after the onset of symptoms. The most common initial complaints were fever and chills or rigors. Upper respiratory tract symptoms such as rhinorrhea and sore throat were present in a minority of patients. At the time of examination, abnormal auscultatory findings were present in 19 (38%) [8].

Chest x-ray finding abnormalities are usually absent during the initial phase of illness, but findings become progressively abnormal during the lower respiratory illness phase. Initially this is characterized by early focal interstitial infiltrates progressing to more generalized infiltrates. ARDS has occurred in many patients who become very seriously ill.

Laboratory abnormalities most often associated with SARS include absolute lymphopenia, mild neutropenia, and thrombocytopenia. Mild to moderately elevated creatine phosphokinase, lactate dehydrogenase, and transaminase levels were seen in 30–80% of cases (Table 3).

Lee et al. found that advanced age, male sex, a high peak creatine phosphokinase value, a high lactate dehydrogenase level, a high initial neutrophil count (i.e., 4.6 vs. 3.7×10^{-9}/L), and a low serum sodium level were significant predictive factors for ICU admission and death [12]. On multivariate analysis, the only factors that were predictive of an adverse outcome were advanced age, a high peak lactate dehydrogenase level, and a higher absolute neutrophil count.

TABLE 2 Symptoms of Patients with SARS at Presentation (%)

Symptoms	Peiris[a] (50)	Lee[b] (138)	Poutanen[c] (10)
Fever	100	100	100
Chills	74	73	—
Cough	62	57	100
Myalgia	54	61	20
Rhinorrhea	24	23	—
Diarrhea	10	20	50
Headache	20	56	30

( )=number of patients.
[a] Ref. 8.
[b] Ref. 12.
[c] Ref. 10.

TABLE 3 Laboratory Abnormalities on Presentation of Patients with SARS (%)

Laboratory test	Pieris[a]	Lee[b]	Poutanen[c]
Lymphopenia	68	70	89
Thrombocytopenia	40	45	33
Elevated CPK	26	32	56
Elevated LDH	—	71	80
Elevated transaminases	34	23	78

The percentage is based on the number of patients who had the test performed.
CPK=creatine phosphokinase.
LDH=lactate dehydrogenase.
[a] Ref. 8.
[b] Ref. 12.
[c] Ref. 10.

Characteristics of the initial patients reported to the CDC with either suspect or probable SARS in the United States are shown in Table 4. As of the end of April 2003, the overall worldwide mortality rate of probable cases was 6.5%; however, at that time there had been no reported deaths in the United States.

DIAGNOSIS

At the time of this writing, there were no specific diagnostic tests available in general laboratories for the novel coronavirus strain. However, several laboratories, including the CDC and WHO, were working to develop a variety of methods, including PCR-based and serological tests. Information from a limited number of samples tested for serology suggests that antibodies may not be detectable by ELISA or indirect fluorescence until a couple of weeks after the onset of symptoms [6].

TREATMENT

At the time of this writing, there is no specific therapy recommended. A variety of treatments have been attempted, but there are no controlled data. Most patients have been treated throughout the illness with broad-spectrum antimicrobials, supplemental oxygen, I.V. fluids, and other supportive measures. Some clinicians have advocated a combination of ribaviran and corticosteroids, but the efficacy of these drugs has not been established. Early testing of ribaviran and other antiviral compounds against the novel coronavirus had not produced evidence of in vitro activity [13].

TABLE 4 Characteristics of SARS Cases in the United States (as of April 29, 2003)

Characteristic	Probable cases (N=56) No. (%)	Suspect cases (n=233) No.(%)
Age		
0–4	7 (13)	36 (15)
5–17	3 (5)	14 (6)
18–64	33 (59)	159 (68)
≥65	12 (21)	21 (9)
Unknown	1 (2)	3 (2)
Sex		
Female	24 (43)	115 (49)
Male	30 (54)	117 (50)
Unknown	2 (4)	1 (0)
Race		
White	26 (46)	131 (56)
Black	0 (0)	5 (2)
Asian	25 (45)	83 (36)
Unknown	4 (7)	14 (6)
Exposure		
Travel[a]	54 (96)	213 (91)
Close contact	1 (2)	16 (7)
HCW[b]	1 (2)	4 (2)
Hospitalized >24 hr		
Yes	37 (66)	9 (22)
No	18 (32)	178 (76)
Unknown	1 (2)	4 (2)
Required ventilator		
Yes	2 (4)	1 (0)
No	53 (95)	228 (98)
Unknown	1 (2)	4 (2)
Deaths	0 (0)	0 (0)
SARS-assoc coronavirus findings		
Confirmed	6 (11)	0 (0)
Negative	13 (23)	41 (18)
Undetermined[c]	37 (66)	192 (82)

[a] to Mainland China, Hong Kong, Hanoi, Singapore, Toronto.
[b] Health care worker.
[c] Collection and/or laboratory testing has not been completed.
Source: CDC. Updated interim U.S. cases. Available at http://www.cdc.gov/ncidod/sars/casedefinition.htm.

PREVENTION

Because the causative agent of SARS is contagious, prevention measures center on avoidance of exposure and infection control strategies for suspected cases and contacts. Guidelines for infection control have been published and should be consulted for updated recommendation [14]. Health care workers encountering a possible case of SARS (suspected or probable) should take meticulous safety precautions and should seek advice from an expert in SARS infection control. Hospitalized patients with suspected SARS should be isolated in negative pressure rooms; health care workers should wear masks (N-95 respirator such as used for tuberculosis) to prevent air-droplet and airborne acquisition. Because coronaviruses can survive on environmental surfaces, good hand washing is highly recommended as well. Figure 2 represents a checklist used at our hospital to evaluate patients for the possibility of SARS.

SUMMARY

Because a new virus causes SARS, it is very difficult to predict the eventual significance of this infection. However, at the time of this writing, there is great concern about its future impact. It has had enormous economic and political impact on the affected areas of the world. Although significant progress has been made concerning the etiology, epidemiology, and prevention of this virus, many important questions remain: Why do some people develop severe illness and others have only mild symptoms? Is there a large segment of infected patients with subclinical infection? How long do patients shed the virus? Will there be specific antiviral therapy? Will a vaccine be effective? Without answers to some of these questions, the eventual outcome of SARS remains unclear.

REFERENCES

1. WHO. Case definitions for surveillance of severe acute respiratory syndrome SARS). http:/www.who.int/csr/sars/casedefinition/htm
2. CDC. Updated interim U.S. case definition of severe acute respiratory syndrome (SARS). http:/www.cdc.gov/ncidod/sars/casedefinition/htm
3. WHO. Cumulative Number of Reported Probable Cases of Severe Acute Respiratory Syndrome (SARS). Vol. 2003. WHO, 2003.
4. Outbreak of severe acute respiratory syndrome—Worldwide, 2003. JAMA 2003; 289:1775–1776.
5. Update: Outbreak of severe acute respiratory syndrome—worldwide, 2003. MMWR Morb Mortal Wkly Rep 2003; 52:241–246, 248.
6. Ksiazek TG, Erdman D, Goldsmith C, et al. A novel coronavirus associated with severe acute respiratory syndrome. N Engl J Med 2003; 10:10.

7. Drosten C, Gunther S, Preiser W, et al. Identification of a novel coronavirus in patients with severe acute respiratory syndrome. N Engl J Med 2003; 10:10.
8. Peiris JSM, Lai ST, Poon LLM, Yam LYC, et al. Coronavirus as a possible cause of severe acute respiratory syndrome. Lancet 2003. Published online April 8, 2003. http:/image.thelancet.com/extras/033477web.pdf.
9. Tsang KW, Ho PL, Ooi GC, et al. A cluster of cases of severe acute respiratory syndrome in Hong Kong. N Engl J Med 2003; 11:11.
10. Poutanen SM, Low DE, Henry B, et al. Identification of severe acute respiratory syndrome in Canada. N Engl J Med 2003; 10:10.
11. Preliminary clinical description of severe acute respiratory syndrome. Morb Mortal Wkly Rep 2003; 52:255–256.
12. Lee N, Hui D, Wu A, Chan P, Cameron P, et al. A major outbreak of severe acute respiratory syndrome in Hong Kong. N Engl J Med 2003. Published at www.nejm.org on April 7, 2003.
13. CDC. Severe acute respiratory syndrome (SARS) and coronavirus testing—United States, 2003. Morb Mortal Weekly Rep 2003; 53:297–302.
14. Outbreak of severe acute respiratory syndrome—worldwide, 2003. MMWR Morb Mortal Wkly Rep 2003; 52:226–228.

Index

About the Editors

CHARLES H. NIGHTINGALE is Vice President for Research and Director of the Institute for International Healthcare Studies at Hartford Hospital, Connecticut, as well as Research Professor at the University of Connecticut School of Pharmacy, Storrs. The author of approximately 500 journal articles, numerous book chapters, and 238 published abstracts, Dr. Nightingale is a Fellow of the American College of Clinical Pharmacology and the Infectious Disease Society of America, as well as a member of the American Society for Clinical Pharmacology and Therapeutics, among others. An editorial board member for numerous publications, Dr. Nightingale received the B.S. degree (1961) from Fordham University, Bronx, New York, the M.S. degree (1966) from St. John's University, Jamaica, New York, and the Ph.D. degree (1970) from the State University of New York at Buffalo.

PAUL G. AMBROSE is Director of the Division of Infectious Diseases, Cognigen Corporation, Buffalo, New York, Assistant Clinical Professor of the University of the Pacific School of Pharmacy, Stockton, California, as well as a member of the Buffalo Pharmacometrics Study Unit, State University of New York at Buffalo. The author or coauthor of over 50 books, book chapters, and journal articles, Dr. Ambrose serves on the editorial boards of *Antimicrobial Agents and Chemotherapy, Antibiotics for Clinicians, and the Journal of Infectious Disease Pharmacotherapy*. Additionally, Dr. Ambrose is a member of the Infectious Disease Society of America and the Society of Infectious Disease Pharmacists. Dr. Ambrose received the Pharm.D. degree (1992) from the University of the Pacific, Stockton, California.

THOMAS M. FILE, JR. is Chief of the Infectious Disease Service and Director of HIV Research, Summa Health System, Akron, Ohio, as well as Professor of Internal Medicine and Master Teacher, Northeastern Ohio Universities College of Medicine, Rootstown, Ohio. He is the author of more than 200 articles, textbook chapters, and abstracts and is on the editorial board of the *Journal of Respiratory Disease*. Holding many professional society memberships, Dr. File is a Fellow of the American College of Physicians, the Infectious Diseases Society of America (IDSA), and the American College of Chest Physicians, and is a member of the American Thoracic Society. He is also on IDSA and American Thoracic Society committees for guidelines on community-acquired pneumonia. Dr. File received the B.A. degree (1968) from Albion College, Michigan, the M.D. degree (1972) from the University of Michigan Medical School, Ann Arbor, and the M.S. degree (1997) in Medical Microbiology from The Ohio State University, Columbus.

ISBN 0-8247-4698-8

90000

9 780824 746988